A Guide to Dissection of the

HUMAN BODY

A Guide to Dissection of the
HUMAN BODY

F P Lisowski

LRCPI, LRCSI, LM (Rotunda), PhD (Birmingham, UK)

Emeritus Professor University of Hong Kong

Division of Anatomy and Physiology,
University of Tasmania

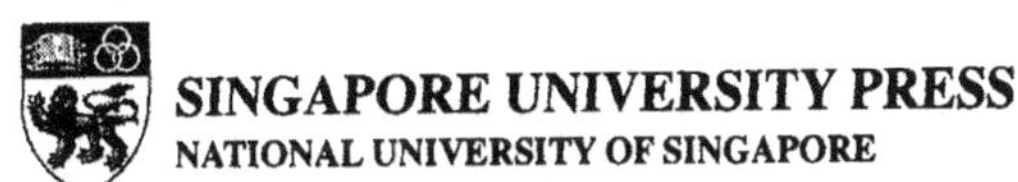

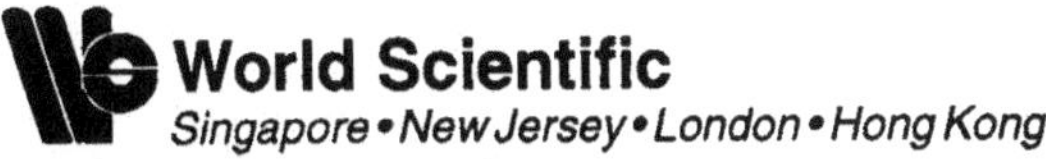

Published by

Singapore University Press
Yusof Ishak House, National University of Singapore
10 Kent Ridge Crescent, Singapore 119260

and

World Scientific Publishing Co. Pte. Ltd.
5 Toh Tuck Link, Singapore 596224
USA office: Suite 202, 1060 Main Street, River Edge, NJ 07661
UK office: 57 Shelton Street, Covent Garden, London WC2H 9HE

British Library Cataloguing-in-Publication Data
A catalogue record for this book is available from the British Library.

A GUIDE TO DISSECTION OF THE HUMAN BODY

ISBN-13 978-981-02-3528-4
ISBN-10 981-02-3528-3
ISBN-13 978-981-02-3569-7 (pbk)
ISBN-10 981-02-3569-0 (pbk)

This guide to dissection is dedicated to
past medical students of
Liverpool, Birmingham, Addis Ababa, Hong Kong and Tasmania
whom it has been a privilege and pleasure to teach.

Seeing once is better than hearing many times
Doing once is better than seeing many times

— *ancient Chinese saying*

The beginning of wisdom is the investigation of things.

— *from the* Daxue, *originally part of the* Book of Rites

PREFACE

The *Guide to Dissection* arose out of the original *A New Approach to Dissection of the Human Body* by R. Kanagasuntheram, A. Krishnamurti and P. Sivanandasingham.* It is an entirely rewritten and altered text. Considerable changes and additions have been introduced to conform with the current shorter dissecting courses which have been implemented. The author of the present *Guide to Dissection* herewith wishes to acknowledge with grateful thanks the early work undertaken by Professor R. Kanagasuntheram, Professor A. Krishnamurti and Dr P. Sivanandasingham and their encouragement.

One has to recognise that there is no substitute for dissection if one wants to learn gross anatomy; it is a three-dimensional approach which is fundamental to understanding the normal function of the human body. Gross anatomy is essentially a visual discipline and deals only with the kind of anatomy that can be demonstrated and learnt in the dissecting laboratory. All matters irrelevant to this purpose have, as far as possible, been excluded. The principle is to give directions for dissection and examination from which the student should be able to make his/her own observations and discoveries. The sequence of dissections that is described covers the entire body and can be adapted to practical courses of any desired duration.

*Kanagasuntheram, R., Krishnamurti, A. and Sivanandasingham, P.: *A New Approach to Dissection of the Human Body*. 2nd ed. (Singapore, Singapore University Press, 1980), now out of print.

Knowing that the average student soon forgets the mass of anatomical detail he/she is sometimes enjoined to learn, and with the object of encouraging the kind of study which provides a three-dimensional idea of the structure of the body, details have been eliminated which have no apparent scientific or educational value, or which have little obvious clinical significance.

This guide is a manual intended to facilitate and guide human anatomical dissections. *It is not a replacement for a textbook.* Since recent medical curricula have reduced the number of hours available for gross anatomical studies, it is the objective of the guide to save time whenever possible. Consequently, the text is concise.

The manual is programmed in such a way that the dissection of the whole human body can be completed in 110 to 160 actual hours of dissection. This is essential at a time when the teaching of gross anatomy in most medical schools has been drastically reduced from some 350 hours in the 1970s.

The guide comprises the following programme:

1. It commences with a *General Introduction* and a brief section on *Terminology* that should be read by both students and their tutors.
2. Each *Anatomical Region* under consideration for dissection has:
   (a) a brief *Introduction* which explains the disposition of the structures on the basis of embryology and evolution;
   (b) an *Overview* of the section to be dissected where the relevant features are mentioned and which can be usefully discussed by the tutor before the commencement of the dissection. This also enables the student to familiarise him/herself with the necessary terminology even before attending the class. The use of various audiovisual aids will enable the student to comprehend the structures of the section he/she will be dissecting during the particular session;
   (c) a *Dissection Schedule* which guides the student through a set of instructions. These are given serially and in short steps so as to expose all the relevant important features. *All the practical instructions are highlighted in italics*;
   (d) a *Summary* which highlights the salient features of the part dissected;
   (e) a list of *Objectives*, the purpose of which is to encourage students to form discussion groups to ensure that they learn those aspects which

will be required in their clinical years. The objectives should also be discussed and clarified with the help of a tutor after the student has completed a particular dissection schedule.

The dissecting instructions set out in this guide are designed for the study of the parts of the body in the following order: Upper Limb, Lower Limb, Thorax, Abdomen, and Head and Neck. However, each of the five anatomical regions stands alone as an independent unit. Thus, anatomical dissection may be carried out in any sequence desired and as specified by the tutor. The teaching staff may choose to delete certain parts of this guide from the class assignment. However, additional dissection projects may be desirable, particularly for students on special assignment or elective rotations.

The terminology used is mostly according to the latest anatomical nomenclature available.

The provision of diagrams or illustrations has been deliberately avoided so as to encourage the student to be more self-reliant. There are excellent anatomical atlases which should be used in conjunction with the dissecting guide and with the dissection. The dissection of the brain is omitted since it is dealt with in neuroscience courses.

The present format is a result of experimentation over several years. The success of this method has prompted the compilation of this manual. It is to be hoped that this guide will be accepted and found useful in teaching institutions.

It is with great pleasure that the author acknowledges the advice and comments of Professor Colin C. Wendell Smith, University of Tasmania, on the latest anatomical nomenclature; Professor R. Kanagasuntherum, Singapore; Professor Charles E. Oxnard, University of Western Australia; Dr. Patricia P. H. Chow-Cheong, Chinese University of Hong Kong; Dr. O. Wai-Sum, University of Hong Kong; and Associate Professor Colin Hinrichsen, University of Tasmania, for their comments and helpful suggestions. I am also grateful to Professor Norman Saunders, University of Tasmania, for his sustained support.

In particular I wish to thank Miss Sandra Kellett, Mrs. Sharon Monk and Mrs. Tracey Walls for their patience and kindness in word processing the various drafts of this manual.

I am deeply indebted to Dr. K. K. Phua, the Editor-in-Chief, Ms. Lim Sook Cheng, the Scientific Editor, and Ms. Joy Marie Tan, Editor, of World Scientific Publishing Co.; and to their staff for their kind help and guidance. Similarly, I wish to express my appreciation to Ms. Patricia Tay and Singapore University Press for their assistance.

I owe warm thanks to my wife Ai Yue for her encouragement, support and interest throughout this enterprise.

FPL
Hobart, 1998

ACKNOWLEDGEMENT

Grateful acknowledgement is made to Oxford University Press for granting permission to use certain extracts from the sections dealing with terminology, the anterior abdominal wall and the eyeball in Zuckerman, S., Darlington, D. and Lisowski, F. P. *A New System of Anatomy: A Dissector's Guide and Atlas*. 2nd ed. (Oxford: Oxford University Press, 1981).

CONTENTS

Introduction

GENERAL

Gross anatomy is largely clinically oriented and in a sense can be termed *clinical anatomy*. A true understanding of gross anatomy depends upon the basic science of human structure; it depends upon knowing how apparently complex gross anatomy results from the very simple anatomy of the early embryo; how that apparently complex anatomy is related to function, e.g. biomechanical function; and how complex anatomy is related to evolution. Gross anatomy forms the foundation for procedures in diagnosis and treatment, radiology, surgery, obstetrics and other medical fields.

Every practitioner who sees a patient makes a *physical examination* of the patient's anatomy. Since the examiner's sensory nervous system works by analogue methods, physical examination consists of comparing the possibly abnormal with a mental image of the normal.

Though gross anatomy is concerned with practical work in the dissecting laboratory, it also includes *imaging anatomy* and *living* or *surface anatomy*. It is a science of the living, not of the dead, and though our knowledge is, perforce, acquired from the cadaver it is in terms of the living that you must think. It also teaches something about human and constitutional variations — no two bodies are ever alike — and about the plasticity of the human form and biological variation of living populations.

The intent of this guide is not to teach clinical practice but to guide you in learning and appreciating the anatomy of the human body, the anatomical language and principles that will be needed in your medical career. The guide helps to make anatomy rational, interesting and directly applicable to the clinical problems encountered in the health professions. If anatomy is simply memorised and not understood, it will soon be forgotten. The practice of good medicine requires a significant knowledge of anatomy.

Dissecting material is both scarce and immensely valuable. Therefore, you must always scrupulously follow the instructions given by the department, tutor and dissecting manual concerning the care of the dissection and the procedure to be followed, otherwise much time and effort may be wasted.

At any time only two to four members of a dissecting table group are able to dissect and two will read out aloud from the instruction manual. Those that do not dissect should follow both the text and dissection, make appropriate reference to atlases and textbooks, and see to it that the dissectors carry out their work properly. It is essential that each one of you takes his/her proper turn in dissection. The practice of medicine demands both knowledge and manual dexterity and it is during the anatomy course that this good habit is acquired.

Before you follow a particular dissection schedule you should always study the relevant *Overview* in the guide and the relevant section in the textbook in order to become familiar with the major features that you will encounter.

A good dissection should display clearly and cleanly the main features of the region. You should be as neat and accurate as you can — for a slovenly dissector will be a slovenly doctor. There must be no blind dissection, you must always have a preliminary session with the manual to find out what main structures to look for, and where to find them.

During dissection, in addition to reading the dissecting instructions and dissecting, you should at all times be discussing and questioning with your fellow students and with your tutors matters such as the relation of the anatomy that is being dealt with to development, function, and the related practical importance.

The manual gives clear and explicit instructions on how to get the best view of the part. It is quite astonishing how many find themselves in trouble because they have either failed to read the dissecting instructions or have failed to understand them. There is no excuse for this. A failure to take in and understand written or verbal instructions can be immensely dangerous in medical practice, and now is the time for the student to train himself/herself to be meticulous.

Dissection is something more than merely following instructions, nor is it a purely mechanical task. It is a kind of original visuotactile method of investigation; nobody has ever investigated the particular body you are working on, and it is individual and unique. What you find out for yourself sticks in your mind much better than what is shown to you by somebody else. Dissection provides plenty of mental problems on which you ought to sharpen your wits.

Many make the mistake of believing that gross anatomy can be satisfactorily studied for examination purposes from the textbook alone. These people are readily recognisable at the practical and oral examinations. Gross anatomy is a practical and functional subject, not a theoretical subject, and when you are qualified your patients will not be satisfied with your ability to recite little lists of relationships, but will demand someone who knows how and where to find these relationships and how they function within their own bodies.

In the dissection tutorial you learn to understand the structural relationships and the structure-function inter-relationship, and you learn to cultivate the visual memory. It is upon these that you will constantly depend upon in your clinical work.

You have to consider how the anatomy of soft parts in the region you dissected must change when the part is moved in the living body. How would you attempt to locate the main arteries and nerves from the surface of the living body? What results would follow if the main nerve of a region were cut? Or if the main artery were tied? Questions such as these help to fix the important features of the region firmly in the mind.

In every dissection it is helpful to build your knowledge of the region as a whole round a framework provided by certain key structures. These may be muscles, nerves, ligaments or arteries. It is preferable to select those key structures which are of intrinsic functional or professional significance. And thinking should be systematised.

There are three points of view that should be applied to every region of the body: the functional, the clinical and the conceptual.

(a) The *functional aspect*: You should mentally stand back from the details of the dissection and try to take a broad view of the functions of the part upon which you are working. Thus, if you are studying the foot, which takes a leading part in walking, running and jumping, it ought to at once occur to you that one of the most important things about it must be the bony, muscular and ligamentous mechanisms by which the weight of the body is supported and transferred.

(b) The *clinical aspect*: You should adopt a more specifically professional point of view and consider the anatomy of common injuries, infections and other diseases which may occur in the region under consideration. Thus, the relationships of the middle ear are of little functional significance, but are of great practical importance because an infection within the middle ear may endanger hearing or even life.

(c) The *conceptual aspect*: You will find it valuable to remember that the key to a dissection may lie not in an individual structure, but in an idea. Therefore, one of the most important aids to the understanding of the disposition of the abdominal viscera is a knowledge of the local embryology. And the understanding of the evolutionary development of humans as primates is of importance in studying humans structurally and functionally.

In the dissection tutorial facts, principles and their relation to function are discussed. These are the keys to solving problems of an anatomical-clinical nature. The dissection tutorial plays the role that bedside teaching plays in the clinical years.

With regard to the value of dissection *versus* a study of prepared (prosected) parts, there is no doubt as to which is the more rewarding. From experience it is clear that the knowledge gained from dissecting a cadaver is retained longer and more vividly than that gained from examining prepared specimens. Dissection of the body is an essential basis for the understanding of human structure, organisation and function. It is a visuotactile method of learning and is of value as a discipline and as a training in observation and investigation. It often comes as a salutary shock to discover during dissection that the body does not agree with the textbook.

Dissection is itself a basic research method in application for the student which is carried out nowhere else in the preclinical course — you do your own investigation and confirm or contradict the description in the literature, i.e. actual research in the proper sense, and you use a technique that is analytical in nature. One cannot teach locomotion or the limits of joint movement until the student has dissected the relevant parts. He/she cannot otherwise understand what is happening.

DISSECTION

The Cadaver

When you are assigned to a cadaver, you assume responsibility for its proper care. You will find that the body has already been embalmed with a suitable preservative fluid. Occasionally, the arteries have been injected with a red colouring dye.

The whole body has been kept moist by adequate wrappings. Uncover only those parts of the body to be dissected. Inspect every part periodically, and renew and moisten the wrappings as the occasion demands. Do not leave any part exposed to the air needlessly. Give special attention to the face, hands, feet and external genitalia. Once a part is allowed to become dry and hard, it can never be fully restored, and further dissection is impossible. Plastic bags are particularly useful to prevent drying.

Do not be surprised if it turns out that someone has a better-preserved body to dissect than you have (or vice versa). A large number of factors influence the way preservation fluid flows through the body.

Your main concern will necessarily be the cadaver which you are dissecting, but always allow colleagues who are working on other bodies to see what you are doing, and, whenever possible, check your own findings on their dissections.

Anatomy departments in countries where the expectation of life is high, that is to say about 70 years or more, will as a rule receive only senile cadavers. The senile body not only differs from the body of a young person in lacking teeth and having atrophied muscles, but also in the relative proportions of various other structures. Some bodies may be emaciated, others may have a lot of subcutaneous and other fat. Not surprisingly, many of the bodies which come to the dissecting room reveal marks of previous disease. You may even find that the cadaver you are dissecting is that of a person who died of cancer. In that case you may have to study the affected parts on some other body.

While the general arrangements of the muscles, vessels, and nerves which make up the body follow the same pattern you will discover during the course of your dissection that anatomical details vary considerably from one individual to another. So do not be surprised, for example, if in the cadaver you are dissecting, an artery arises from some main trunk differently from the way described.

Another point worth noting is that the appearance of the tissues in the cadaver is very unlike that of the same tissues in the living body. For example, arteries are differentiated more easily from veins in the living body than in the dead; different planes of fascia are separable more readily on the operating-table than you will find possible in the cadaver you are dissecting; and organs and muscles are more fixed in position in the cadaver. Their colour, texture, and surface-markings are also different in the living as compared with the body prepared for dissection by the injection of fixatives. Note, too, that the degree of distension of different parts of the alimentary canal are bound to differ in the cadaver you dissect from what would be expected in a healthy person.

You must always remember that former living persons have donated their bodies for medical studies in good faith. Therefore, the cadaver must be treated with respect and dignity. Improper behaviour in the dissecting laboratory cannot be tolerated.

Working conditions

You must protect your clothing by wearing a long laboratory coat. At the samc time you must wear disposable latex gloves when handling dead (or living) human material. Adequate light is essential for efficient dissection. And make use of wooden blocks to stabilise parts of the cadaver wherever necessary.

Instruments

The following dissecting instruments should be procured:

1. A *scalpel* designed for detachable knife blades. The scalpel handle should be made of metal. The blade should be about 4 cm long and its cutting edge should be somewhat curved. The blades should be changed frequently. No one can do good work with a blunt scalpel. Therefore, a sufficient supply of blades will be needed.
2. Two pairs of *forceps*:
   (a) One pair with blunt and rounded ends whose gripping surfaces should be serrated; and
   (b) a fine pair with sharp-pointed ends for delicate work.

3. Two pairs of *scissors*:
   (a) One large pair about 15 cm in length, with blunt ends; and
   (b) a fine pair with sharp points for delicate dissection.
4. A metal *probe* or seeker with a blunt tip.

Other instruments which you will occasionally need, such as bone forceps, various saws and a long-bladed knife, will be provided as part of the equipment of the dissecting laboratory.

Techniques of dissection

Before you begin to dissect, it is *essential* that you read these instructions:

Reflection of skin

You are given the exact position of every skin incision you have to make. Cut through the skin, remembering that it is rarely more than 2 mm thick. A decrease in resistance as you cut will tell you that you have reached the subcutaneous tissue.

To detach the skin from the subcutaneous tissue, use stout forceps to grip the angle where two incisions meet, and cut with your scalpel between the skin and the underlying subcutaneous tissue or fascia. As you lift the skin away (this is called *reflecting the skin*) pull on it, and continue cutting close to, and parallel with its under-surface, keeping the flap tense as you reflect it away. Most of your reflections will be made so that the flap you lift is left attached by one edge. The skin can then be replaced, between periods of dissection, over the part you are studying.

Reflection of fascia

The subcutaneous tissue between the skin and whatever structure it overlies (usually muscle) consists of fatty connective tissue known as **superficial fascia**, and a deeper layer of non-fatty membranous fascia called the **deep fascia**. The cutaneous nerves and vessels ramify in the superficial fascia, having pierced the deep fascia. Using a scalpel and forceps, the superficial fascia is then reflected from one of the edges of the area laid open by the reflection of skin.

Cleaning muscles, nerves and arteries

By *cleaning* a muscle, a nerve or a vessel, one means completely removing the connective tissue and fat or fascia by which it is ensheathed. This is done with forceps and scalpel, where necessary piecemeal. When you dissect, do not hesitate to remove small veins.

When you are asked to *define* a nerve or artery, or a muscle, you are meant to carry on with the process of cleaning until the whole structure is clearly and cleanly exposed. The same is implied in the word *following* a nerve or artery.

Any tissue that is removed from the body should be put into a receptacle so that it can eventually be buried.

Most of your dissection will be made with a sharp scalpel and forceps.

Blunt dissection refers to the process of isolating a structure without using the blade of a knife. Blunt dissection often involves pulling a nerve or artery to one side, so it must be carried out with care. One can, for example, separate a vessel which is bound by connective tissue to a nerve by pushing the points of closed forceps or scissors between them and then gently opening the blades, or one can separate them by pushing gently with the handle of a scalpel.

Do not be rough, but never be afraid to use your fingers to feel the structures which you have to clean and isolate. If, for example, it is necessary to cut through a muscle, be quite certain that you can define its edges, and if possible first insinuate a finger between it and the structures on which it is lying. As a preliminary to inserting your finger, it may be necessary to push gently with the handle of a scalpel.

You may sometimes find that some of the muscles you are dissecting are unexpectedly friable and that they tear. All you can do to overcome this shortcoming is to examine the muscle or part concerned on somebody else's dissection.

Never regard your examination of a particular part or region as completed until you have really exposed the structures described in the text.

Bones

You will find it useful to have at hand the bones of the particular part on which you are working. The bones of the limbs help you to understand the action of the muscles that rise from and become inserted into them, while those of the pelvis and skull help you to understand the position of different soft structures, and the points of emergence of vessels and nerves.

Care of the dissection

After each period of study it is essential that any individual part that is being dissected should be wrapped up in order to prevent loss of moisture and hardening of the specimen. Also, from time to time moisten the parts that you are dissecting.

Structures that cannot be adequately dissected

You will have no difficulty in dissecting the muscles, the visceral organs, and the main vessels and nerves of the body. Some anatomical structures that are important functionally cannot, however, be studied adequately by the straightforward methods of dissection which you will be using. The main one is the **lymphathic system**. This consists of a network of minute channels and associated nodes that are found in most parts of the body. All you will see, and then only in some of your dissections, are well-defined solid lumps of matted tissue of varying shape, usually embedded in fascia. These are lymph nodes. When you dissect the thorax you will also come across the main collecting duct of the whole lymphatic tree. But this is about all you will see of the system.

Your dissection will also fail to reveal some of the more detailed parts of the **nervous system** of the body. The brain and spinal cord, which comprise the **central nervous system**, are dealt with in Neuroscience courses. Another major part of the nervous system, the **autonomic nervous system**, cannot be adequately dissected.

STRUCTURES ENCOUNTERED DURING DISSECTION

Having studied the techniques of dissection it will be useful to you to note some of the structures that you will encounter during dissection. In dissecting the human body you will come across various structures such as skin, superficial fascia, deep fascia, muscles, tendons, blood vessels, lymph vessels and nodes, nerves, bones, joints and organs.

Skin

The skin forms the outer covering of the body and is composed of a superficial layer, the **epidermis**, and a deep layer, the **dermis**. The skin is slightly thicker over the extensor than over the flexor surface. However, it is extremely thick over the palms and soles, which are, in fact flexor surfaces.

Superficial fascia

The superficial fascia is deep to the skin. Within this layer lie the superficial nerves, blood vessels and lymphatics. The superficial fascia consists of loose areolar tissue and is filled with fat. In some situations like the anterior abdominal wall and gluteal region (buttock), there is a large accumulation of fat. Since fat is an insulator, the superficial fascia acts as retainer of body heat.

Deep fascia

Deep to the superficial fascia lies the deep fascia. This is a tough connective tissue tunic which covers the underlying muscles. Sometimes the muscles are attached to this fascia. The deep fascia also sends in septa between muscles providing a covering for them as well as sheaths for blood vessels and nerves. Occasionally, the deep fascia sends extensions between different functional groups of muscles. These extensions which gain attachments to bones are called **intermuscular septa**. The deep fascia is also extremely thickened in the region of the wrist and ankle where they form well defined transverse bands extending across bony prominences. These bands are called the **retinacula**. With the underlying bone they form osteofascial tunnels providing a passage for tendons, which are thus prevented from springing out during contraction of the muscles.

Muscle

When the deep fascia has been cleared away you will be on to muscle. This is commonly known as voluntary, skeletal or striated muscle. The muscles contribute to about 50 per cent of the body weight. They are composed of muscle fibres. The fibres in individual muscles are arranged in different ways so that the muscles are often described as **strap-like** when the individual fibres are long and arranged in parallel; **fusiform** when a fleshy belly tapers towards both ends, often ending in a tendon; and **pennate** when there is a resemblance to a feather. Pennate muscles are described as *unipennate*, *bipennate* or *multipennate*. These various types will be encountered during dissection. Muscles are usually connected at their ends to skeletal elements. These attachments of a muscle are usually described as its **origin** and **insertion**. The origin is generally the proximal attachment and is usually the fixed point from which the muscle acts so that the skeletal element into which it is inserted distally is able to move. Usually the origins of muscles are fleshy and their insertions tendinous. The tendons are formed by condensations of fibrous tissue and possess great tensile strength. Sometimes a tendon may be flat and thin and forms a broad sheet when it is called an *aponeurosis*.

Contraction of muscles in the living can be seen and felt. This can be *tested by making a muscle contract against resistance*. Muscles have a rich blood and nerve supply. The point of entry of these into a muscle is called the **neurovascular hilus**. The innervation of muscles is both motor and sensory. The stimulation of the motor nerve causes a contraction of the muscle. The sensory nerve carries information about the nature of the force of contraction, the degree of stretch, etc, of the muscle it innervates.

Blood vessels

Blood vessels are of three major types — **arteries, veins** and **capillaries**. Arteries are thick-walled vessels which carry blood away from the heart to the tissues. Veins return the blood from the tissue to the heart. Intervening between the arterial and venous sides of the circulation are minutes vessels called capillaries. In the cadaver, the arteries appear paler and are palpably thicker, while the veins have thin walls and are bluish or dark in colour. Veins superficial to the deep fascia often run alone while those deep to the deep fascia accompany arteries and are called **venae comitantes**.

In the living, arteries are pulsatile and their pulsations are visible when they lie close to the surface. Such arteries are usually *palpated against an underlying bone*, e.g. pulsations of the radial artery are felt by compressing it against the radius (a *pressure point*).

Lymphatics

The cells comprising the tissue of the body are bathed in fluid called **tissue fluid**, which is derived from **blood plasma**. Tissue fluid provides a medium for the transport of nutrients to cells as well as for the removal of their waste products. Part of the tissue fluid re-enters the blood circulation but the remainder (**lymph**) is drained by a system of extremely thin-walled channels called **lymph capillaries**. They unite to form **lymph channels** which accompany blood vessels. The lymphatic channels lying superficial to the deep fascia generally accompany the superficial veins, while the deeper vessels accompany arteries. *Lymph vessels are not normally seen during dissection*. During their course they are interrupted by **lymph nodes** which contain discrete aggregations of lymphocytes which are a type of white blood cells. Tissue fluid in the lymph channels after filtering through lymph nodes is carried by lymphatic channels of increasing calibre which ultimately enter the large veins in the neck.

Bones

Bones form the major part of the human skeleton and provide the supporting framework for the body. Although they appear to be rigid, they are extremely plastic. During growth and repair this plasticity is easily seen. Even at normal times there is a continuous turnover of the constituents of bone. Bone is in fact an organ and not merely a tissue since it has in its matrix, nerves, blood vessels and lymphatics like any other organ of the body.

Bones are generally classified according to their shapes. **Long** and **short** bones are peculiar to the limbs; **flat** bones are generally found in the girdles of the limbs, ribs and vault of the skull; **irregular** bones are peculiar to the vertebral column and base of the skull. **Sesamoid** bones are those that are developed in some tendons. The knee cap or patella is a good example of a sesamoid bone.

Each long bone has a shaft or **diaphysis** and two ends or **epiphyses**. The diaphysis and the epiphysis are developed from separate ossification centres. The ossification of the diaphysis invariably begins before birth, whereas the centres for the epiphyses *usually* form after birth. The epiphyses unite with the diaphysis at different times. The epiphysis which begins ossifying *first usually unites with the diaphysis later*. Since this end of the diaphysis continues to grow in length after the opposite end has ceased its growth, it is called the *growing end* of the bone.

The shaft of a typical long bone usually presents a prominent foramen somewhere about its middle. This is called the **nutrient foramen** as it transmits fairly large blood vessels called the nutrient vessels which supply the shaft.

The canal for the nutrient artery is invariably directed *away* from the growing end of the bone.

Most of the bony surfaces provide attachments for muscles. Fleshy attachments of muscles usually leave no marks on the bone. Tendinous attachments if flattened or aponeurotic leave rough markings. Thick tendons are usually attached to smooth areas which are either depressed or raised. Admixture of tendon and muscle fibres invariably leave very rough markings on bones.

Joints

Junctional regions between bones develop into joints. Joints can be classified as **fibrous, cartilaginous** or **synovial**, depending on the type of tissue present between the articular ends of the bones. Generally, fibrous joints permit very little movement, while synovial joints provide the greatest degree of freedom of movement. The cartilaginous joints form an intermediate group. However, there are exceptions to these general statements.

Terminology

For the purpose of description the body is considered to be in the **anatomical position**. In this position the subject is assumed to be standing, with the feet together, the arms to the side, and with the head and eyes and the palms of the hands facing forward. To ensure consistency of description it is important to keep this anatomical position constantly in mind.

The position of structures relative to each other in the body is defined in relation to the following planes:

The **Median Plane**: This is the back-to-front vertical plane which cuts through the body in the midline. This plane bisects the body into symmetrical right and left halves.

A **Sagittal Plane**: This is any vertical plane parallel to the median plane.

A **Frontal Plane** or **Coronal Plane**: This is any vertical plane at right angles to the median plane.

A **Transverse Plane**: This is any **horizontal plane** through the body at right angles to both the sagittal and frontal planes.

Any structure lying closer than another to the midline of the body is said to be **medial** to it, and any further from the midline **lateral**. Every structure automatically has a medial and a lateral aspect. A point or plane in space closer than another to the head-end of the body is said to be **superior** to it, and, conversely, the point or plane further away is **inferior**. The terms **cranial** and **caudal** replace the terms 'superior' and 'inferior' in descriptions of the embryo, and they are also sometimes replaced by the terms **rostral** and **caudal** in descriptions of the brain. The terms **proximal** and **distal** are used in describing parts of the limbs which are closer to, or further from, the attachment of the limbs to the trunk.

The front surface of the body, or of any structure in the body, is called its **anterior** surface, and conversely the back of any surface is denoted by the term **posterior**. The terms **ventral** and **dorsal** are synonymous with 'anterior' and 'posterior'.

The term **supine** refers to the body lying on its back, i.e. dorsal surface. The term **prone** refers to the body lying on its face, i.e. ventral surface. The hand is said to be **supinated** when the **palmar** surface faces forward as in the anatomical position. When the hand is rotated so that the palmar surface faces posteriorly it is said to be **pronated**. The sole of the foot is known as the **plantar** surface. When the plantar surface is turned medially, the foot is **inverted**; when laterally, **everted**.

Structures which lie near to the surface of the body are described as **superficial** to others which lie on a **deep** plane. The term **external** describes the structures outside an area, space, or structure, and the term **internal** describes those within.

When referring to structures of the wrist and hand, the terms **radial** and **ulnar** are often used instead of 'lateral' and 'medial'. This avoids any confusion due to the fact that when the hand is pronated its lateral border (i.e. the side of the thumb) lies 'medial' to the side of the little finger, which in the supinated position is medial. And in the leg and foot the terms **tibial** and **fibular** are often used instead of 'medial' and 'lateral'.

The term **flexor surface** generally refers to the ventral aspect of the body while the dorsal aspect is referred to as the **extensor surface**; but the lower limb is an exception in that the extensor surface has become ventral, owing to the fact that it has undergone rotation during fetal life. The terms **pre-axial** and **post-axial** borders are used in reference to the margins of the limbs. The pre-axial border is in relation to the thumb (pollux) and first toe (hallux), while the post-axial border is in relation to the little finger and fifth toe.

Section 1

UPPER LIMB

Introduction

Human beings belong to the Order Primates. This group of mammals are more renowned for their adaptability than for their adaptation. Thus, they have avoided the pitfalls of specialisation and consequently have become the most flourishing group of mammals in the past 50 to 60 million years. Most primates are arboreal. This arboreal habitat has not only given them security from enemies but it has also improved their sense of vision. With this improvement in visual perception there has been a corresponding reduction of their olfactory sense organs, the latter having become unimportant in an arboreal environment. This reduction of the olfactory apparatus has been accompanied by a recession of the snout which is the region of exquisite tactile sensibility in macrosmatic animals. In the human species this tactile function is taken over chiefly by the upper limbs which have become emancipated from the burden of weight-bearing. Such tactile sensibility has become specially marked towards the distal parts of the upper limb, i.e. digits.

Moreover, humans have also inherited the prehensile or grasping function of the upper limbs from their arboreal ancestry. Superimposed on to the more primitive prehensile function of the hand is the evolution of finer precision movements. Thus, the hand has developed into a prehensile organ possessing strength, stability, mobility, a high degree of neuromuscular coordination, and sensory discrimination. This, together with the specialised development of the human brain, i.e. the combination of the human hand and mind, has culminated in the manufacture and use of tools, thus giving birth to the rich human cultural activities of arts and crafts. Consequently, the human hand is both a sensory and a motor apparatus. Also, one has to be aware that although over the past 50 million years there has been little change in the *structure* of the skeleton and muscles of the hand, the changes in *function* have been profound. For example, the opposability of the thumb to the index finger is a unique human trait and it is important to realise that functionally the thumb represents one half of the hand. And in connection with the functional aspect, the clinical importance of the hand is obvious since 45 per cent of all industrial injuries are associated with the hand.

In the study of the upper limb as well as other parts of the body, you must bear in mind the functional correlates of the morphological structures that you encounter during the dissection sessions.

Overview of Schedule 1

Before you begin dissection note:

PECTORAL REGION AND AXILLA

Relevant skeletal features:

thoracic cage — sternum; costal cartilages; ribs and thoracic vertebrae;
sternum — manubrium; body; xiphoid process; jugular notch; sternal angle;
first rib — surfaces; borders; ends;
clavicle — medial end; shaft; lateral end;
scapula — surfaces; borders; processes (spine, acromion, coracoid);
humerus — head; greater and lesser tubercles; crests of the greater and lesser tubercles; intertubercular groove; surgical neck.

Subcutaneous structures:

mammary gland; supraclavicular nerves; anterior and lateral cutaneous branches of intercostal nerves and accompanying arteries; cephalic vein.

Deep fascia:

pectoral; clavipectoral; axillary.

Muscles:

pectoralis major; obliquus externus abdominis; serratus anterior; pectoralis minor; subclavius; subscapularis; teres major; latissimus dorsi; coracobrachialis; short head of biceps; long head of triceps; deltoid.

Boundaries of axilla

Nerves:

roots, trunks, divisions and cords of *brachial plexus.*

Arteries:

axillary artery and its branches.

Veins:

axillary vein and its tributaries.

Lymph nodes:

axillary groups.

Surface anatomy:

axillary artery.

Clinical anatomy:

injuries to brachial plexus; lymph drainage of breast.

Dissection Schedule 1

PECTORAL REGION AND AXILLA

1. *With the body on its back make the following incisions:*
   (a) *a median incision extending from the* **jugular notch** *to the* **xiphoid process**;
   (b) *from the jugular notch along the* **clavicle** *to the* **acromion process of the scapula**. *Continue the cut down the lateral side of the arm to its middle*;
   (c) *a transverse incision from the lower end of incision* (b) *to the medial side of the arm*;
   (d) *from the xiphoid process horizontally to the* **posterior axillary line**;
   (e) *encircle the* **nipple**.
   Reflect the skin flaps.

2. *As you dissect you may come across the following cutaneous nerves, but do not spend time searching for them*:
   (a) the cutaneous **medial**, **intermediate** and **lateral supraclavicular nerves** which descend over the clavicle. These nerves are branches of the cervical plexus and supply the skin of the upper pectoral and shoulder regions;
   (b) the **anterior cutaneous branches** of the intercostal nerves which are accompanied by **perforating branches** of the **internal thoracic artery**. These nerves and vessels emerge about 3 cm from the midline;
   (c) the **lateral cutaneous branches** of the **intercostal (thoracic) nerves** which emerge along the **midaxillary line** and divide into anterior and posterior branches.

3. *Examine the extent of the* **female breast** *lying in* the superficial fascia and note that there is an extension of the breast tissue into the axilla (**axillary tail**). *Make a transverse cut across the breast passing through the nipple. Try to identify some of the lobes and ducts of the gland.* Note the **suspensory ligaments**, which are *fibrous strands* passing from the nipple and skin of the breast to the deeper layer of superficial fascia.

4. *Remove the breast and the remains of the superficial fascia* and note the underlying **pectoralis major muscle** which is covered by deep fascia

known as the **pectoral fascia**. Below and lateral to the pectoralis major *you will see* the interdigitating slips of origin of the **obliquus externus abdominis** and **serratus anterior muscles**. *Remove the deep fascia covering the pectoralis major.*

5. *Identify the clavicular part of the pectoralis major* and note that the **cephalic vein** lies in a groove between it and the **deltoid muscle (deltopectoral groove)**.

6. Note that the pectoralis major arises from: (a) the medial half of the anterior surface of the clavicle, (b) the sternum, and (c) the upper six costal cartilages. *Cut the muscle close to its origins and reflect it laterally.* The **lateral** and **medial pectoral nerves** supply the pectoralis major and the underlying **pectoralis minor muscle**. Note that the pectoralis major muscle is inserted into the **crest of the greater tubercle of the humerus**.

7. *Define the underlying* **clavipectoral fascia** which lies between the clavicle and the upper border of the pectoralis minor. This fascia splits above to enclose the **subclavius muscle** lying below the clavicle and the pectoralis minor below. *Clean the subclavius* which passes from the first rib to the inferior surface of the clavicle.

8. *As you clean away the fascia* note that the cephalic vein pierces the clavipectoral fascia in the **infraclavicular fossa** and drains into the **axillary vein**.
9. *Next clean the pectoralis minor* and note its origin from ribs 3, 4, 5 and its insertion into the **coracoid process of the scapula**.

Note that the pectoralis major, clavipectoral fascia, subclavius and the pectoralis minor form the **anterior wall of the axilla**.

10. *Clean the* **axillary fascia** which is a continuation of the pectoral fascia. This fascia forms the **base of the axilla**. Embedded within the fascia *you may find the* **axillary lymph nodes** which are arranged as follows:
    (a) a **pectoral** or **anterior group** along the lower border of the pectoralis minor;
    (b) a **brachial** or **lateral group** along the lower part of the axillary vein;
    (c) a **central group** in relation to the central part of the axillary vein;

(d) an **apical group** along the axillary vein at the apex of the axilla; and
(e) a **subscapular** or **posterior group** along the **subscapular** vessels.

11. *Reflect the pectoralis minor from its origin. Identify the* **axillary artery** and note that the pectoralis minor divides the course of this vessel into three parts. The *first part* is proximal to the muscle, the *second part* lies behind the muscle while the *third part* is distal to the muscle. *At the same time clean the axillary vein.*

12. *Now examine the part of the* **brachial plexus** *lying in the axilla.* Note that the brachial plexus lies partly in the neck, partly behind the clavicle and partly in the axilla. The plexus is made up of **roots, trunks, divisions, cords** and **branches.**

    The *roots* are the anterior primary rami of C5,6,7,8 and T1 and communications from C4 and T2. The roots lie in the neck.

    The *trunks* are **upper, middle** and **lower**. They also lie in the neck.

    The *divisions* lie behind the clavicle.

    The *cords* are **lateral, posterior** and **medial** and lie in the axilla. These cords are associated with the first and second parts of the axillary artery and give rise to *branches* that are associated with the third part of the axillary artery.

13. *Now proceed to clean the branches of the cords in relation to the third part of the axillary artery*:
    (a) the **medial cutaneous nerve of arm** lying medial to the axillary vein. This supplies the medial side of the arm (*do not waste time searching for it*);
    (b) the **medial cutaneous nerve of forearm** running superficially between the vein and the artery. This supplies the medial side of the forearm;
    (c) the **ulnar nerve**, lying between the vein and the artery but in a deeper plane to the medial cutaneous nerve of forearm;
    (d) the **median nerve** lying lateral to the artery. Observe that this nerve has two roots, the **medial root** which crosses in front of the artery to join the **lateral root** lying lateral to the artery;

(e) the **musculocutaneous nerve** situated lateral to the median nerve and supplying the coracobrachialis, biceps and brachialis muscles. *Trace the medial cutaneous nerve of forearm and ulnar nerve proximally to their origins from the* **medial cord** of the brachial plexus *and the musculocutaneous nerve to its origin from the* **lateral cord**. Note that the medial root of the median nerve arises from the medial cord and the lateral root of the nerve from the lateral cord of the plexus. Observe that the *medial cord is medial* to the *second part* of the axillary artery while the *lateral cord* is *lateral* to the artery;

(f) the **axillary** and **radial nerves** situated behind the artery. *Trace them to their origins from the* **posterior cord** of the brachial plexus which lies *behind* the *second part* of the axillary artery.

The three cords of the brachial plexus are in fact named according to their relationship to the *second part* of the axillary artery.

14. *Identify the* **subscapularis, teres major** and **latissimus dorsi muscles** which form the *posterior wall of the axilla. Trace the* **thoracodorsal nerve** which is accompanied by the **subscapular vessels**. Note the entry of the nerve and vessels into the latissimus dorsi muscle at its **neurovascular hilus**. The subscapularis and teres major muscles are supplied by the **subscapular nerves**.

15. The axillary artery has numerous branches. One of the major branches is the **subscapular artery**. *Clean the artery* and note that it lies along the posterior wall of the axilla. Another set of branches are the **circumflex humeral arteries** that supply the shoulder joint.

16. *Trace and observe that the axillary nerve passes through the* **quadrilateral space** bounded by the subscapularis above, teres major below, **long head of triceps** medially and the upper end of the humerus laterally.

17. *Clean the latissimus dorsi and teres major muscles close to their insertions into the floor of the* **intertubercular groove** *and* **crest of the lesser tubercle of the humerus**, *respectively*. Note that the *lateral wall of the axilla* is narrow due to the convergence of the anterior and posterior walls towards the intertubercular groove. Between the converging walls lie the **short head of the biceps** and **coracobrachialis muscles**.

18. Note that the **serratus anterior muscle** takes origin from the upper eight ribs and is inserted into the medial border of the **scapula**. It forms the *medial wall of the axilla. Secure the* **long thoracic nerve** on the lateral side of the thorax. It arises from the nerve roots of C5, 6, 7 and supplies the muscle on its external surface.

Summary

The axilla may be regarded as a three-sided pyramid whose truncated apex is situated between the clavicle, the upper border of the scapula and the outer border of the first rib. Nerves supplying the upper limb descend from the lower part of the neck through the apex of the axilla. These nerves form the brachial plexus. The plexus supplies the entire upper limb musculature with the exception of the trapezius and the levator scapulae.

The brachial plexus is formed by the ventral rami of C5, 6, 7, 8 and T1 nerves. It has the following stages:

roots:	C5, 6, 7, 8, T1
trunks:	**upper trunk** formed by the union of C5, 6 **middle trunk** formed by C7 **lower trunk** formed by the union of C8, T1
divisions:	each trunk divides into an **anterior** and a **posterior division**
cords:	**lateral cord** formed by the anterior divisions of the upper and middle trunks (C5, 6, 7) **medial cord** formed by the anterior division of the lower trunk (C8, T1) **posterior cord** formed by the posterior divisions of the upper, middle and lower trunks (C5, 6, 7, 8 [T1]).

The *roots* and *trunks* of the plexus are found *in the neck*, the *divisions* of the trunks *behind the clavicle*, and the *cords* and *branches* in the *axilla.*

The nerves forming the plexus lie behind the plane of the vessels in the neck and subsequently undergo re-arrangement in the axilla so that the medial, lateral and posterior cords assume their respective positions around the *second part* of the **axillary artery**. Distal to this, the lateral cord and its branches lie above and lateral to the artery, the medial cord and its branches are below and medial to the artery, and the posterior cord and its branches lie posterior to the artery. Moreover, whenever nerves arising from the medial or lateral cords cross the artery they usually do so in front of the artery, while those arising from the posterior cord cross behind the vessel.

It must be borne in mind that the anterior divisions of the brachial plexus supply the muscles forming the anterior wall of the axilla and the flexor muscles of the free upper limb, while the posterior divisions supply the muscles forming the posterior wall of the axilla and the extensor muscles of the free upper limb.

Lymphatic Drainage of the Breast

This is of importance in understanding the spread of breast cancer. The lymph vessels of the breast generally follow the course of blood vessels. They follow: (a) along the lower border of pectoralis minor and drain mainly into the **pectoral group of axillary lymph nodes**, (b) along the internal thoracic artery to the **internal thoracic lymph nodes** and (c) the posterior intercostal arteries to the **posterior intercostal nodes**. Rarely lymphatics from the breast may pass into the abdomen between the xiphoid process and the costal margin to end in the **diaphragmatic nodes**. They may even communicate with the lymphatics of the opposite breast.

Objectives for Dissection Schedule 1

1. Topic: Pectoral region and axilla

General objective 1

Comprehend the arrangement of the muscles in relation to the axilla.

Specific objectives

1. Explain the pectoral region as a link between the trunk and mobile upper limb.
2. Demonstrate the actions of pectoralis major and minor.
3. Define the muscles contributing to the formation and contour of the anterior and posterior axillary folds.
4. Define the medial and lateral walls of the axilla.

General objective 2

Comprehend the arrangement of the nerves and blood vessels of the axilla.

Specific objectives

1. Explain how the apex of the axilla forms the highway for nerves and blood vessels between the neck and upper limb.
2. Surface mark the axillary artery and define its extent.
3. Identify the roots, trunks, divisions and cords of the brachial plexus in prosected specimens.
4. Illustrate the functional aspects of the divisions of the plexus.
5. Explain this functional subdivision by taking individual nerves in turn.
6. Surface mark the pectoralis minor muscle and discuss why it is the key structure of the region.

2. Topic: The mammary gland

General objective

Comprehend the general anatomy of the breast and the clinical importance of this knowledge.

Specific objectives

1. Define the muscles forming the "bed" of the adult female breast.
2. Define the base of the gland and the axillary tail.
3. Outline the blood supply of the organ.
4. Outline the routes of lymph drainage of the breast.
5. Discuss the clinical importance of the knowledge of the blood supply and lymphatic drainage of the breast.

Overview of Schedule 2

Before you begin dissection note:

FRONT OF ARM AND CUBITAL REGION

Relevant skeletal features:

humerus — deltoid tuberosity; supracondylar ridges; epicondyles;
radius — head; radial tuberosity;
ulna — coronoid process.

Subcutaneous structures:

medial cutaneous nerves of arm and forearm; upper and lower lateral cutaneous nerves of arm; lateral and posterior cutaneous nerves of forearm; cephalic, basilic and median cubital veins; cubital lymph nodes.

Deep fascia:

medial and lateral intermuscular septa; flexor and extensor compartments.

Muscles:

biceps brachii; brachialis; coracobrachialis; pronator teres; brachioradialis.

Boundaries of cubital fossa

Nerves:

musculocutaneous; ulnar; median; radial.

Arteries:

brachial artery and its branches; radial and ulnar arteries.

Veins:

venae comitantes of brachial artery.

Surface anatomy:

brachial artery.

Clinical anatomy:

suitability of antecubital veins for intravenous injections and taking blood for analysis and for transfusion.

Dissection Schedule 2

FRONT OF ARM AND CUBITAL REGION

1. *Make the following incisions:*
   (a) *from the lateral end of the transverse incision (c) of Dissection Schedule 1, make a vertical incision along the lateral side of the upper limb to about the middle of the forearm.*
   (b) *carry this incision horizontally across the front of the forearm to its medial border.*

   Reflect the skin flap.

2. *Clean the* **cephalic** *and* **basilic veins** lying in the superficial fascia lateral and medial to the biceps brachii muscle, respectively. The termination of the cephalic vein into the axillary vein has already been identified. Note that the basilic vein pierces the deep fascia about the middle of the arm and becomes the **axillary vein** at the lower border of the teres major. Observe the connections between the cephalic and basilic veins in the cubital fossa.

3. *Find the* **lateral cutaneous nerve of forearm** on the lateral side of the biceps in the cubital region. This is a continuation of the musculocutaneous nerve.

4. *Incise the deep fascia along the length of the arm in the midline. Make transverse cuts at the upper and lower ends and reflect the flaps. As you do so, observe the* **medial** *and* **lateral intermuscular septa** which are attached to the **medial** and **lateral supracondylar ridges** of the humerus, respectively. These septa divide the arm into an anterior *flexor* and a posterior *extensor* compartment.

5. *Clean the* **biceps brachii** *and* **coracobrachialis muscles**. Note that the tendon of the **long head of biceps** arises from the **supraglenoid tubercle** of the scapula. *Expose the part of the tendon which lies in the intertubercular groove by cutting through the fascial expansion from the pectoralis major. Observe the origin of the* **short head of biceps** *and coracobrachialis from the coracoid process of the scapula. Follow the coracobrachialis to its insertion* into the middle of the medial side of

the shaft of the humerus. Note that the musculocutaneous nerve enters the coracobrachialis in its upper part.

6. *Trace the median and ulnar nerves from the axilla into the arm. Observe* that the median nerve accompanies the **brachial artery**. *Secure the ulnar nerve* which accompanies the brachial artery in its upper part and then pierces the medial intermuscular septum at the mid-humeral level to enter the posterior compartment of the arm.
7. *Clean the brachial artery* and note that it has numerous branches.
8. *Trace the tendon of insertion of the biceps into the* **radial tuberosity** *and into the deep fascia of the forearm via the* **bicipital aponeurosis.**
9. *Divide the bicipital aponeurosis* and note the division of the brachial artery into **radial** and **ulnar arteries.**
10. *Trace the median nerve to its entry into the forearm* between the two heads of the **pronator teres muscle**. *Preserve the branches arising from the nerve.*
11. *Cut transversely across the middle of the biceps muscle and draw the two halves apart.* The musculocutaneous nerve will now be seen lying on the **brachialis muscle** which it supplies. Note the origin of the brachialis from the lower half of the anterior surface of the shaft of the humerus and its insertion into the **coronoid process of the ulna**.
12. In the distal fourth of the arm, *identify the radial nerve lying between the brachialis and* **brachioradialis muscles**. The nerve sends branches to these muscles.
13. Note the triangular **cubital fossa**. Its base is an imaginary line between the **medial** and **lateral epicondyles of the humerus**. The brachioradialis forms the lateral boundary and pronator teres forms the medial boundary of the fossa. The floor is formed by the brachialis above, which separates it from the **elbow joint**, and below by the **supinator muscle**. *Review the contents of the fossa*, from lateral to medial they are the tendon of biceps; the brachial artery with its terminal branches: radial and ulnar arteries; and the median nerve.

Summary

It will be observed that the anterior compartment of the arm contains the flexor muscles, i.e. coracobrachialis, biceps and brachialis, which are innervated by the musculocutaneous nerve. The biceps muscle passes over both the shoulder and elbow joints and consequently has actions on both these joints, whereas the brachialis, crossing only the elbow, has its action solely on the elbow joint.

The **brachial artery** which commences at the lower border of the teres major lies in the groove between the flexor and extensor muscles down to the middle of the arm. The artery lies medial to the humerus in the upper part of the arm and in front of it lower down. The division of the brachial artery into **radial** and **ulnar arteries** usually occurs in the cubital fossa opposite the neck of the radius.

Objectives For Dissection Schedule 2

Topic: Front of arm and cubital region

General objective

Comprehend the principles of the arrangement of the muscles, nerves and blood vessels of the region.

Specific objectives

1. Describe the formation of the flexor and extensor compartments of the arm.
2. Illustrate the actions of individual muscles of the flexor compartment.
3. Define the position of the neurovascular bundle (median nerve and brachial artery) in the upper and lower parts of the arm and their relationship to the humerus.
4. Discuss the effects of lesion of the nerves supplying the flexor group in terms of segmental innervation of the elbow joint.
5. Surface mark the brachial artery and illustrate the points of arterial compression, the site for recording blood pressure and the vulnerability of the brachial artery in fractures of the lower end of the humerus (supracondylar fractures).
6. Understand the vulnerability of: (a) the median nerve in supracondylar fractures, and (b) the ulnar nerve in fracture of the medial epicondyle.
7. Review the boundaries and contents of the cubital fossa.

Overview of Schedule 3

Before you begin dissection note:

SUPERFICIAL DISSECTION OF BACK OF TRUNK, SCAPULAR REGION AND BACK OF ARM

Relevant skeletal features:

skull — mastoid process; superior nuchal line; external occipital protuberance;
vertebral column — spines of vertebrae; vertebra prominens C7 (or T1); sacrum; coccyx;
hip bones — iliac crest; posterior superior iliac spine at the level of S2 spine;
scapula — medial, superior and lateral (axillary) borders; scapular notch; spine of scapula; supra- and infraspinous fossae; spinoglenoid notch; glenoid cavity; infraglenoid tubercle; superior angle at the level of T2 spine; inferior angle at the level of T7 spine;
humerus — greater and lesser tubercles; deltoid tuberosity; radial groove;
ulna — olecranon process.

Subcutaneous structures:

cutaneous branches of dorsal rami; posterior cutaneous nerve of arm.

Deep fascia:

thoracolumbar fascia.

Ligaments:

ligamentum nuchae; supraspinous ligaments; coracoacromial ligament; superior transverse scapular ligament.

Muscles:

trapezius; latissimus dorsi; levator scapulae; rhomboid minor and major; deltoid; supraspinatus; infraspinatus; teres major and minor; inferior belly of omohyoid; subscapularis; serratus anterior; triceps brachii; anconeus.

Boundaries of quadrangular space

Nerves:

accessory; suprascapular; axillary; other nerves supplying muscles.

Arteries:

transverse cervical; suprascapular; subscapular; anatosmoses around scapula; circumflex humeral.

Surface anatomy:

axillary nerve; radial nerve.

Clinical anatomy:

fracture of the neck of the humerus; fracture of the middle of the shaft of the humerus.

Dissection Schedule 3

SUPERFICIAL DISSECTION OF BACK OF TRUNK, SCAPULAR REGION AND BACK OF ARM

1. *With the body in the prone position make the following incisions*:
   (a) *a midline incision from about the spine of T1 down to the tip of the* **coccyx**;
   (b) *from the tip of the coccyx curving upwards and laterally along the* **iliac crest** *to the mid-axillary line* (*if not already done*);
   (c) *from the spine of L1 vertebra laterally to the* **midaxillary line**;
   (d) *from the spine of T1 laterally to about 2 cm above the lateral end of the clavicle*;
   (e) *cut transversely across the middle of the back of the forearm to its medial border.*

   Reflect the skin flaps.

2. At the back of the neck and trunk note the **posterior primary rami of the cervical, thoracic** and **lumbar nerves** which may be accompanied by small vessels. These will be seen piercing the deep fascia about 3–4 cm from the midline.

3. *Remove the superficial and deep fasciae to expose the first layer of muscles of the back of the trunk,* i.e. **trapezius** and **latissimus dorsi**. Note the origin of the trapezius from the **occipital bone** to the **spine** of the twelfth **thoracic vertebra** and its insertion into the **clavicle, acromion process** and the **crest of the spine of the scapula**. Similarly, *define the origin of the latissimus dorsi* from the lower thoracic spines, **thoracolumbar fascia, iliac crest**, lower ribs and **inferior angle of the scapula** and its insertion into the **intertubercular groove of the humerus**.

4. *Divide the trapezius vertically about 2 cm from the midline working from below upwards to the level of the horizontal skin incision* (d). *Clean and preserve the descending* **accessory nerve** entering the deep surface of the lateral portion of the divided muscle. *Then cut the trapezius horizontally along the skin incision* (d) *and from its attachment to the clavicle and acromion and turn the lower cut part of the trapezius laterally.*

5. Note the second layer of muscles lying deep to the trapezius. They are from above downwards the: (a) **levator scapulae**, (b) **rhomboid minor**, and (c) **rhomboid major**. They are inserted serially along the medial border of the scapula *above*, *at* and *below* the spine. *Divide the three muscles close to the* **medial border of the scapula**.

6. *Clean the* **deltoid muscle** arising from the anterior aspect of the lateral third of the clavicle, the lateral border of the **acromion** and the crest of the spine of the scapula. Note the insertion of the muscle into the **deltoid tuberosity** of the humerus. *Examine* the direction of the anterior, middle and posterior fibres of the muscle.

7. *Cut the deltoid muscle close to its origin and push the muscle downwards and secure the* **axillary nerve** *lying on its deep surface*. It supplies the deltoid and **teres minor** muscles.

8. *Identify the* **subacromial bursa** situated partly below the acromion process and partly below the **coracoacromial ligament** (arch). Deep to the bursa is the supraspinatus tendon.

9. *Clean the* **supraspinatus** *and* **infraspinatus muscles** arising from the **supra-** and **infraspinous fossae** of the scapula. They are inserted into the upper and middle facets on the **greater tubercle of the humerus**. These two muscles are supplied by the **suprascapular nerve**.

10. *Divide the latissimus dorsi vertically below the inferior angle of the scapula and separate the two parts of the muscle*. The three muscles attached along the **axillary** (lateral) **border of the scapula** can now be seen. These are from below upwards: the **teres major**, **teres minor** and **long head of triceps**.

11. *Feel the origin of the* **subscapularis muscle** on the anterior surface of the scapula and its insertion into the **lesser tubercle of the humerus**. *Quickly review the insertions of the* supraspinatus, infraspinatus, teres minor and subscapularis tendons. Note their intimate relationship to the capsule of the shoulder joint thus forming the **rotator cuff**.

12. *Examine the slips of origin of the serratus anterior* passing from the upper eight ribs to the whole length of the medial border of the scapula, the last

four slips passing to the inferior angle. *Divide the serratus anterior vertically along the medial border of the scapula.*

Back of Arm

13. *In order to examine the radial nerve* which gives branches to the **long, lateral** and **medial heads of the triceps muscle**, *cut the long head of triceps close to its origin from the* **infraglenoid tubercle of the scapula** *and displace it medially. Follow the radial nerve distally* between the lateral and medial heads of the triceps where it enters the **groove for the radial nerve** on the posterior surface of the humerus. *Detach the lateral head of triceps from its origin from the upper part of the posterior surface of the humerus.* The medial head arises from the posterior surface of the humerus below the groove. Note that the radial nerve also supplies the **anconeus muscle** which is situated behind and lateral to the elbow joint.
14. *Define the common insertion of the triceps on the* **olecranon process** of the ulna.
15. *Follow the radial nerve* from the groove for the radial nerve towards the lateral side of the arm where it pierces the lateral intermuscular septum. *Observe* that the nerve subsequently lies on the brachialis and is overlapped by the **brachioradialis** and **extensor carpi radialis longus**. The radial nerve supplies all three muscles. *Observe* the division of the radial nerve into **superficial** and **deep branches** just above the elbow.

Summary

The muscles of the back of the trunk are arranged in layers. The superficial two layers are chiefly concerned in attaching the upper limb girdle to the trunk. Consequently, the majority of the muscles such as the trapezius, rhomboids and levator scapulae act only on the shoulder girdle. However, the latissimus dorsi which passes from the trunk to the humerus has actions both on the girdle and the shoulder joint.

The different parts of the trapezius may act together or independently. Thus, the upper fibres of the muscle may act independently in shrugging the shoulder or they may act in concert with the lower fibres as in rotating the scapula so that the glenoid cavity faces upwards and forwards during abduction of the arm. Although the trapezius produces the latter action, it is the serratus anterior which is the chief muscle in rotating the inferior angle of the scapula outwards and upwards. This muscle also holds the scapula to the thoracic wall during the excursions of this bone which is acted upon by a number of muscles attached to it.

In the back of the arm, the radial nerve gives off most of its branches before it enters the groove for the radial nerve of the humerus while only the lower lateral cutaneous nerve of arm and the posterior cutaneous nerve of forearm are given off as the nerve lies in the groove. Since the nerve is intimately related to the bone in this part of its course, fractures of the humerus about the middle of the shaft may damage the nerve. However, in the resultant paralysis the triceps is unaffected.

The axillary nerve may be injured in dislocation of the shoulder joint and in fractures of the surgical neck of the humerus with resultant loss of abduction of the arm.

Objectives for Dissection Schedule 3

Topic: Superficial dissection of back of trunk, scapular region and back of arm

General objective 1

Comprehend the arrangements of the muscles of the regions.

Specific objectives

1. Define the attachments of the first and second layers of the back muscles.
2. Define the attachments of the muscles on the ventral and dorsal surfaces of the scapula.
3. Define the attachments of the muscles on the medial and lateral borders of the scapula.
4. Define the three heads of the triceps brachii and its actions.
5. Illustrate the boundaries of the quadrangular space and the structures passing through it.

General objective 2

Comprehend the arrangements of the nerves and blood vessels of the regions.

Specific objectives

1. Appreciate the segmental innervation of the skin of the back of the trunk by dorsal rami.
2. Explain the significance of the innervation of most of the scapular muscles by the posterior divisions of the brachial plexus.
3. Discuss the clinical importance of the segmental nerve supply of the elbow joint.
4. Surface mark the radial and axillary nerves in the arm.
5. Deduce the effects of lesion of: (a) the axillary nerve in fracture of the neck of the humerus, (b) the radial nerve in a mid-shaft fracture.

Overview of Schedule 4

Before you begin dissection note:

1. JOINTS OF THE SHOULDER REGION

1.1 Sternoclavicular Joint

Relevant skeletal features:

manubrium; medial end of clavicle; first costal cartilage.

Muscles in relation to capsule of joint:

pectoralis major; sternocleidomastoid; subclavius.

Capsule:

attachments.

Ligaments:

anterior and posterior sternoclavicular; interclavicular; costoclavicular.

Synovial membrane:

reflection.

Intraarticular structures:

articular disc.

Articular surfaces:

size of sternal and clavicular articular surfaces.

Movements:

gliding; rotation.

Nerve supply:

medial supraclavicular; nerve to subclavius.

1.2 Acromioclavicular Joint

Relevant skeletal features:

lateral end of the clavicle; acromion process of the scapula.

Muscles in relation to capsule of joint:

trapezius; deltoid.

Capsule:

attachments.

Ligaments:

coracoclavicular.

Synovial membrane:

reflection.

Intraarticular structures:

articular disc (sometimes present).

Movements:

gliding; rotation.

Nerve supply:

suprascapular; lateral pectoral.

Clinical anatomy:

dislocation.

1.3 Shoulder Joint

Relevant skeletal features:

glenoid cavity; head of humerus.

Muscles in relation to capsule of joint:

deltoid; rotator cuff muscles; long head of biceps; long head of triceps.

Capsule:

attachments.

Ligaments:

coracoacromial; coracohumeral; glenohumeral.

Intracapsular structures:

tendon of long head of biceps.

Synovial membrane:

reflection.

Articular surfaces:

humeral and glenoidal articular surfaces; labrum glenoidale.

Movements:

flexion; extension; abduction; adduction; medial and lateral rotation; circumduction.

Nerve supply:

suprascapular; axillary; lateral pectoral.

Clinical anatomy:

dislocation.

2. BACK OF FOREARM AND HAND

Relevant skeletal features:

radius — posterior surface; dorsal tubercle; styloid process;
ulna — supinator crest; posterior surface; head; styloid process;
carpus, metacarpus and phalanges.

Subcutaneous structures:

posterior cutaneous nerve of forearm; superficial branch of radial nerve; dorsal branch of ulnar nerve.

Deep fascia:

extensor retinaculum; osteofascial compartments.

Muscles:

brachioradialis; extensor carpi radialis longus and brevis; extensor digitorum; extensor digiti minimi; extensor carpi ulnaris; supinator; abductor pollicis longus; extensor pollicis longus; extensor indicis.

Nerves:

deep branch of radial; posterior interosseous.

Arteries:

posterior interosseous; dorsal carpal arch and branches.

Veins:

dorsal venous arch; basilic and cephalic veins.

Clinical anatomy:

radial nerve palsy; fracture of lower end of radius (Colles' fracture).

Dissection Schedule 4

JOINTS OF SHOULDER REGION AND BACK OF FOREARM AND HAND

Turn the body onto its back and examine:

1. The **sternoclavicular joint**: *Detach the tendinous* **sternal head** *of the* **sternocleidomastoid muscle**. Note the capsule. *Detach the subclavius from its costal origin. Look for the important* **costoclavicular ligament** that extends from the inferior surface of the medial end of the clavicle to the first rib and costal cartilage. This is an accessory ligament of the joint. It prevents excessive forward and backward movement and also upward displacement of the medial end of the clavicle. *Cut downwards through the upper part of the capsule close to the sternum and slightly pull the clavicle laterally* to see the **articular disc**. Note that the disc is attached to the upper part of the medial end of the clavicle above, to the first costal cartilage below, and anteriorly and posteriorly to the capsule.

2. *Cut through the middle of the clavicle with a saw.*

3. The **acromioclavicular joint**: Note this joint and its capsule. *Look for the* **coracoclavicular ligament** stretching between the inferior surface of the clavicle and the superior surface of the **coracoid process**. This ligament is an accessory ligament. *Observe* the **coracoacromial ligament** extending from the horizontal part of the coracoid process to the apex of the **acromion process**.

4. The **shoulder joint**: *Define the capsule* and note the tendons of the rotator cuff which are fused to it. *Cut the subscapularis medial to its insertion, reflect the two parts and identify the* **subscapular bursa** *deep to the subscapularis tendon* and note that it communicates with the shoulder joint. *Detach the short head of biceps and coracobrachialis from their origin on the coracoid process. Identify the tendon of the long head of the biceps lying deep to the* **transverse humeral ligament** which stretches across the upper part of the **intertubercular groove**. Note that the **coracohumeral ligament** extends from the root of the coracoid process (above the **supraglenoid tubercle**) towards the **greater tubercle of the humerus**. This strengthens the upper part of the capsule. Observe the laxity of the

capsule of the joint and note its attachment to the **anatomical neck** of the humerus, except inferiorly where it passes down for 1 cm on to the shaft of the bone. This is the weakest and least protected part of the capsule. *Carefully cut the remaining rotator cuff muscles around the shoulder joint.*

(a) *Make a vertical incision through the posterior part of the capsule and rotate the head of the humerus medially. Try to view the* **glenohumeral ligaments** passing from the anterior margin of the **glenoid cavity** towards the anatomical neck of the humerus. *Now cut through the anterior part of the capsule and identify the origin of the long head of the biceps* from the supraglenoid tubercle of the scapula. Note the difference in the size of the humeral and scapular articular surfaces.

(b) *Identify the* **labrum glenoidale** attached to the margins of the glenoid cavity.

(c) *Remove the upper limb by cutting through the remains of the capsule and long head of biceps, and cut any remaining structures so as to free the limb.*

BACK OF FOREARM AND HAND

1. *Having removed the free upper limb from the trunk, make the following incisions on the posterior aspect of the forearm and hand:*
   (a) *a median incision from the middle of the forearm down to the root of the middle finger;*
   (b) *a transverse incision across the wrist;*
   (c) *a curved incision at the level of the heads of the metacarpal bones;*
   (d) *a longitudinal incision along the middle of each digit to the nail bed.*
   Reflect the skin flaps.

2. *Clean the* **dorsal venous arch** which lies over the posterior aspect of the metacarpal region and note the commencement of the **basilic** and **cephalic veins** from the ulnar and radial sides of the arch, respectively.

3. Note that the **dorsal branch of the ulnar nerve** pierces the deep fascia above the wrist on the medial side of the forearm. This nerve supplies the medial one and a half digits. The **superficial branch of the radial nerve** supplies the remaining digits. It can be seen in the lower lateral part of the forearm.

4. *Define the* **extensor retinaculum** which is attached to the lower end of the **radius** laterally and the **pisiform** and **triquetral** medially. It retains the tendons in their position. *Remove the deep fascia and open the extensor retinaculum with a scalpel.*

5. *Define the three marginal muscles of the forearm*: (a) **brachioradialis** arising from the upper part of the **lateral supracondylar ridge** of the humerus and gaining insertion into the lower lateral end of the radius; (b) **extensor carpi radialis longus** passing from the lower part of the lateral supracondylar ridge to the base of the second metacarpal bone; (c) **extensor carpi radialis brevis** extending from the **lateral epicondyle of the humerus** to the base of the third metacarpal. Note, once again, the nerve supply from the trunk of the **radial nerve** to the first two muscles and to the extensor carpi radialis brevis from the **deep branch of the radial nerve** which you will see later.

6. *Now examine the three superficial extensors*: (a) **extensor digitorum**, (b) **extensor digiti minimi** and (c) **extensor carpi ulnaris**. These three muscles have a common origin from the lateral epicondyle of the humerus. *Trace the extensor digitorum into the hand* where it splits into four tendons for the medial four digits. Note that the extensor digiti minimi fuses with the extensor digitorum tendon for the little finger. *Next trace the extensor carpi ulnaris to its insertion into the base of the fifth metacarpal bone.*

7. *Divide the extensor digitorum, extensor digiti minimi and extensor carpi ulnaris midway between their origin and insertion to bring into view the deep group of five muscles. Study their attachments and follow them to their insertion.* From above downwards these are:
   (a) the **supinator**, passing from the lateral epicondyle of the humerus and **supinator crest of the ulna** to the upper third of the radius. Note how the muscle winds round the posterior surface of the radius;
   (b) **abductor pollicis longus** taking origin from the upper posterior surfaces of both radius and ulna and gaining insertion into the base of the first metacarpal;
   (c) **extensor pollicis brevis** arising from the posterior surface of the radius and inserting into the base of the proximal phalanx of the thumb;

Observe that the tendons of the last two muscles run side by side on the lateral aspect of the wrist:

(d) **extensor pollicis longus** taking origin from the posterior surface of the ulna and gaining insertion into the base of the terminal phalanx of the thumb; note that the tendon passes medial to the **dorsal tubercle of the radius** on the posterior aspect of the distal end of the radius;

(e) **extensor indicis** originating from the lower part of the posterior surface of the ulna and fusing with the extensor digitorum tendon for the index finger.

8. *Trace the deep branch of the radial nerve through the supinator* and note that it continues as the **posterior interosseous nerve**. In its lower part the nerve accompanies the **posterior interosseous artery**. The posterior interosseous nerve supplies the superficial and deep extensor muscles.

9. *Again trace the extensor tendons as they pass under the extensor retinaculum.* Note that they lie in their separate osteofascial compartments. As they lie in these compartments, they are covered by **synovial sheaths**.

10. *Identify once again the tendons of the extensor digitorum.* Note that the tendons to the index and little fingers are joined by the tendons of the extensor indicis and extensor digiti minimi, respectively. *Observe* that the tendons begin to expand towards the digits where they form the **extensor expansions**. These expansions also receive contributions from the **lumbrical** and **interossei** muscles in the hand. *Trace the slips from the expansions to their insertions into the bases of the intermediate and distal phalanges.*

11. *Near the wrist find the* **radial artery** passing backwards beneath the tendons of the abductor pollicis longus, extensor pollicis brevis and extensor pollicis longus to enter the palm from behind between the two heads of the **first dorsal interosseous muscle** in the first intermetacarpel space.

Summary

The **sternoclavicular joint**, though classified as a saddle joint, permits varying types of movements of the clavicle such as elevation, depression, forward and backward movements, as well as rotation. The strength of this joint depends largely on the strength of the ligaments. In particular, the costoclavicular ligament and the interarticular disc check the upward displacement of the medial end of the clavicle. Consequently, dislocation of the medial end of the clavicle does not usually occur.

The **shoulder joint** is a ball and socket joint in which mobility is greatly increased at the expense of stability. The strength of the joint depends chiefly on the rotator cuff muscles which are fused to the capsule of the joint. The joint is least protected inferiorly and consequently dislocations commonly occur here.

The *plane of the joint* is set obliquely so that the arm is carried forwards and medially during flexion and backwards and laterally during extension. Abduction is initiated by the supraspinatus and further carried out by the deltoid. As abduction proceeds towards a vertical position, the humerus is rotated laterally.

It must also be borne in mind that during movements of the shoulder joint, simultaneous movements occur at the sternoclavicular and acromioclavicular joints. Consequently, any restriction of movements of these joints will indirectly affect the movements of the shoulder joint. Moreover, movements of the shoulder joint are assisted by an excursion of the scapula on the thoracic wall. Therefore, any paralysis of muscles which move the scapula will restrict the range of movement at the shoulder joint. Indeed in abduction of the arm through a possible 180°, scapular rotation by itself contributes to about a third of the total movement.

The muscles of the back of the forearm can be classified into superficial and deep groups. The *superficial* set comprises the brachioradialis, extensor carpi radialis longus and brevis which are situated laterally (marginal group) and the extensor digitorum, extensor digiti minimi and extensor carpi ulnaris which occupy the dorsal aspect of the forearm. The *deep group* is formed by the supinator, abductor pollicis longus, extensor pollicis brevis, extensor pollicis longus and the extensor indicis. All these muscles are supplied by the radial nerve or its branches. Consequently, in cases of injury to the radial nerve, the extensor muscles will be paralysed leading to a condition known as **wrist drop**.

Objectives for Dissection Schedule 4

1. Topic: Joints of the shoulder girdle

General objective 1

Comprehend the arrangement of the osteoligamentous structures of the joints of the shoulder girdle.

Specific objectives

1. Orientate the sternum, clavicle, scapula and humerus.
2. Articulate the clavicle with the sternum and first costal cartilage and compare the clavicular and sternal articular surfaces.
3. Describe the ligaments of the sternoclavicular joint.
4. Assign a functional role to the articular disc of the sternoclavicular joint.
5. Articulate the clavicle with the acromion.
6. Describe the ligaments of the acromioclavicular joint.
7. Assign the functional role to the coracoclavicular ligament.
8. Articulate the humerus with the scapula.
9. Compare the articular surfaces of the shoulder joint.
10. Describe the attachments of the capsular, transverse and coracohumeral ligaments of the shoulder joint.
11. Identify the anatomical and the surgical neck of the humerus.
12. Define the axes and movements of the shoulder joint.
13. Discuss the stability of the shoulder joint.
14. Analyse the innervation of the shoulder joint based on Hilton's law.
15. Explain how movements of the shoulder joint are associated with movements of the acromioclavicular and sternoclavicular joints.
16. Interpret X-rays of these joints.

General objective 2

Comprehend the arrangement of the muscles acting on the joints of the shoulder girdle.

Specific objectives

1. Classify the muscles acting on the shoulder joint into flexors, extensors, abductors, adductors and rotators.
2. Outline the role of the rotator cuff muscles.
3. Explain the effects of paralysis of the deltoid, supraspinatus and serratus anterior.
4. Explain the role of serratus anterior, trapezius, rhomboids and levator scapulae in scapular rotation.

2. Topic: Back of the forearm and hand

General objective 1

Understand the disposition of the muscles in the region.

Specific objectives

1. Enumerate the muscles of the superficial and deep extensor groups.
2. Define the osteofascial compartments on the back of the wrist and enumerate the tendons passing through each compartment.
3. Define the formation and termination of the extensor expansions to each digit.
4. Comment on the tendons to the thumb, index finger and little finger.

General objective 2

Comprehend the arrangement of the nerves and blood vessels of the region.

Specific objectives

1. Define the muscles supplied by the radial nerve and its branches.
2. Indicate the segmental innervation of the wrist joint and the joints of the fingers.

3. Explain wrist drop in anatomical terms.
4. Analyse the cutaneous innervation and dermatomic pattern of the region.
5. Trace the origin, course and termination of the basilic and cephalic veins.

Overview of Schedule 5

Before you begin dissection note:

FRONT OF FOREARM AND HAND

Relevant skeletal features:

humerus — medial epicondyle; medial supracondylar ridge;
radius — head; surfaces; borders; styloid process;
ulna — surfaces; borders; head; styloid process;
carpus — hook of hamate; tubercle of scaphoid; pisiform; tubercle and groove of trapezium.
metacarpus and phalanges.

Subcutaneous structures:

medial cutaneous nerve of forearm; lateral cutaneous nerve of forearm; palmar cutaneous branch of ulnar nerve; palmar cutaneous branch of median nerve; digital nerves and vessels; cephalic, basilic and median cubital veins.

Deep fascia:

flexor retinaculum; palmar aponeurosis; fascial septa of the hand; fibrous flexor sheaths.

Ligaments:

deep transverse metacarpal ligaments.

Muscles:

flexor carpi ulnaris; palmaris longus; flexor carpi radialis; pronator teres; flexor digitorum superficialis; flexor digitorum profundus; flexor pollicis longus; pronator quadratus; thenar and hypothenar muscles; lumbricals; adductor pollicis; interossei.

Synovial sheaths of long flexor tendons.

Nerves:

median; ulnar; superficial radial.

Arteries:

radial and ulnar arteries and their branches; superficial and deep palmar arches.

Surface anatomy:

radial and ulnar arteries; median nerve near the wrist.

Clinical anatomy:

Volkmann's ischaemic contracture; Dupuytren's contracture; fascial spaces of hand.

Dissection Schedule 5

FRONT OF FOREARM AND HAND

1. *Make the following incisions on the anterior aspect of the forearm and hand*:
   (a) *a median incision from the middle of the forearm to the root of the middle finger*;
   (b) *a transverse incision across the wrist*;
   (c) *a curved incision across the roots of all five digits*;
   (d) *a longitudinal incision along the middle of each digit down to its distal end.*

   Reflect the skin flaps.

2. *Clean the portions of the* **cephalic** *and* **basilic veins** *in the front of the forearm.*

3. *Clean the deep fascia of the forearm and define the* **flexor retinaculum** *at the wrist* which is a thick, quadrangular band of deep fascia bridging the **carpal canal**. This will be examined later.

4. *Expose the superficial group of muscles of the forearm by removing the deep fascia* which not only covers them but also gives them partial origin. From medial to lateral, these muscles are the **flexor carpi ulnaris, palmaris longus, flexor carpi radialis** and the **superficial head of the pronator teres**. All of these arise from the **medial epicondyle of the humerus**, the common flexor origin, except the superficial part of the pronator teres which has its origin from the **medial supracondylar ridge**.

5. *Trace the flexor carpi ulnaris tendon from the common flexor origin and from the upper part of the posterior border of the ulna to the* **pisiform bone**. The slender palmaris longus passes distally to insert into the flexor retinaculum and **palmar aponeurosis**. This muscle may be absent. The flexor carpi radialis runs towards the flexor retinaculum where it passes through the retinaculum in a separate compartment to insert into the bases of the second and third metacarpal bones (see later). The **pronator teres** is a short muscle which runs laterally and downwards to be inserted into the middle of the lateral side of the shaft of the radius.

6. *Cut the superficial group of muscles about the middle of their muscle bellies and reflect them.* The nerve supply to the pronator teres, flexor carpi radialis and palmaris longus comes from the **median nerve**. The flexor carpi ulnaris is supplied by the **ulnar nerve**. *Verify* that the ulnar nerve runs *behind* the medial epicondyle and enters the forearm between the two heads of the flexor carpi ulnaris.

7. *Identify the* **flexor digitorum superficialis** *and the* **deep head of the pronator teres** which lie deep to the superficial group of muscles. *Preserve the median nerve* as it passes down between the two heads of the pronator teres and deep to the flexor digitorum superficialis. The latter muscle has a broad origin from the medial epicondyle of the humerus, **coronoid process of the ulna** and **anterior border of the radius**. Note the fibrous arcade which overlies the median nerve and ulnar artery as they pass beneath this muscle. *Observe the tendons of the superficialis as they lie near the wrist* and note that they pass to the **index, middle, ring** and **little fingers**.

8. *Identify the median nerve* just proximal to the flexor retinaculum emerging from beneath the flexor digitorum superficialis and lying between the tendons of palmaris longus and flexor carpi radialis.

9. *Cut the flexor digitorum superficialis muscle in its middle and reflect the two parts.* Note the innervation from the median nerve. *Observe* that the neurovascular structures comprising the median nerve, ulnar artery and ulnar nerve lie on the deep group of muscles.

10. *Trace the* **ulnar artery**, which runs downwards from the cubital fossa, deep to the deep head of the pronator teres, towards the medial side of the wrist where it lies *superficial* to the **flexor retinaculum**. The artery gives off numerous branches, the most important being the **common interosseous artery** which arises at the level of the radial tuberosity high up in the forearm and divides into **anterior** and **posterior interosseous branches**.

11. *Define the palmar aponeurosis* which lies immediately deep to the skin of the palm and trace the four slips passing from it to the roots of the medial four fingers. *Trace the* **digital branches** *of the median and ulnar nerves* as they pass down between these slips accompanied by digital arteries.

12. *Examine the* flexor retinaculum which is attached laterally to the **tubercle of the scaphoid** and lips of the groove on the **trapezium** and medially to the pisiform and **hook of the hamate**. Note the **palmaris brevis**, a small subcutaneous muscle running transversely from the retinaculum towards the **hypothenar eminence**, and *remove it. Identify the ulnar nerve and artery lying superficial to the flexor retinaculum.*

13. *Carefully reflect the palmar aponeurosis downwards* and note the fascial septa passing from the palmar aponeurosis to the first and fifth metacarpal bones and separating the flexor tendons from the **thenar** and **hypothenar muscles.**

14. *Next trace the distal part of the ulnar artery into the palm* where it continues as the **superficial palmar arch** which lies in front of the superficial tendons. This arch is reinforced by the **palmar branch of the radial artery**. Note that lateral to the pisiform bone the ulnar artery gives off a small **deep palmar branch** which accompanies the **deep branch of the ulnar nerve**. The superficial palmar arch gives off four **common palmar digital branches** to the medial three-and-a-half digits. The radial side of the index and both sides of the thumb are supplied by the radial artery (see later).

15. *Trace the ulnar and median nerves from the wrist into the palm where the origin of their digital branches can be seen.* Note that the median nerve reaches the palm *deep* to the flexor retinaculum by passing through the carpal tunnel. The nerve supplies the three thenar muscles.

16. *Clean the thenar muscles. Identify the laterally placed* **abductor pollicis brevis** *and the more medially situated* **flexor pollicis brevis**. Note the origin of both these muscles from the flexor retinaculum, the scaphoid and the trapezium. Both are inserted into the lateral side of the base of the **proximal phalanx** of the thumb. *Trace their nerve supply from the median nerve. Cut the two muscles in the middle, reflect them and define the more deeply placed* **opponens pollicis** passing from the flexor retinaculum and trapezium to the shaft of the **first metacarpal bone**.

17. *Next turn your attention to the hypothenar muscles. Identify and cut the* **abductor digiti minimi** *and* **flexor digiti minimi brevis** *in the middle and identify the* **opponens digiti minimi** *muscle.* They arise from the flexor

retinaculum, the pisiform bone and the hook of the hamate. *Identify the insertions of the abductor and flexor into the medial side of the base of the proximal phalanx of the fifth digit and the opponens into the shaft of the fifth metacarpal bone.* The nerve supply to these muscles comes from the deep branch of the ulnar nerve which passes between the abductor and flexor digiti minimi to enter the deep aspect of the palm. Note that the branch is accompanied by the deep palmar branch of the ulnar artery. *Try to find them.*

18. *Now clean the following deep structures on the front of the forearm*:
    (a) laterally **flexor pollicis longus muscle** arising from the anterior surface of the radius and interosseous membrane;
    (b) medially **flexor digitorum profundus muscle** arising from the interosseous membrane as well as from the anterior and medial surfaces of the ulna;
    (c) below **pronator quadratus muscle** extending between the distal fourth of the ulna and radius and lying deep to the deep flexor tendons. It is the principal pronator;
    (d) the **anterior interosseous nerve** from the median nerve supplying the above three muscles with the exception of the medial part of flexor digitorum profundus which receives its innervation from the ulnar nerve. The anterior interosseous nerve lies on the interosseous membrane between flexor digitorum profundus and flexor pollicis longus and terminates in the pronator quadratus. The nerve is accompanied by the anterior interosseous artery.

19. *Trace the radial artery deep to the brachioradialis. Divide the brachioradialis muscle in its middle and reflect it so as to identify the artery and the accompanying superficial branch of the radial nerve. Follow the radial artery* down to the **styloid process of the radius**. Note the structures on which this artery lies. Its branches in this region are:
    (a) the **superficial palmar artery** arising above the wrist and descending to join the superficial palmer arch;
    (b) the **arteria princeps pollicis** which supplies the thumb;
    (c) the **arteria radialis indicis** which supplies the index finger;
    (d) and branches to the neighbouring muscles.

20. *Make a vertical incision down the middle of the flexor retinaculum. Observe* the arrangement of the tendons of the flexor digitorum superficialis, flexor digitorum profundus, flexor pollicis longus and flexor carpi radialis as they pass under the retinaculum and the relationship of the median nerve to these tendons. *Below the retinaculum identify the four* **lumbrical muscles** arising from the tendons of the flexor digitorum profundus. These muscles are inserted into the radial side of the extensor expansion. Note that the medial two lumbricals receive their innervation from the deep branch of the ulnar nerve and the lateral two lumbricals from the median nerve.

21. Note that the tendons of the flexors digitorum superficialis and profundus are covered by **synovial sheaths**. *Trace these tendons from the palm to one of the digits by incising the* **fibrous flexor sheath** *covering them. You will see* that the superficialis tendon *splits* into two bundles which pass around the profundus tendon and insert *into the sides* of the **middle phalanx** and that the profundus tendon inserts into the **base of the distal phalanx**. *Then trace flexor pollicis longus to its insertion into the base of the distal phalanx of the thumb. Next cut the tendons of the flexor digitorum profundus and flexor pollicis longus just above the wrist and turn them and the superficialis tendons downwards. Also, cut through the middle of the superficial palmar arch and the accompanying nerve so as to get a better view of the deep aspect of the palm.*

22. *Now turn your attention to the deep intrinsic group of muscles which lie beneath the flexor tendons. Clean the* **adductor pollicis**. Its **transverse head** arises from the shaft of the third metacarpal bone while its **oblique head** arises from the bases of the second and third metacarpals and **capitate**. Both heads are inserted into the medial side of the base of the proximal phalanx of the thumb. Note that the potential **fascial spaces (palmar spaces)** of the hand are situated deep to the flexor tendons and superficial to the adductor pollicis and **interossei**.

23. *Identify the radial artery* emerging between the transverse and oblique heads of the adductor pollicis. *Reflect the oblique head from its origin. Observe* that the **deep palmar arch** is formed by the continuation of the radial artery and the deep branch of the ulnar artery. Note that the **palmar**

metacarpal arteries arise from the deep palmar arch and join the digital branches from the superficial palmar arch.

24. *Clean the deep branch of the ulnar nerve* which supplies the medial two lumbricals, adductor pollicis and all the interossei muscles. *Reflect the transverse head of adductor pollicis from its origin.* Note that the **four palmar interossei** arise from the corresponding metacarpal bones and the **four dorsal interossei** from the adjacent metacarpal bones. The palmar interossei are inserted into the extensor expansion and the dorsal interossei are inserted into the bases of the proximal phalanges and the extensor expansion. Primarily all the interossei and the lumbricals are *flexors* of the metacarpophalangeal joints; in addition, the palmar interossei *adduct* the digits towards the middle finger and the dorsal interossei *abduct* the digits and the middle finger. In consequence of their insertions into the extensor expansions these three sets of muscles are able in certain conditions to *extend* the middle and distal phalanges.

Summary

The muscles of the front of the forearm can be subdivided into: (a) those muscles passing to the digits, i.e. digital flexors, and (b) those concerned with flexion of the wrist. The tendons of the flexor digitorum superficialis are inserted into the intermediate phalanges whereas those of the flexor digitorum profundus and flexor pollicis longus gain insertion into the distal phalanges. It is noteworthy that the presence of separate flexor tendons for the intermediate and distal phalanges increases the grasping efficiency of the hand. The actions of these slips on the interphalangeal joints are opposed by the slips of insertion of the extensor expansions. However, the action of the flexors is more powerful than that of the extensors.

The presence of a separate flexor pollicis longus for the thumb and an early separation of the tendon from the flexor digitorum profundus to the index finger provide a greater degree of freedom of movement to these digits. A similar specialisation of the extensor tendons for the thumb and index has already been noted.

The thenar muscles of the hand also exhibit a certain amount of specialisation. The large size of the opponens pollicis and the presence of a special adductor for the thumb are features peculiar to the thumb. Moreover, the thumb is capable of rotation so that its palmar surface can be opposed towards the pulps of the other digits.

The flexor carpi radialis and flexor carpi ulnaris are usually flexors of the wrist. But they can also function together with their corresponding antagonistic extensors in producing radial or ulnar deviation of the wrist. For example, the flexor and the extensor carpi ulnaris act together in producing ulnar deviation of the wrist.

The *muscles of the front of the forearm* are innervated by the median nerve or its anterior interosseous branch except the flexor carpi ulnaris and the medial portion of the flexor digitorum profundus which receive their nerve supply from the ulnar nerve. The *intrinsic muscles of the hand* are supplied by the ulnar nerve except the thenar muscles and the lateral two lumbricals which are innervated by the median nerve. *The nerves which supply the intrinsic muscles of the hand are derived from the T1 segment of the brachial plexus.*

The median nerve may be compressed within the carpal tunnel giving rise to the **carpal tunnel syndrome**. Similarly, the ulnar nerve may be compressed as it lies behind the medial epicondyle of the humerus. Damage to the median nerve produces a condition known as the **simian hand** while damage to the ulnar nerve produces a **claw hand**.

The radial and ulnar arteries are the principal vessels of the forearm. In their course, they lie between the radial and ulnar nerves. The ulnar artery continues as the superficial palmar arch while the radial artery continues into the more proximally situated deep palmar arch.

Objectives for Dissection Schedule 5

Topic: Front of forearm and hand

General objective 1

Comprehend the arrangement of the muscles of the region.

Specific objectives

1. Enumerate the superficial, intermediate and deep flexors of the forearm.
2. Define the attachments of the superficial group of flexors.
3. Define the attachments and surface mark the flexor retinaculum.
4. Enumerate the order of structures superficial and deep to the retinaculum.
5. Describe the formation of the thenar and hypothenar compartments and their contained muscles.
6. Indicate the actions of the thenar and hypothenar muscles.
7. Define the fibrous flexor sheaths, synovial sheaths and terminations of long flexor tendons.
8. Describe the origins and insertions of the lumbricals and interossei.
9. Outline the actions of the flexor, lumbrical and interossei muscles.

General objective 2

Comprehend the arrangement of the nerves and blood vessels of the region.

Specific objectives

1. Define the neurovascular plane of the forearm.
2. Describe the course and distribution of the radial and ulnar arteries.
3. Demonstrate the formation of the superficial and deep palmar arches and surface mark them.
4. Analyse the nerve supply to the flexor compartment of the forearm.
5. Define the dermatomic pattern of the region.

6. Deduce the effects of lesion of the ulnar and median nerves at the elbow and wrist.
7. Discuss the importance of the arrangement of the digital vessels and nerves in local anaesthesia.
8. Recognise the clinical importance of the palmar spaces.

Overview of Schedule 6

Before you begin dissection note:

JOINTS OF FREE UPPER LIMB

1. Elbow Joint

Relevant skeletal features:

humerus — trochlea; capitulum; radial, coronoid and olecranon fossae;
ulna — trochlear notch; coronoid and olecranon processes;
radius — head; neck; tuberosity.

Muscles in relation to capsule of joint:

brachialis; biceps; triceps; anconeus.

Capsule:

attachments.

Ligaments:

ulnar collateral; radial collateral.

Synovial membrane:

reflection.

Articular surfaces:

shape; carrying angle.

Movements:

flexion; extension.

Nerve supply:

musculocutaneous; radial.

Blood supply:

anastomosis around elbow.

Clinical anatomy:

dislocations; fractures.

2. Proximal, Middle and Distal Radioulnar Joints

Relevant skeletal features:

radius — head; ulnar notch; interosseous border;
ulna — radial notch; head; interosseous border.

Capsule:

attachments.

Ligaments:

annular (proximal joint).
interosseous membrane.

Intraarticular structures:

articular disc (distal joint).

Synovial membrane:

reflection.

Movements:

pronation; supination; axis of movement.

3. Wrist Joint

Relevant skeletal features:

distal end of radius; articular disc; scaphoid; lunate; triquetrum.

Capsule:

attachments.

Ligaments:

palmar radiocarpal and palmar ulnocarpal; dorsal radiocarpal; radial and ulnar collateral.

Synovial membrane:

reflection.

Articular surfaces:

shape.

Movements:

flexion; extension; adduction; abduction; circumduction.

4. Intercarpal, Midcarpal, Carpometacarpal, Metacarpophalangeal and Interphalangeal Joints

Relevant skeletal features:

carpus; metacarpus; phalanges.

Capsule:

attachments.

Ligaments:

dorsal and palmar; collateral; interosseous.

Synovial membrane:

reflection.

Movements:

flexion, extension (all joints); adduction, abduction (midcarpal joint, metacarpophalangeal joints and carpometacarpal joint of thumb); rotation and circumduction (carpometacarpal joint of thumb).

Dissection Schedule 6

JOINTS OF FREE UPPER LIMB

1. Elbow and Proximal Radioulnar Joints

These joints are described together as they have a common capsule and synovial cavity.

1.1. Note the intimate relationships of the brachialis and triceps muscles to the anterior and posterior parts of the **elbow joint**, respectively, and the supinator to the proximal radioulnar joint. *Remove these muscles and then remove the flexor and extensor muscles from their epicondylar origins. Take care so as not to damage the* **capsule of the elbow joint** *and the* **annular ligament**; the latter surrounds the head of the radius and is attached to the margins of the **radial notch of the ulna**.

1.2. *Define the* **ulnar collateral ligament** *of the elbow joint*. This is composed of three distinct bands: **anterior, posterior** and **oblique**. The anterior band passes between the medial epicondyle of the humerus and the coronoid process of the ulna; the posterior band passes between the medial epicondyle and the olecranon process of the ulna; and the oblique band passes between the coronoid and olecranon processes.

1.3. *Define the triangular-shaped* **radial collateral ligament** *of the elbow joint* which extends fanwise from the lateral epicondyle to the annular ligament.

1.4. *Observe* that the anterior and posterior parts of the capsule of the elbow joint are weak. *Make a transverse cut through the anterior part of the joint capsule and examine the articular surfaces.*

1.5. Note that the **annular ligament** of the **proximal radioulnar joint** is somewhat funnel-shaped, being wider superiorly. The ligament passes around the head of the radius and is attached to the anterior and posterior margins of the radial notch of the ulna.*Cut through the annular ligament on its lateral aspect and verify its shape.* This joint is part of the elbow joint.

2. Interosseous Membrane

Next examine the **interosseous membrane** which forms a bond between the radius and ulna. *Remove the muscles, nerves and vessels in order to see the interosseous membrane.*

3. Distal Radioulnar and Wrist Joints

These two joints are considered together because the **inferior radioulnar joint** cannot be studied without cutting through the capsule of the **wrist joint**.

3.1. *Review the flexor and extensor tendons related to the wrist joint.*

3.2. *Define the capsule of the wrist joint and observe the* **palmar radiocarpal** *and* **palmar ulnocarpal ligaments**; *the* **dorsal radiocarpal ligament**; *and the* **radial** *and* **ulnar collateral ligaments**.

3.3. *Cut through the dorsal part of the capsule of the wrist joint and expose the articular surfaces. Look at the triangular* **articular disc** whose apex is attached to the root of the **styloid process of the ulna** and its base to the lower margin of the **ulnar notch of the radius**.

4. Intercarpal, Midcarpal, Carpometacarpal, Metacarpophalangeal and Interphalangeal Joints

4.1. *Remove the muscles related to these joints* and note the **palmar, dorsal** and **intersseous ligaments** at the **intercarpal joints**. *Open the midcarpal joint from the dorsal aspect and examine the articular surfaces.*

4.2. **Carpometacarpal joint of the thumb.** *Examine the loose capsule. Open the capsule posteriorly and examine the shape of the articular surfaces.* What movements are possible at this joint?

4.3. *Next examine the strong* **palmar** *and* **collateral ligaments** *of the* **metacarpophalangeal joints**. Note that the **deep transverse metacarpal ligaments** connect the medial four **palmar ligaments**.

4.4. The **interphalangeal joints.** Note the strong **palmar** and **collateral ligaments**.

Summary

The **elbow joint** is a **hinge joint** in which movements of flexion and extension take place. To facilitate these movements the anterior and posterior parts of the capsule are thin. However, the collateral ligaments are strong to provide stability to the joint. The axis of movement is not entirely transverse and consequently the forearm tends to deviate outwards to produce the so-called carrying angle when the forearm is fully extended *in the supine position*. This angle disappears during pronation of the forearm and during flexion of the elbow.

The **radioulnar joints**. The movements occurring at these joints are pronation and supination. The axis for these movements passes through the centre of the head of the radius and the root of the styloid process of the ulna. Pronation and supination are most effective when the elbow is semiflexed. In this position the elbow joint is most stable.

The **wrist joint** is an **ellipsoid joint** in which the articular surface of the carpus extends more on to the dorsal than the palmar aspect. This explains why extension of the wrist is more than flexion. However, it should be noted that movement of the wrist joint involves simultaneous movements at the midcarpal joint. In flexion of the wrist, there is more movement taking place at the midcarpal joint than at the wrist joint. Furthermore, the range of adduction at the wrist is more than abduction.

The **carpometacarpal joint** of the thumb is a **saddle joint** between the trapezium and the first metacarpal bone. *Abduction* and *adduction* occur at right angles to the plane of the palm while flexion and extension take place in a plane parallel to the palm. In addition, rotation also occurs at this joint.

Opposition of the thumb is the movement whereby the palmar surface of the thumb is brought into apposition with the palmar surfaces of the other digits.

Objectives for Dissection Schedule 6

1. Topic: Elbow joint

General objective

Comprehend the arrangement of the osteoligamentous structures of the joint and the disposition of the muscles around it.

Specific objectives

1. Identify the trochlea; capitulum; coronoid, radial and olecranon fossae of the humerus.
2. Articulate the radius and ulna with the humerus.
3. Demonstrate the attachments of the capsular ligament and the radial and ulnar collateral ligaments.
4. Discuss the muscles involved in flexion and extension.
5. Discuss the clinical importance of segmental innervation of the joint.
6. Indicate the types of dislocation and sites of common fractures around the joint.
7. Interpret X-rays of these conditions as well as those of normal joints.

2. Topic: Radioulnar joints

General objective

Comprehend the movements of pronation and supination of the forearm.

Specific objectives

1. Define the articulating surfaces of the proximal and distal radioulnar joints.
2. Demonstrate pronation and supination and the axis for these movements.
3. Discuss the line of pull of the biceps, supinator, pronator teres, pronator quadratus and brachioradialis muscles in relation to this axis.
4. Assign functional roles to the anconeus muscle; annular ligament and articular disc.

5. Discuss the segmental innervation of the joints.
6. Interpret X-rays of the forearm and hand in pronation and supination.

3. Topic: Wrist and midcarpal joints

General objective

Comprehend the structural and functional aspects of the joints.

Specific objectives

1. Define the articulating surfaces, capsules and synovial reflections of the joints.
2. Enumerate the primary flexors and extensors of the wrist.
3. Identify the tendons around the wrist in the living.
4. Define the movements at the wrist in terms of its ellipsoid articular surfaces.
5. Discuss the range of movements at the wrist and associated movements occurring at the midcarpal joint.
6. Assign functional roles to the muscles acting on the joints in terms of prime movers, antagonists, synergists and fixation muscles.
7. Discuss the segmental innervation of the joints.
8. Interpret X-rays of normal joints and those with fractures around the wrist.

4. Topic: Small joints of the hand

General objective

Evaluate the functional anatomy of the hand.

Specific objectives

1. Classify the carpometacarpal joint of the thumb, the metacarpophalangeal and interphalangeal joints according to the shape of the articulating surfaces.

2. Review the modes of insertion of the long flexors and extensors of the forearm; the lumbricals and interossei.
3. Explain the increased freedom of movement of the index and little fingers and the specialised movements peculiar to the thumb.
4. Comprehend the anatomical basis of power, precision, hook and pinch grips.
5. Demonstrate the position of rest and the working position of the hand.
6. Analyse the contributions of the skin and subcutaneous structures in the performances of manual skills.
7. Outline the segmental innervation of the smaller joints of the hand.
8. Interpret the X-rays of the hand.

Additional Objectives for Upper Limb

1. Topic: Nerves of the upper limb

General objective

Understand the disposition of the nerves of the upper limb and the clinical importance of this knowledge.

Specific objectives

1. Illustrate the formation of the brachial plexus and its distribution.
2. Demonstrate the ulnar, median, musculocutaneous, radial and axillary nerves, mentioning their root values.
3. Surface mark the above nerves and place them in relation to the relevant bones.
4. Demonstrate tendon jerks and discuss their anatomical basis.
5. Demonstrate the anatomical principles in testing sensory loss.
6. Explain the anatomical basis for the causation and manifestation of Erb's and Klumpke's paralyses; crutch palsy and wrist drop; claw hand; cervical rib and carpal tunnel syndromes.

2. Topic: Blood vessels and lymphatics of the upper limb

General objective

Understand the principles of the blood supply and lymphatic drainage.

Specific objectives

1. Identify the subclavian, axillary, brachial, radial and ulnar arteries.
2. Indicate the extent of these arteries, their surface marking, the points for feeling the pulse and the site for recording blood pressure in the upper limb.
3. Illustrate the concept of the *neurovascular plane*.
4. Illustrate the principles of collateral circulation and peri-articular anastomoses.

5. Explain the arrangement of superficial and deep veins.
6. Demonstrate manoeuvres for displaying superficial veins and the presence of valves in them.
7. Define the routes of venous drainage and the extent of the cephalic, basilic, median cubital, and axillary veins.
8. Discuss the selection of the cubital fossa as the site for intravenous infusions.
9. Indicate the routes of drainage of superficial and deep lymphatics.
10. Describe the regional lymph nodes and attempt to palpate them in the living.
11. Discuss the anatomical basis of Volkmann's ischaemic contracture and Dupuytren's contracture.

3. Topic: Skeletal framework of the upper limb

General objective

Understand basic anatomical principles in the study of the bones of the upper limb.

Specific objectives

1. Exemplify short, long, flat, membrane and cartilage bones using the bones of the upper limb.
2. Describe the ossification of a long bone using the humerus as an example.
3. Discuss common sites of fractures in relation to the line of transmission of stress and the changes in the contour of the bones.
4. Analyse radiographs of long bones in children and adults pointing out the importance of a sound knowledge of epiphyseal lines and the arrangement of bony lamellae along lines of stress.
5. Discuss the relative importance of periosteal, epiphyseal, metaphyseal and nutrient arteries in the vascularisation of a typical long bone.
6. Discuss the genesis and adult structure of the marrow cavity and its clinical importance.

4. Topic: Joints of the upper limb

General objective

Comprehend the classification of synovial joints.

Specific objectives

Exemplify the features of a ball and socket, pivot, ellipsoid, plane, condyloid, saddle and hinge joints based on the joints of the upper limb.

5. Topic: Muscles of the upper limb

General objective

Comprehend the various actions of groups of muscles in the upper limb.

Specific objectives

1. Demonstrate the muscle actions in the pectoral, shoulder, arm, forearm and hand regions.
2. Consider the nerve supply of the various muscle groups.

Section 2

LOWER LIMB

Introduction

Human beings are unique among the primates in that they have adopted a bipedal mode of locomotion which has produced a substantial advantage over the older, more stable, quadrapedal gait. Bipedalism brings the advantage of a greater range of vision and frees the hands for use and for making tools and carrying food. As a result of bipedal locomotion, the weight of the body is transmitted to the lower limb via the pelvis. This has brought about several specialisations in the architecture of the skeleton, joints and muscles of the lower limb. These specialisations will have to be examined as you proceed with the dissection of the lower limb.

Since the lower limb is an outgrowth from the lateral aspect of the lower part of the trunk, its nerves and blood vessels are drawn out from within the abdomen and pelvis. Consequently, the nerves and vessels entering the front of the thigh pass beneath the **inguinal ligament**; those to the medial side of the thigh issue through the **obturator canal**; and those entering the gluteal region traverse the **greater sciatic foramen**.

It must also be borne in mind that the lower limb has undergone rotation during development. Thus the original (embryonic) *extensor or dorsal surface has shifted to the anterior or ventral aspect in the adult.* Therefore, the extensor muscles which are now in the anterior compartment of the thigh are supplied by **dorsal divisions of the lumbar plexus** (femoral nerve L2, 3, 4). Similarly, the adductor muscles which lie on the medial side of the thigh developmentally belong to the flexor compartment and are hence supplied by **ventral divisions of the lumbar plexus** (obturator nerve L2, 3, 4). The pure flexor muscles which are now at the back of the thigh are called the **hamstring muscles.** These are supplied by **ventral divisions of the sacral plexus** via branches from the tibial component of the sciatic nerve. In the *thigh*, the anterior (extensor), medial (adductor) and posterior (flexor) compartments are separated by the medial, posterior and lateral intermuscular septa. Of these the lateral intermuscular septum is the most well defined. However, all three septa fade away in the lower part of the thigh.

As in the thigh, the muscles of the *leg* are also arranged as broad functional groups separated by intermuscular septa. Both the anterior compartment containing the extensor muscles and the lateral compartment containing the fibular (peroneal) muscles belong developmentally to the extensor group.

Consequently, the common fibular (peroneal) nerve which supplies them is derived from the **dorsal divisions of the sacral plexus**. Note that the muscles in the posterior compartment are supplied by the tibial nerve.

The *foot* and hand have many similarities, but the hand is a tactile, grasping organ, whereas the functions of the foot are support and locomotion. The foot has evolved from a prehensile ape foot into the sprung arches of humans — one of the most specialised features in the human species.

Overview of Schedule 7

Before you begin dissection note:

ANTERIOR AND MEDIAL ASPECTS OF THE THIGH

Relevant skeletal features:

hip bone —pubic tubercle; anterior superior iliac spine; iliac crest; tubercle of iliac crest;
femur —head; neck; greater and lesser trochanters; linea aspera; condyles; epicondyles; adductor tubercle; supracondylar ridges;
patella
tibia —condyles; tibial tuberosity.

Subcutaneous structures:

great saphenous vein, its tributaries with accompanying arterial branches; cutaneous nerves of the thigh; saphenous nerve; superficial inguinal lymph nodes.

Deep fascia:

fascia lata; iliotibial tract; intermuscular septa; compartments of the thigh.

Muscles:

sartorius; iliopsoas; quadriceps femoris; pectineus; adductors.

Boundaries of femoral triangle and adductor canal

Nerves:

femoral and obturator nerves and their branches.

Arteries:

femoral artery and its branches.

Veins:

femoral vein and its tributaries.

Deep lymph nodes:

deep inguinal nodes.

Surface anatomy:

femoral artery.

Clinical anatomy:

injury to femoral artery; disuse atrophy of extensors; femoral hernia.

Dissection Schedule 7

ANTERIOR ASPECT OF THE THIGH

1. *Make the following incisions*:
   (a) *a curved incision along the fold of the groin from the anterior superior iliac spine to the pubic tubercle*;
   (b) *a vertical incision along the medial aspect of the limb from the pubic tubercle to a point 10 cm below the level of the knee*;
   (c) *extend the lower end of incision* (b) *across the front of the leg to its lateral border.*

   Reflect the skin.

2. *Clear away the superficial fascia. As you do so identify the* **great saphenous vein** behind the medial condyle of the femur and trace it upwards to its entry into the **femoral vein.** Note that some of the tributaries that drain into the great saphenous vein in the region of the groin are accompanied by superficial arteries arising from the **femoral artery**.

3. Note that the **superficial inguinal lymph nodes** are disposed as follows:
   (a) in a horizontal set below the **inguinal ligament**; and
   (b) in a vertical chain along the upper end of the great saphenous vein.

4. Note that the cutaneous nerves which supply the front and medial aspect of the thigh come from the **femoral nerve**.

One cutaneous branch of the femoral nerve that you should *try to find* is the **saphenous nerve** which runs along with the great saphenous vein, behind the medial condyle of the femur.

5. Note that the membranous layer of the superficial fascia of the lower anterior abdominal wall extends into the thigh and fuses with the deep fascia along a horizontal line passing laterally from the **pubic tubercle**. *Remove the remains of the superficial fascia* in order to expose the deep fascia of the thigh known as the **fascia lata**. Note the attachments of this fascia to the inguinal ligament and **iliac crest** in front and on the lateral side. Identify the **iliotibial tract**, a well-defined thickening of this fascia

on the lateral side of the thigh. *Define its extent* between the **tubercle of the iliac crest** and the **lateral condyle of the tibia**.

6. *Observe a deficiency* in the deep fascia around the region of entry of the great saphenous vein into the femoral vein. This deficiency is known as the **saphenous opening** and is covered by a sieve-like fascia termed the **cribriform fascia**. *Clear away this fascia* and note the sharp crescentic margins of the saphenous opening. The centre of this opening lies 3 cm below and lateral to the pubic tubercle.

7. *Remove the deep fascia* in order to expose the muscles of the front of the thigh but *preserve the iliotibial tract. Make an attempt to identify the* **medial** and **lateral intermuscular septa**.

8. *Define the inguinal ligament and identify the muscles below it.* From lateral to medial, these are: **iliopsoas**, **pectineus**, and **adductor longus**. The triangular area bounded by the inguinal ligament above, the **sartorius** laterally and the medial border of the adductor longus medially is referred to as the **femoral triangle**. *Clean the following structures within the triangle*:
   (a) the **femoral nerve** in the groove between the muscular **iliacus** and the tendinous **psoas**;
   (b) the **femoral artery** lying 1 cm medial to the *femoral nerve* on the psoas tendon;
   (c) the **femoral vein** lying immediately medial to the artery.

Note that the upper 3–4 cm of the femoral vessels are enclosed in a fascial covering called the **femoral sheath**; this is a funnel-shaped prolongation of the **fascia iliaca** posteriorly and the **fascia transversalis** anteriorly.

Within the femoral sheath, on the *medial side of the femoral vein look for a space known as the* **femoral canal**. This has a blind lower end and contains only fat and a lymph node. *Examine* the boundaries of the mouth of the canal which is known as the **femoral ring**. *Verify* that the inguinal ligament is anterior, the **lacunar ligament** is medial, the **pecten pubis** is posterior and the femoral vein is lateral to the ring. Clinically the femoral canal is important since it is the site for **femoral hernia**.

9. *Clean the sartorius and study its attachments.* Note that it arises from the **anterior superior iliac spine** and is inserted into the **medial surface of the tibia** close to the upper end of the bone. *Clean the femoral nerve* and note that it supplies the sartorius and pectineus muscles.

10. *Turn your attention to the femoral artery* and note that it has several superficial branches. A major branch is the **profunda femoris** which arises from the lateral side of the femoral artery 4–5 cm below the inguinal ligament.

11. *Trace the profunda femoris artery* running behind the adductor longus towards the apex of the femoral triangle where it lies deep to the femoral vessels.

12. *Cut the sartorius muscle in its middle* so as to expose the **adductor canal**. Note that the adductor canal is a groove between the **vastus medialis** anteriorly and the **adductor longus** and **adductor magnus** posteriorly, and is bridged by the sartorius which forms the roof of the canal. *Identify the following contents of the canal*:
    (a) femoral artery and vein;
    (b) saphenous nerve;
    (c) **nerve to the vastus medialis**.

13. *Trace the femoral artery and vein downwards* and note that they pass through an opening in the adductor magnus to enter the **popliteal fossa**.

14. *Now turn your attention to the extensor muscles* which lie in the front of the thigh. *Clean them.* These are:
    (a) the **rectus femoris** arising from the **anterior inferior iliac spine** and from above the **acetabulum**;
    (b) the **vastus medialis** and **vastus lateralis** lying on either side of the rectus femoris and arising from the medial and lateral aspects of the shaft of the femur;
    (c) the **vastus intermedius** which lies deep to the rectus femoris and taking origin from the upper two thirds of the anterior and lateral surfaces of the shaft of the femur. *Divide the rectus in the middle and turn it apart* to see the vastus intermedius.

Observe that the extensor muscles are partly inserted into the **patella** and partly continued down as the **ligamentum patellae** which is attached to the **tibial tuberosity**. The extensor muscles are supplied by the femoral nerve.

MEDIAL SIDE OF THE THIGH

1. *Identify and clean the* **gracilis** which is a strap-like muscle passing from the pubic bone to the medial side of the upper end of the tibia. *Next detach the gracilis muscle from its origin and reflect it downwards.*
2. *Now turn your attention to the adductor muscles* which are arranged in three layers. The **pectineus** arises from the **superior ramus of the pubis** and is inserted into the back of the femur below the **lesser trochanter**. The **adductor longus** arises by a tendon from the **body of the pubis** and is inserted into the **medial lip of the linea aspera**. *Observe* that these two muscles lie edge to edge and constitute the superficial layer.
3. *Cut the pectineus and adductor longus* close to their origin from the pubic bone and *turn them downwards taking care to preserve the* **anterior division of the obturator nerve**, *which lies on the* **adductor brevis**. This muscle forms the middle layer.

Study the attachments of the adductor brevis muscle. It arises from the body and **inferior ramus of the pubis** and is inserted into the upper half of the linea aspera. *Detach the adductor brevis from its origin and reflect it downwards.*

4. *Find the* **posterior division of the obturator nerve** *lying on the* **adductor magnus muscle** which forms the deepest layer. *Trace the posterior division of the obturator nerve proximally* and note that it enters the adductor compartment by piercing the **obturator externus muscle**.
5. Note that the obturator nerve supplies all the adductor muscles as well as the obturator externus and gracilis.
6. *Study the attachments* of the adductor magnus and obturator externus muscles:
   (a) The adductor magnus, which is a composite muscle, arises from the ischiopubic ramus and the **ischial tuberosity**. From here the muscle fibres fan out to gain insertion into the back of the femur along the

medial lip of the linea aspera and the **medial supracondylar ridge** down to the **adductor tubercle**. The upper horizontal portion forms the true adductor part while the lower fibres which mainly arise from the ischial tuberosity and run vertically downwards to the adductor tubercle constitute the hamstring part. This part of the muscle is supplied by the **tibial part of the sciatic nerve** (see later).

(b) The obturator externus arises from the external surface of the **obturator membrane** and the adjoining bone. Its insertion will be seen later.

7. *Follow the* **iliopsoas** *towards its insertion into the* **lesser trochanter of the femur**.

8. *Trace the passage of the profunda femoris artery between the pectineus and adductor longus and subsequently deep to the adductor longus* where it gives off **perforating arteries** as it lies on the adductor brevis and adductor magnus.

Summary

The musculature of the anterior and medial aspects of the thigh consists chiefly of the extensor and adductor groups. The **quadriceps femoris** belonging to the extensor group comprises the rectus femoris, vastus medialis, vastus intermedius and vastus lateralis. They cover the anterior, lateral and medial sides of the shaft of the femur. The quadriceps as well as the sartorius and pectineus are innervated by the femoral nerve arising from the **dorsal divisions of L2, 3, 4**.

Why are the extensors, i.e. quadriceps, well developed in humans?

The *adductor muscles* comprise an anterior layer formed by pectineus and adductor longus, a middle layer formed by the adductor brevis and a posterior layer consisting of the adductor magnus. In addition to these, the gracilis and obturator externus are also included in this group as they are all supplied by a common nerve, i.e. obturator nerve derived from the **ventral divisions of L2, 3, 4**. It will be observed that the anterior division of the obturator nerve lies between the superficial and middle layers while the posterior division lies between the middle and posterior layers, i.e. the two divisions are separated by the adductor brevis.

The femoral and obturator nerves do not proceed beyond the thigh region. However, the saphenous nerve might be regarded as a continuation of the femoral nerve into the medial side of the leg and foot. The femoral nerve lies *lateral* to the femoral artery in the femoral triangle and the saphenous nerve accompanies the artery in the adductor canal.

The femoral artery runs from the **midinguinal point** towards the apex of the femoral triangle where the femoral artery, the femoral vein, profunda vein and profunda artery lie in this order from before backwards. In its further course the femoral artery lies in the adductor canal which is in fact a groove between the vastus medialis and the adductors. The artery then leaves the canal to enter the popliteal region through an opening in the tendon of the adductor magnus. It is also noteworthy that the profunda femoris artery and its branches provide the major arterial supply to the thigh.

Objectives for Dissection Schedule 7

Topics: Anterior and medial aspects of the thigh

General objective 1

Comprehend the arrangement of the blood vessels and lymphatics of the region.

Specific objectives

1. Outline the principles of the venous drainage by classifying veins into superficial and deep.
2. Identify the great saphenous vein, its tributaries and its termination into the femoral vein.
3. Identify the superficial and deep inguinal lymph nodes and outline the principles of lymph drainage.
4. Define the boundaries of the femoral triangle and adductor canal.
5. Demonstrate the femoral sheath, femoral artery, femoral vein, femoral canal and femoral ring.
6. Analyse the boundaries of the femoral canal and its relation to femoral hernia; distinguish femoral from inguinal hernia.
7. Identify the course and extent of the femoral artery and indicate the common sites of injury.
8. Outline the territory of supply of the profunda femoris artery.

General objective 2

Understand the significance of muscular compartments and the distribution of nerves.

Specific objectives

1. Describe the fascia lata and the intermuscular septa passing from it to the femur.
2. Evaluate the concept of muscular compartments.
3. Evaluate the actions of the muscles of this region in the living subject.

4. Revise the principles of formation of the lumbar plexus with special reference to the femoral and obturator nerves.
5. Evaluate the cutaneous innervation and dermatomic pattern of the region.
6. Discuss the effects of lesions of the femoral and obturator nerves and outline clinical tests for these.

Overview of Schedule 8

Before you begin dissection note:

GLUTEAL REGION AND POSTERIOR ASPECT OF THE THIGH

Relevant skeletal features:

bone — gluteal surface; sciatic notches and foramina; iliac crest, tubercle and spines; ischial spine and tuberosity;

sacrum

coccyx

femur — greater trochanter; trochanteric fossa; trochanteric crest; quadrate tubercle; gluteal tuberosity; linea aspera;

tibia — condyles and shaft;

fibula — head.

Subcutaneous structures:

cutaneous nerves.

Muscles:

gluteus maximus, medius and minimus; tensor fasciae latae; piriformis; obturator internus and gemelli; quadratus femoris; hamstring muscles including the ischial part of the adductor magnus.

Nerves:

sciatic nerve and its divisions; inferior gluteal nerve; nerve to quadratus femoris; nerve to obturator internus; pudendal nerve; superior gluteal nerve.

Arteries:

superior and inferior gluteal arteries; arterial anastomoses.

Surface anatomy:

posterior superior iliac spine; greater trochanter; gluteal fold; sciatic nerve.

Clinical anatomy:

site for intramuscular injection.

Dissection Schedule 8

GLUTEAL REGION AND POSTERIOR ASPECT OF THE THIGH

1. *With the body in the prone position make the following incisions:*
   (a) *a curved incision from the anterior superior iliac spine along the iliac crest to the posterior superior iliac spine (if not already made);*
   (b) *from the posterior superior iliac spine to the midline and then vertically down to the tip of the coccyx;*
   (c) *from the tip of the coccyx curving downwards and laterally to the middle of the lateral border of the thigh;*
   (d) *a horizontal incision across the back of the leg 10 cm below the knee;*
   (e) *a vertical incision along the midline of the back of the thigh extending between incisions* (c) *and* (d).

   Reflect the skin flaps.

2. Note that the superficial fascia in the gluteal region is much more heavily laden with fat, particularly in the female — this being a secondary sex characteristic. *Observe* the pad of fibrofatty tissue over the **ischial tuberosity** which acts as a cushion in the sitting posture.

3. As you dissect you will come across numerous cutaneous nerves. Do not spend time on them. However, note the **posterior femoral cutaneous nerve** lying along the midline of the thigh; *trace this nerve* from the lower posterior part of the knee upwards towards the gluteal fold.

4. *Remove the fatty superficial fascia over the gluteal region* and observe the large **gluteus maximus muscle** covered by deep fascia. *Clean this muscle and study its attachments.* This muscle arises from the posterolateral surface of the **sacrum** and the adjoining posterior surface of the **ilium** and **sacrotuberous ligament**. Its major part is inserted into the posterior part of the iliotibial tract and its smaller deep part into the **gluteal tuberosity of the femur**.

5. Note that the lower border of gluteus maximus descends obliquely across the horizontally disposed gluteal fold. *Divide the muscle at about the middle between its origin and insertion taking great care not to damage the nerves and vessels and* the **sacrotuberous ligament** *lying deep to it. While reflecting the muscle, observe* the ligament and the **inferior gluteal nerve**

and vessels as well as branches of the **superior gluteal artery** entering the deep surface of the muscle. *Now identify the* **piriformis** which is the key muscle in the dissection of this region. Using a skeleton, *review its origin* from the front of the middle three pieces of the sacrum. Note its insertion into the upper border of the **greater trochanter** of the femur.

6. *Carefully clean the structures in relation to the piriformis muscle. Identify the large* **sciatic nerve** as it emerges from the middle of its *lower border* to course down the middle of the back of the thigh. Lying on it is the posterior femoral cutaneous nerve. *Clean the inferior gluteal nerve and vessels* lying medial to the sciatic nerve. Other structures which are medial to the sciatic nerve are the **nerve to obturator internus**, the **internal pudendal** vessels and the **pudendal nerve**. These vessels and nerves pass across the **ischial spine** and **sacrospinous ligament** to enter the **lesser sciatic foramen**. *Observe* the extent of the sacrotuberous ligament.

7. *Clean the structures that lie caudal to the piriformis.* These are from above downwards:
   (a) tendon of **obturator internus** with the **gemellus superior** and **inferior muscles** lying above and below it; follow the obturator internus tendon to its insertion into the medial surface of the greater trochanter of the femur;
   (b) the **quadratus femoris**; note its attachments to the lateral border of the ischial tuberosity and the **quadrate tubercle of the femur**. Note also that the **nerve to quadratus femoris** supplies that muscle on its deep surface;
   (c) the upper border of the adductor magnus.

8. *Now proceed to examine the structures above the piriformis.* The muscle seen immediately above the piriformis is the **gluteus medius** and the muscle lying partly under cover and partly in front of it is the **gluteus minimus**. Passing between these two muscles are the **superior gluteal nerve** and a branch of the superior gluteal artery. *Study the attachments* of the gluteus medius. It arises from the posterior surface of the ilium and is inserted into the lateral surface of the greater trochanter. *Detach the gluteus medius from its insertion and trace the superior gluteal nerve* which after supplying the medius and the minimus accompanies the deep branch of

the superior gluteal artery towards the anterior superior iliac spine where the nerve ends by innervating the **tensor fasciae latae muscle**.

9. *Study the attachments* of the gluteus minimus and tensor fasciae latae. The gluteus minimus arises from the posterior surface of the ilium below and anterior to the gluteus medius and is inserted into the front of the greater trochanter. The tensor fasciae latae takes origin from the anterior part of the iliac crest and is inserted into the upper anterior part of the iliotibial tract. *Cut the gluteus minimus at its insertion and the tensor fasciae latae from its origin.*

10. *First cut the tendon of the obturator internus and the gemelli muscles. Next cut the piriformis and then the quadratus femoris vertically. Reflect the cut ends so as to expose the obturator externus deep to the latter muscle.*

11. *Remove the deep fascia over the back of the thigh and clean the hamstring muscles* consisting of the **semimembranosus, semitendinosus, long head of biceps femoris** and **ischial portion of the adductor magnus**. Observe that these muscles arise from the ischial tuberosity. Their insertion will be seen later. *Trace the nerve supply to these muscles* from the **tibial** *part* of the sciatic nerve. *Clean the* **short head of the biceps femoris** arising from the region of the linea aspera and *secure its nerve supply from the* **common fibular** (peroneal) *part* of the sciatic nerve.

12. *Identify the profunda femoris artery*, where it was seen previously behind the adductor longus and in front of adductor brevis and adductor magnus, and *trace its perforating branches*. Note that the upper arteries pierce the adductor brevis and magnus while the lower ones pierce only the magnus muscle. *Trace these vessels* towards the vastus lateralis where they form an anastomosis with one another and supply the posterior (flexor) group of muscles.

13. *Now detach the semimembranosus, semitendinosis, biceps femoris and ischial portion of the adductor magnus from the ischial tuberosity and cut the remainder of the adductor magnus from the ischiopubic ramus. Also cut the sciatic nerve at this level.*

Summary

The most prominent feature of the gluteal region is the massive size of the gluteus maximus which is one of the largest muscles in the human body. Both the large size of the muscle and its insertion into the iliotibial tract are to be associated with the erect posture in humans and their bipedal mode of progression. This large muscle is supplied by the inferior gluteal nerve.

It must also be appreciated that the gluteus maximus, medius and minimus are found in three different planes from superficial to deep. At their origins, the maximus is most posterior and the minimus is most anterior with the medius in between. A similar relationship is maintained at their insertions.

The small muscles at the back of the hip joint are the piriformis, the two obturators, the two gemelli, and the quadratus femoris. All except the quadratus femoris are inserted into the greater trochanter. As the capsule of the hip joint is weak *posteriorly*, these muscles at the back of the hip provide some support for the joint. These muscles form a rotator cuff similar to that around the shoulder joint. Note that they are all lateral rotators of the thigh.

The hamstring muscles arising from the ischial tuberosity receive their innervation from the *tibial portion* of the sciatic nerve. The short head of biceps femoris which arises from the linea aspera is supplied by the *common fibular* component of the sciatic nerve.

The semitendinosus is inserted into the medial surface of the upper part of the shaft of the tibia while the semimembranosus gains insertion into the **medial condyle of the tibia**. The ischial part of the adductor magnus is attached to the **adductor tubercle** of the femur while the biceps femoris has its insertion on to the **head of the fibula**. These insertions will be seen later.

The *sciatic nerve* innervates not only the hamstring muscles of the thigh but also the *entire* leg and foot musculature. It is also noteworthy that this nerve is covered only by the gluteus maximus in the gluteal region and by the long head of biceps femoris in the thigh.

The superior and inferior gluteal arteries are distributed chiefly to the gluteal region. The gluteal arteries take part in various anastomoses which can provide a collateral circulation when the femoral artery is obstructed.

Objectives for Dissection Schedule 8

Topic: Muscles, nerves and blood vessels of the gluteal region

General objective 1

Appreciate the arrangement of the muscles and their functions.

Specific objectives

1. Orientate the anatomical position of the pelvic girdle, hip bone and femur.
2. Identify the crest, tubercle, spines and gluteal lines of the ilium.
3. Identify the tuberosity, spine and ramus of the ischium.
4. Identify the crest, tubercle, body and superior and inferior rami of the pubis.
5. Identify the head, neck, greater and lesser trochanters, trochanteric line and crest, trochanteric fossa and the linea aspera of the femur.
6. Appreciate the arrangement of the muscles of the region in three strata.
7. Evaluate the actions of the gluteal muscles.
8. Evaluate the actions of the small muscles at the back of the hip.
9. Evaluate the actions of the hamstring muscles.
10. Analyse the double nerve supply of the adductor magnus and biceps femoris muscles.

General objective 2

Analyse the arrangement of the nerves and blood vessels of the region.

Specific objectives

1. Explain the formation of the greater and lesser sciatic foramina.
2. Enumerate the structures traversing the sciatic foramina.
3. Explain why the piriformis is considered the key muscle of the region.
4. Appreciate the functional subdivisions of the sciatic nerve.
5. Outline the course of the pudendal nerve and vessels.

6. Outline the distribution of the superior gluteal nerve.
7. Surface mark the course of the sciatic nerve.
8. Explain the site selected for administration of intramuscular injections.

Overview of Schedule 9

Before you begin dissection note:

HIP JOINT, POPLITEAL FOSSA AND BACK OF LEG

1. HIP JOINT

Relevant skeletal features:

acetabulum — developmental components; head of femur.

Muscles in immediate relation to capsule of joint:

iliopsoas; pectineus; obturator externus; short lateral rotators; gluteus minimus; reflected head of rectus femoris.

Capsule:

attachments.

Thickening of capsule:

iliofemoral, pubofemoral, ischiofemoral ligaments.

Intraarticular structures:

ligamentum teres.

Synovial membrane:

reflection.

Articular surfaces:

articular cartilage; acetabular labrum; transverse ligament.

Movements:

flexion; extension; abduction; adduction; medial and lateral rotation; circumduction.

Nerve supply:

application of Hilton's law.

Blood supply:

to joint and head of femur.

Clinical anatomy:

dislocation of hip; fractures of femoral neck.

2. POPLITEAL FOSSA AND BACK OF THE LEG

Relevant skeletal features:

femur — popliteal surface; condyles;
tibia — condyles; upper end of medial surface; posterior surface; soleal line; medial malleolus;
fibula — posterior surface; lateral malleolus;
calcaneus — attachment of flexor retinaculum.

Subcutaneous structures:

saphenous nerve and other cutaneous nerves; small saphenous vein.

Deep fascia:

osteofascial compartments; transverse fascial septum; flexor retinaculum.

Muscles:

semitendinosus; semimembranosus; biceps femoris; gastrocnemius; plantaris; soleus; popliteus.
Boundaries of popliteal fossa
flexor digitorum longus; flexor hallucis longus; tibialis posterior.

Nerves:

sciatic nerve; tibial nerve; common fibular nerve.

Arteries:

popliteal; posterior tibial; anterior tibial; fibular.

Veins:

popliteal vein and its formation.

Lymph nodes:

popliteal.

Surface anatomy:

popliteal artery; posterior tibial artery.

Clinical anatomy:

recording of blood pressure in the lower limb.

Dissection Schedule 9

HIP JOINT, POPLITEAL FOSSA AND BACK OF LEG

HIP JOINT

1. *With the body still in the prone position* note that the iliopsoas muscle lies in front and below the hip joint while the short lateral rotators are at the back of the joint. *Follow the tendon of the obturator externus* as it curves upwards and laterally along the back of the neck of the femur deep to the quadratus femoris to reach the **trochanteric fossa**. *Cut the obturator externus.*

2. *Remove the remaining muscles on the posterior aspect of the hip joint and clean the capsule.* Note that the capsule covers only the medial two-thirds of the neck of the femur posteriorly, while anteriorly it is attached to the **intertrochanteric line**.

3. *Turn the body on to its back, cut the tendon of the iliopsoas just below the hip joint and reflect it. Next examine the anterior part of the capsule. Define the* **iliofemoral ligament** extending from the upper margin of the acetabulum to the intertrochanteric line of the femur. Note the two thickened bands, lateral and medial, attached to the upper and lower ends of the intertrochanteric line, respectively.

4. *Define the* **pubofemoral ligament** attached above to the superior ramus of the pubic bone adjoining the acetabulum and blending below with the medial band of the iliofemoral ligament.

5. *Identify the* **ischiofemoral ligament** attached to the ischium below and behind the acetabulum and passing upwards and laterally to fuse with the posterior part of the capsule. Why do the three ligaments of the hip show an increasing degree of twist? When do these ligaments get taut?

6. *Open the joint by cutting obliquely from above downwards and medially across the capsule.*

7. *Pull the head of the femur out of the acetabulum* and observe that the **ligament of the head of the femur (ligamentum teres)** resists its separation from the acetabulum. *Cut the ligamentum teres and withdraw*

the head of the femur from the acetabulum. Note that the fibrocartilaginous **acetabular labrum** which is attached to the margin of the acetabulum also resists the withdrawal of the head of the femur. Why?

8. *Identify the* **acetabular notch** on the inferior margin of the acetabulum and note that this notch is bridged across by the **transverse ligament**. *Verify the attachment of the ligamentum teres* passing from a pit in the head of the femur to the margins of the acetabular notch and to the transverse ligament.

9. *Cut any remaining structures and free the limb from the pelvis.* The lower limb has now been seperated from the body.

POPLITEAL FOSSA AND BACK OF LEG

1. *In the free lower limb make the following incisions*:
   (a) *a vertical incision in the midline of the back of the leg down to the heel*;
   (b) *a transverse incision connecting the two malleoli across the back of the ankle.*

   Reflect the skin flaps.

2. *As you clear away the superficial fascia* you will find several cutaneous nerves. Note that the saphenous nerve accompanies the great saphenous vein on the medial side of the leg.

3. *Examine the deep fascia of the leg* which forms a complete covering for the musculature of the leg. It also sends septa to the anterior and posterior margins of the fibula thus separating the leg muscles into *three compartments*, namely, anterior (extensor), lateral (fibular) and posterior (flexor) compartments. Note that the medial surface of the tibia is subcutaneous.

4. *Define the* **flexor retinaculum** extending between the **medial malleolus of the tibia** and the **medial process of the tuber calcaneus**.

5. *Remove the deep fascia behind the knee and trace the hamstring muscles to their insertions.* Observe that the biceps femoris tendon is inserted into the **head of the fibula** together with the attachment of the **fibular ligament of the knee joint**. *Follow the semitendinosus to its insertion* into the upper

end of the medial surface of the shaft of the tibia behind the insertions of the sartorius and gracilis. *Trace* the main insertion of the semimembranosus into the groove on the posteromedial aspect of the medial condyle of the tibia. Note that it gives expansions which form the **oblique popliteal ligament** of the knee and the fascia covering the **popliteus muscle**.

6. *Identify the boundaries of the* **popliteal fossa**. These are:
   (a) semitendinosus and semimembranosus above and medially;
   (b) biceps femoris above and laterally;
   (c) **medial head of the gastrocnemius muscle** below and medially;
   (d) **lateral head of the gastrocnemius** supplemented by the **plantaris muscle** below and laterally.

7. *Study the origins of the calf muscles.* Note that the lateral head of the gastrocnemius arises from the lateral surface of the lateral condyle of the femur while the medial head arises from the **popliteal surface of the femur** just above the medial condyle. The plantaris arises from the popliteal surface of the femur just above the lateral condyle of the femur.

8. *Clean the contents of the popliteal fossa. Trace the termination of the* **small saphenous vein** *into the* **popliteal vein**. *Identify* the division of the sciatic nerve into the **tibial** and **common fibular** (peroneal) **nerves** in the upper part of the fossa. Both branches give off genicular and muscular branches.

9. *Note that the common fibular nerve runs* along the medial margin of the biceps tendon.

10. *Proceed to clean the* **popliteal** *vessels*, the continuation of the femoral vessels. Note that the vein lies deep to the tibial nerve. *Identify the artery* which lies deep to the vein directly on the popliteal surface of the femur. Note the presence of **popliteal lymph nodes** in relation to the popliteal vessels (these are deep lymph nodes).

11. Note that the **popliteal artery** gives off genicular branches that accompany the corresponding genicular nerves.

12. *Detach the two heads of the gastrocnemius muscle and the plantaris muscle from their origins.*

13. *Study the attachments of the* **popliteus**. Note that it is attached proximally by a short rounded tendon to the anterior part of the **popliteal groove** on the lateral femoral condyle (it is also attached to the **posterior cruciate ligament** and the posterior part of the **lateral meniscus**, see later). The popliteus tendon which lies within the capsule of the knee joint issues out of the capsule to gain attachment below to the posterior surface of the tibia above the **soleal line**.

14. *Identify the large* **soleus muscle** lying beneath the gastrocnemius. It arises from the upper part of the posterior surface of the fibula and the soleal line of the tibia.

15. *Find* the combined tendons of the gastrocnemius, soleus and plantaris below forming the **tendocalcaneus** which is inserted into the posterior aspect of the **calcaneus**.

16. *Separate the soleus from the fibula and tibia and from the fibrous arcade* covering the **posterior tibial** vessels and nerve. You can now see the **transverse fascial septum** of the leg covering the deep layer of calf muscles.

17. *Trace the popliteal artery downwards and identify its terminal branches*, the **anterior** and **posterior tibial arteries**, at the lower border of the popliteus muscle.

18. *Observe* the neurovascular bundle lying between the superficial flexors which have been reflected and the deep group. The tibial nerve gives muscular branches to the gastrocnemius, soleus, and the deep flexors. *Clean these muscles and note the origin of*:
    (a) the **flexor digitorum longus** from the tibia;
    (b) the **flexor hallucis longus** from the fibula; and somewhat deeper
    (c) the **tibialis posterior** from both bones and the intervening **interosseous membrane**.

19. *Follow the posterior tibial artery downwards and secure its most important branch* — the **fibular** (peroneal) **artery** which runs downwards and laterally deep to the flexor hallucis longus to supply the fibular muscles and the fibula.

20. Turn your attention to the region of the flexor retinaculum and *identify the following structures lying beneath this retinaculum.* From medial to lateral these are:
    (a) tendon of tibialis posterior;
    (b) tendon of flexor digitorum longus;
    (c) posterior tibial vessels;
    (d) tibial nerve; and
    (e) flexor hallucis longus tendon.

Note that the tendon of the flexor digitorum longus crosses the tendon of the tibialis posterior a short distance above the ankle.

Summary

The **hip joint** exhibits both stability and mobility. The stability of the joint can be gauged by:

(a) the congruence of the articular surfaces lined by articular cartilage;
(b) the depth of the acetabular cavity; and
(c) the strength of the muscles and ligaments.

The role of the ligaments in the upright posture must be understood. This can be inferred from the fact that the centre of gravity of the trunk falls behind a line joining the centres of the femoral heads. Moreover, all the ligaments become increasingly taut during extension until the full congruence of the articular surfaces is brought about. This is the most stable or 'locked' position of the joint.

The **ligamentum teres** was originally a part of the fetal capsule which has been pushed into the joint so that the synovial membrane tends to enclose it. In the child, the blood vessels passing through the ligamentum teres constitute the main source of blood supply to the head of the femur while in the adult, the branches of the profunda femoris take over this function. What will be the effect of a fracture of the neck of the femur in a child and in an adult?

The **popliteal fossa** is a diamond-shaped hollow behind the knee where the main vessels and nerves passing from the anterior and posterior aspects of the thigh come together and are subsequently rearranged and distributed to the leg and foot. The sciatic nerve divides in the upper part of the popliteal fossa into its *two functional components* — the common fibular and tibial nerves. The common fibular nerve supplies the anterior (extensor) and lateral (fibular) compartments as well as the dorsum of the foot. The tibial nerve supplies the posterior compartment of the leg and the muscles of the sole of the foot.

The **popliteal artery**, a continuation of the femoral artery at the opening in the adductor magnus, divides into anterior and posterior tibial arteries at the lower border of the popliteus. The anterior tibial artery after passing through the interosseous membrane supplies the anterior compartment of the leg and the dorsum of the foot. The posterior tibial artery supplies the back of the leg and sole of the foot while the fibular artery, a branch of the posterior tibial artery, supplies branches to the fibular compartment.

The muscles of the back of the leg can be divided into a *superficial group* comprising the gastrocnemius, plantaris and soleus and a *deep group* consisting of the flexor digitorum longus, flexor hallucis longus and tibialis posterior. These muscles are plantar flexors, in addition tibialis posterior is also an invertor. The superficial and deep groups are separated by a **transverse fascial septum** and the neurovascular plane lies between these two groups of muscles.

Objectives for Dissection Schedule 9

Topic: Hip joint

General objective 1

Comprehend the essential features of: (a) the articulating bones; and (b) the ligaments around the joint.

Specific objectives

1. Define the articulating surfaces of the hip joint in the skeleton.
2. Identify the different developmental parts of the hip bone and their contribution to the acetabulum.
3. Describe the attachments of the ligaments of the hip joint and analyse their functional significance.
4. Demonstrate the different kinds of movement possible at the hip and compare it with the shoulder.
5. Discuss the likely sites for dislocation.
6. Interpret different radiographic views of the hip joint.

General objective 2

Analyse the arrangement and actions of muscle groups around the hip joint.

Specific objectives

1. Identify the muscles on the anterior, medial and posterior aspects of the thigh and recall their attachments and innervation.
2. Arrange the muscles into functional groups as flexors, extensors, abductors, adductors, lateral and medial rotators.
3. Analyse the functional significance of Hilton's law in terms of reflexes arising from receptors in the joint capsule.
4. Deduce the effects of nerve lesions.
5. Illustrate the anatomical basis of the Trendelenburg hip test.

6. Discuss the position of the lower limb in fracture of the neck of the femur and psoas spasm.
7. Explain the importance of the arteries in fractures of the neck of the femur.
8. Conduct an examination of the normal hip joint in the living.

Topic: Popliteal fossa and back of the leg

General objective

Comprehend the arrangement of the muscles, blood vessels and nerves of the region.

Specific objectives

1. Recall insertions of the hamstrings and origins of the calf muscles.
2. Demonstrate the boundaries of the popliteal fossa.
3. Identify the popliteal vessels and division of the sciatic nerve.
4. Demonstrate the changing relationships of the tibial nerve, popliteal vein and artery.
5. Define the attachments of the deep flexor muscles of the leg.
6. Review the areas of supply of the posterior tibial and fibular arteries.
7. Understand the order of the structures passing beneath the flexor retinaculum.

Overview of Schedule 10

Before you begin dissection note:

ANTERIOR AND LATERAL ASPECTS OF THE LEG AND DORSUM OF THE FOOT AND THE KNEE JOINT

Relevant skeletal features:

tibia — borders and surfaces;
fibula — borders and surfaces;
bones of foot — tarsus; metatarsus; phalanges.

Subcutaneous structures:

superficial fibular nerve; cutaneous nerves of calf region such as the saphenous nerve; deep fibular nerve; great saphenous vein; small saphenous vein.

Deep fascia:

osteofascial compartments; extensor retinacula; fibular retinacula.

Muscles:

fibularis longus; fibularis brevis; tibialis anterior; extensor hallucis longus; extensor digitorum longus; fibularis tertius; extensor digitorum brevis.

Nerves:

superficial fibular nerve; deep fibular nerve.

Arteries:

anterior tibial artery; dorsalis pedis.

Clinical anatomy:

dorsalis pedis arterial pulse; intravenous infusion into great saphenous vein.

KNEE JOINT

Relevant skeletal features:

femur — areas for tibia and patella; intercondylar notch;
patella
tibia — condylar articular area; intercondylar eminence and tubercles; tibial tubercle.

Muscles in relation to capsule of joint:

quadriceps; sartorius; gracilis; semitendinosus; semimembranosus; adductor magnus; gastrocnemius; popliteus; fibularis longus.

Capsule:

attachments.

Ligaments:

tibial collateral, fibular collateral; oblique popliteal.

Intraarticular structures:

cruciate ligaments; menisci; popliteus tendon.

Synovial membrane:

reflection; infrapatellar and alar folds; suprapatellar bursa.

Articular surfaces:

articular cartilage.

Movements:

flexion; extension and rotation; 'locking' and 'unlocking' of knee joint.

Nerve supply:

genicular nerves.

Blood supply:

genicular arteries.

Clinical anatomy:

internal derangements.

Dissection Schedule 10

ANTERIOR AND LATERAL ASPECTS OF THE LEG AND DORSUM OF THE FOOT AND THE KNEE JOINT

1. *Make the following incisions*:
   (a) *a vertical incision in the midline of the front of the leg down to the ankle*;
   (b) *extend incision* (a) *along the middle of the dorsum of the foot to the nail bed of the middle toe*;
   (c) *a transverse incision across the front of the ankle connecting the two malleoli*;
   (d) *a transverse incision across the roots of the toes*;
   (e) *midline incisions along the dorsum of the other toes.*

   Reflect the skin flaps and clean away the superficial fascia.

2. Note the **dorsal venous arch** situated opposite the distal ends of the metatarsal bones and note its formation. *Trace:* (a) the **great saphenous vein** commencing from the medial side of the venous arch and passing *in front* of the medial malleolus; and (b) the **small saphenous vein** arising from the lateral side of the arch and running *behind* the lateral malleolus.

Note that there are communications between the great saphenous vein and the **deep veins** in the region of the ankle, knee and adductor canal. Similar communications exist between the small saphenous vein and the deep veins at the level of the ankle. These communicating veins are called **perforating veins**.

3. Note the following nerves:
   (a) **superficial fibular** (peroneal) **nerve** from the **common fibular nerve** piercing the deep fascia about the junction of upper two-thirds with the lower third of the anterior aspect of the leg. *Trace this nerve into the foot* where it divides into medial and intermediate cutaneous branches which supply all the toes except the first interdigital cleft and the lateral side of the little toe;
   (b) **saphenous nerve** along with the great saphenous vein passing in front of the medial malleolus to the medial side of the foot;

(c) the terminal part of the **deep fibular** (peroneal) **nerve**, a branch of the common fibular nerve, piercing the deep fascia in the first intermetatarsal space to supply the first interdigital cleft.

4. *Clean the deep fascia* and note the retinacular bands below which are thickenings in the deep fascia: (a) the **superior extensor retinaculum** which is a transverse band of fascia that extends between the lower ends of the tibia and fibula; and (b) the Y-shaped **inferior extensor retinaculum** lying across the ankle joint.

5. Similarly, *identify the* **superior** and **inferior fibular retinacula.** *Define*: (a) the superior retinaculum passing between the back of the lateral malleolus and the lateral surface of the calcaneus; and (b) the inferior retinaculum stretching between the anterior part of the upper surface of the calcaneus and its lateral surface.

6. *Remove the deep fascia over the anterior and lateral aspects of the leg*, and note the **anterior** and **posterior intermuscular septa** attached to the anterior and posterior borders of the fibula. *Observe* how these septa together with the overlying deep fascia form the anterior (extensor) and lateral (fibular) compartments.

7. *Clean the* **fibularis longus** *and* **fibularis brevis muscles** taking origin from the lateral surface of the fibula, the longus being superficial to the brevis. Note that their tendons pass behind the lateral malleolus with the fibularis longus tendon lying posterior to that of the brevis. *Trace these tendons into the foot and observe* the insertion of the fibularis brevis into the base of the fifth metatarsal bone. The insertion of the longus will be dissected later.

8. *Trace the common fibular nerve round the lateral side of the* **neck of the fibula** *into the fibular compartment. Follow the nerve by cutting through the fibularis longus muscle and secure its terminal branches*, i.e. the **deep** and **superficial fibular nerves**. *Trace the superficial fibular nerve distally.* It supplies the fibularis longus and brevis. *Trace the deep fibular nerve into the extensor compartment.*

9. *Now clean the muscles of the extensor compartment and trace their tendons* which pass beneath the superior extensor retinaculum. From medial to

lateral these muscles are: (a) **tibialis anterior**; (b) **extensor hallucis longus**; (c) **extensor digitorum longus**; and (d) **fibularis tertius**. Tibialis anterior arises from the lateral surface of the tibia and extensor hallucis longus, extensor digitorum longus and fibularis tertius originate from the medial surface of the fibula. Tibialis anterior is inserted into the medial cuneiform and base for the first metatarsal. Extensor hallucis is attached to the terminal phallanx of the first toe. Extensor digitorum divides into four slips which insert into the bases of the intermediate and distal phalanges of the lateral four toes. Fibularis tertius is attached to the dorsum of the fifth metatarsal bone. These four muscles are supplied by the deep fibular nerve.

10. *Divide the superior extensor retinaculum* and identify the **anterior tibial artery** and the **deep fibular nerve** lying between the extensor hallucis and extensor digitorum longus tendons. *Follow the artery and nerve upwards into the leg* and note that they lie between the tibialis anterior and extensor digitorum longus in the upper part of the leg and are crossed by the extensor hallucis longus tendon near the ankle. *Now trace the artery towards the dorsum of the foot* where it continues as the **dorsalis pedis artery** towards the first intermetatarsal space. The continuation of this artery through the first intermetatarsal space into the sole of the foot will be seen later. *Similarly trace the course of the deep fibular nerve* whose medial branch accompanies the dorsalis pedis artery.

11. Note that the lateral branch of the deep fibular nerve enters the deep aspect of the **extensor digitorum brevis muscle**. This muscle arises from the dorsal aspect of the calcaneus. *Clean the four tendons issuing from this muscle* and passing to the medial four toes. Note that the tendon to the first toe is inserted into its proximal phalanx while the other three tendons join the extensor digitorum longus tendons to form the **extensor expansions** over the second, third and fourth toes. *Cut and reflect the long extensor tendons at the level of the ankle joint. Follow the extensor expansions* and note that their slips insert into the intermediate and distal phalanges of the lateral four toes.

12. *Reflect the extensor digitorum brevis from its origin and find the* **arcuate artery**, a branch of the dorsalis pedis artery lying deep to the tendons.

Note that the arcuate artery gives off the **dorsal metatarsal arteries** which become the **dorsal digital arteries**.

13. *Trace the tendon of the fibularis tertius muscle* to its insertion on to the dorsum of the fifth metatarsal bone.

KNEE JOINT

1. *Review the muscles which are closely related to the knee joint.* Note the insertions of the sartorius, gracilis, semitendinosus and semimembranosus tendons into the upper part of the medial surface of the tibia. *Identify the tendon of insertion of the adductor magnus. Now look for the* **tibial collateral ligament** on the medial side of the knee joint and *then find* the cord-like **fibular collateral ligament** on the lateral side. *Find the* **oblique popliteal ligament**, an expansion from the semimembranosus tendon passing upwards and laterally on the posterior aspect of the joint. Note the attachments and relationships of the **popliteus** tendon to the capsule and joint cavity. Remember that the popliteus is important *in unlocking of the knee joint* (initiating flexion).

2. Note that the capsule is deficient anteriorly and is replaced by the tendon of the quadriceps, the patella, and the **ligamentum patellae** in front and by the expansions of the vastus medialis and lateralis on the sides. *Open the joint by cutting transversely through the quadriceps tendon above the patella and by two cuts vertically one on either side of the patella. Draw the patella down and examine the* **synovial infrapatellar fold** in the midline and **alar folds** on either side.

3. *Examine* the opposing articular surfaces of the patella and the femur. Note that it is the *lower part* of the patella which articulates with the femur in full extension. *Observe* that the patella and the medial femoral condyle articulate in full flexion.

4. *Cut transversely across the rest of the capsule and observe the* **posterior** *and* **anterior cruciate ligaments**. *Divide the cruciate ligaments* and note their attachments. *Examine* the **medial** and **lateral menisci** *in situ*. Note the attachment of the popliteus to the posterior aspect of the lateral meniscus. See whether the medial meniscus is attached to the tibial collateral ligament.

Note that the anterior and posterior horns of the menisci are attached anterior and posterior to the **intercondylar eminence** of the tibia, respectively, while the periphery of the menisci is connected to the tibia by **coronary ligaments**.

Summary

The muscles of the extensor and fibular compartments are supplied by the common fibular nerve which reaches the fibular compartment by winding round the neck of the fibula where it is liable to injury. It divides into the superficial fibular nerve supplying the lateral (fibular) compartment and the deep fibular nerve supplying the muscles of the anterior (extensor) compartment. The muscles of the fibular compartment are **evertors**. The muscles of the anterior compartment are **dorsiflexors** of the ankle (physiological extensors). In addition, the tibialis anterior is an **invertor** of the foot while the fibularis tertius assists the fibular muscles in eversion.

The anterior tibial artery reaches the anterior compartment by passing through the interosseous membrane while the deep fibular nerve after piercing the extensor digitorum longus comes to lie on the lateral side of the artery. The anterior tibial artery continues at the level of the ankle joint as the dorsalis pedis whose pulsation can be felt on the dorsum of the foot.

The knee joint is a *modified hinge joint* in which there is considerable freedom of movement. In spite of this, there is also a great degree of stability of the joint which is essential for transmitting the weight of the body. This is provided by strong ligaments and muscles which surround the joint and by the iliotibial tract. Therefore, the functions of the various ligaments and muscles in relation to the knee joint must be studied and understood thoroughly.

The extra-articular area on the medial femoral condyle is used up in the *terminal medial rotation* of the femur *in locking of the knee joint* which occurs in the final stage of extension. What muscle is concerned in unlocking the knee joint?

The synovial infrapatellar and alar folds are due to the invagination of the synovial membrane from the front. They attempt to divide the knee joint into three subdivisions, two between the condyles of the femur and the corresponding condyles of the tibia and the third between the patella and the femur. However, all three joint cavities are continuous as the alar folds are not attached to the femur. The cruciate ligaments invaginate the synovial membrane from the back of the joint and consequently there is no synovial membrane lining the posterior part of the capsule. The attachment of some of the *fibres of the popliteus muscle to the lateral meniscus* and the attachment of the *tibial collateral ligament to the medial meniscus* have opposite effects on the mobility of the menisci.

Objectives for Dissection Schedule 10

1. Topic: Anterior and lateral aspects of the leg and dorsum of the foot

General objective

Comprehend the arrangement and innervation of the muscles in the anterior and lateral compartments of the leg.

Specific objectives

1. Revise the osteofascial compartments of the leg.
2. Identify the structures passing beneath the extensor retinacula.
3. Define the dermatomic pattern of the anterior and lateral aspects in the living.
4. Recollect the course and termination of the common fibular nerve.
5. Define the dermatomic pattern of the anterior and lateral aspects of the leg and dorsum of the foot.
6. Describe the course and termination of the anterior tibial artery.
7. Describe the course of the great saphenous vein.

2. Topic: Knee joint

General objective

Comprehend the arrangement of the osteoligamentous structures of the knee joint.

Specific objectives

1. Identify the condylar and patellar articular surfaces of the femur; examine the groove and pit for the popliteus tendon on the lateral femoral condyle.
2. Enumerate the order of the structures on the upper surface of the tibia from front to back.
3. Demonstrate the attachments of the tibial and fibular collateral and the cruciate ligaments and assign functional roles to them.
4. Recall the actions of the hamstrings, quadriceps and popliteus.

5. Analyse the bony, ligamentous and muscular factors in: (a) 'locking' and 'unlocking'; (b) stability of the patella.
6. Interpret radiographs of the knee.
7. Conduct an examination of a normal knee joint.
8. Discuss the relationship of the hip and knee joints in terms of: (a) maintenance of the erect posture; (b) movements; (c) referred pain.

Overview of Schedule 11

Before you begin dissection note:

SOLE OF FOOT

Relevant skeletal features:

calcaneus — medial and lateral processes of calcaneal tuberosity; sustentaculum tali;
talus
navicular — tuberosity;
cuboid — groove for peroneus longus tendon;
first metatarsal bone
fifth metatarsal bone — tuberosity.

Subcutaneous structures:

medial calcanean nerves and vessels; digital nerves and vessels.

Deep fascia:

plantar aponeurosis; intermuscular septa; muscular compartments.

Muscles:

first layer — abductor hallucis; flexor digitorum brevis; abductor digiti minimi;
second layer — flexor hallucis longus and flexor digitorum longus tendons, lumbricals; quadratus plantae;
third layer — flexor hallucis brevis; adductor hallucis; flexor digiti minimi brevis;
fourth layer — tibialis posterior; fibularis longus tendon; interossei.

Ligaments:

long plantar ligament; plantar calcaneonavicular (spring) ligament.

Nerves:

medial plantar; lateral plantar.

Arteries:

medial plantar artery; lateral plantar artery; plantar arterial arch.

Dissection Schedule 11

SOLE OF FOOT

1. *Make the following incisions on the plantar surface of the foot:*
   (a) *a midline incision from the heel to the tip of the middle toe;*
   (b) *a transverse incision across the roots of the toes;*
   (c) *longitudinal incisions along the middle of the remaining toes.*
   Reflect the skin flaps.

2. *Starting from the heel remove the superficial fascia on the plantar surface* to expose the deep fascia. The deep fascia is thickened to form the **plantar aponeurosis**. Note that the plantar aponeurosis has medial, intermediate and lateral subdivisions. The intermediate (central) part of the plantar aponeurosis, which is strong, is attached behind to the **medial process of the calcaneal tuberosity**. *Follow* its five distal processes passing to the fibrous flexor sheaths of the digits. *Cut the central portion of the plantar aponeurosis transversely near the heel and reflect it.* Note the **medial** and **lateral intermuscular septa** passing deeply from this part of the aponeurosis.

First layer

3. *Remove the rest of the deep fascia* from the medial and lateral sides of the foot and note the *first layer* of muscles comprising the **abductor hallucis, flexor digitorum brevis** and **abductor digiti minimi** from medial to lateral. Note the origin of these muscles from the calcaneal tuberosity. *Trace them towards their insertions.* The abductor hallucis is inserted into the medial side of the base of the proximal phalanx of the first toe. The abductor digiti minimi is inserted into the lateral side of the base of the proximal phalanx of the fifth toe. The flexor digitorum brevis splits into four slips which are inserted into the sides of the middle phalanges of the lateral four toes. Note that these tendons are covered by fibrous flexor sheaths over the digits.

4. *Secure the* **medial plantar nerve** *and* **artery** between the abductor hallucis and flexor digitorum brevis. Note that the nerve supplies cutaneous branches to the medial three and a half toes and motor branches to the

(a) flexor digitorum brevis; (b) abductor hallucis; (c) flexor hallucis brevis; and (d) **first lumbrical**. The medial plantar artery communicates with branches of the **plantar arterial arch** (see later).

5. *Cut the abductor hallucis near its origin and turn it forwards* to expose the commencement of the **medial** and **lateral plantar nerves** and **arteries** which are the terminal branches of the tibial nerve and posterior tibial artery.

6. *Detach the flexor digitorum brevis from its origin and reflect it forwards and trace the lateral plantar nerve and artery towards the lateral side of the foot.*

7. Note that the lateral plantar nerve supplies cutaneous branches to the lateral one and a half toes and muscular branches to the abductor digiti minimi and the remaining plantar muscles that are not supplied by the medial plantar nerve.

Second layer

8. *Cut the abductor digiti minimi at its origin and reflect it.* You will now see the *second layer* which consists of the tendons of **flexor hallucis longus**; **flexor digitorum longus** and the muscles associated with it, i.e. **quadratus plantae** and the four **lumbricals**.

9. *Trace the long flexor tendons to the toes by splitting the fibrous flexor sheaths covering them longitudinally.*

10. *Find the tendon of the flexor hallucis longus* in the groove of the **sustentaculum tali of the calcaneus** and *trace it forwards* to its insertion into the base of the distal phalanx of the first toe.

11. *Observe* that the tendons of the flexor digitorum brevis lie superficial to the tendons of the flexor digitorum longus and both sets of tendons are inserted into the lateral four toes. Note that the brevis tendons split to pass *to the sides of the* **intermediate phalanges** and the longus tendons *pass between the split parts to the* **bases of the distal phalanges**.

12. Note that the **lumbricals**, which arise from the tendons of the flexor digitorum longus insert into the tibial side of the extensor expansion.

13. *Clean the two heads of the origin of the quadratus plantae which arise from the medial and lateral edges of the calcaneus* and observe its insertion into the tendon of the flexor digitorum longus.

Third layer

14. *Divide the two heads of the quadratus plantae and the tendons of the long flexors near the heel and turn them distally* to expose the *third layer* of muscles. These are from medial to lateral:
    (a) **flexor hallucis brevis**;
    (b) **adductor hallucis**;
    (c) **flexor digiti minimi brevis**.

15. *Clean the flexor hallucis brevis and cut it near its origin from the cuboid bone*. Note that it divides into two slips; the medial slip joins the abductor hallucis tendon while the lateral one joins the adductor hallucis to be inserted into the respective sides of the proximal phalanx of the first toe. Note the **sesamoid bones** at these insertions. *Clean the* **oblique** *and* **transverse heads** *of the* **adductor hallucis**. *Note* the origin of the oblique head from the bases of the second, third and fourth metatarsal bones and that of the transverse head from the capsules of the lateral four metatarsophalangeal joints. *Note* the origin of the flexor digiti minimi brevis from the base of the fifth metatarsal bone and *trace it* to its common insertion with the abductor digiti minimi into the lateral side of the proximal phalanx of the fifth toe. *Remove the third layer of muscles* taking care not to damage the lateral plantar nerve and artery.

16. *Clean*:
    (a) the lateral plantar nerve and note that it supplies all the interossei of the four intermetatarsal spaces;
    (b) the lateral plantar artery forming the plantar arterial arch which gives off the **plantar metatarsal** and **plantar digital arteries**.

Note that the arch is reinforced by the dorsalis pedis artery entering the sole through the first intermetatarsal space.

Fourth layer

17. *Now clean the fourth layer* comprising the **interossei** (three **plantar** and four **dorsal**) and the *tendons* of the **tibialis posterior** and **fibularis longus**. *Identify and clean the* **deep transverse metatarsal ligaments** which connect the capsules of all five metatarsal joints. Note again that the lumbricals join the extensor expansions and that the interossei lie in the intermetatarsal spaces and insert into the bases of the proximal phalanges.

Note that the *axial line of the foot passes through the second toe* (c.f. hand).

18. *Identify the tendon of the tibialis posterior and trace its main insertion into the* **tuberosity of the navicular bone**. Other slips pass from this tendon to the bases of the middle three metatarsal bones and to all the tarsal bones except the talus. Note that a slip passes backwards and blends with the **plantar calcaneonavicular** (spring) **ligament**.
19. *Turn to the lateral side of the foot and confirm* the insertion of the **fibularis brevis** into the lateral side of the *base of the fifth metatarsal bone. Trace the fibularis longus tendon* lying in a groove on the inferior surface of the cuboid bone to its insertion into the lateral side of the **medial cuneiform** and **first metatarsal bones**.
20. *Identify the* **long plantar ligament** passing from the **calcaneal tuberosity** to the lips of the groove lodging the fibularis longus tendon. The other deep ligaments will be examined later.

Summary

The plantar muscles of the foot appear to be sandwiched between the deep ligaments of the foot and the superficially placed plantar aponeurosis. Although the muscles of the foot are described in four layers, the arrangement is very much the same as in the hand since the muscles of the first and fifth toes correspond somewhat to those of the thumb and little finger.

The muscles on the lateral side show ligamentous degeneration while those on the medial side of the foot are better developed. This is to be correlated with differences in the functional adaptations of the foot in weight bearing and walking. The shifting of the axial line towards the second toe is also an expression of these functional adaptations. Further confirmation of this is evidenced by the fact that the first toe is placed in the same plane as the other toes and is also intimately connected with the second toe by the deep transverse metatarsal ligament.

The medial plantar nerve corresponds more or less to the median nerve of the hand while the lateral plantar nerve has similarities with the ulnar nerve in its distribution. The medial plantar nerve supplies the abductor and flexor muscles of the first toe and, in addition, the flexor digitorum brevis and the first lumbrical. All the other muscles of the foot are innervated by the lateral plantar nerve.

The lateral plantar artery accompanied by the lateral plantar nerve runs between the first and second layers of muscles towards the lateral side of the foot, and subsequently pursues a recurrent course medially between the third and fourth layers of muscles of the foot. This artery contributes to the plantar arterial arch.

Objectives for Dissection Schedule 11

Topic: Sole of foot

General objective

Comprehend the arrangement of the muscles, nerves and vessels of the sole of the foot.

Specific objectives

1. Define the four conventional muscular layers.
2. Compare the muscles of the first and fifth toes with those of the thumb and little fingers.
3. Compare the long flexors of the foot with those of the hand and explain the actions of quadratus plantae.
4. Explain the actions of the interossei.
5. Define the course and distribution of the medial plantar nerve.
6. Define the course and distribution of the lateral plantar nerve.
7. Illustrate the dermatomic pattern of the sole of the foot.
8. Define the course and distribution of the lateral plantar artery.
9. Define the course and distribution of the medial plantar artery.

Overview of Schedule 12

Before you begin dissection note:

TIBIOFIBULAR JOINTS, ANKLE JOINT AND JOINTS OF THE FOOT

1. ANKLE JOINT

Relevant skeletal features:

lower end of tibia and fibula; talus.

Muscles in immediate relation to capsule of joint:

tibialis anterior; extensor hallucis longus; extensor digitorum longus; fibularis tertius; fibularis brevis; fibularis longus; tibialis posterior; flexor digitorum longus; flexor hallucis longus; tendocalcaneus.

Capsule:

attachments.

Ligaments:

deltoid ligament; lateral ligaments.

Synovial membrane:

reflection.

Articular surfaces:

tibiofibular mortise; posterior tibiofibular ligament; trochlear and malleolar surfaces of talus.

Movements:

dorsiflexion; plantar flexion; side-to-side movement in plantar flexion.

Clinical anatomy:

sprains; avulsion of medial malleolus; Pott's fracture.

2. SUBTALAR, MIDTARSAL AND OTHER JOINTS

Relevant skeletal features:

bones of foot; arches of foot.

Capsule:

attachments.

Ligaments:

plantar calcaneonavicular ligament; plantar calcaneocuboid and long plantar ligaments; deep transverse metatarsal ligaments.

Synovial membranes:

reflection.

Articular surfaces:

between talus and calcaneus; talus and navicular; calcaneus and cuboid.

Movements:

inversion and eversion at subtalar and midtarsal joints; movements at other joints.

Muscles concerned in movements:

invertors and evertors; flexors and extensors.

Clinical anatomy:

fractures of metatarsal bones; club foot.

Dissection Schedule 12

TIBIOFIBULAR JOINTS, ANKLE JOINTS, AND JOINTS OF FOOT

TIBIOFIBULAR JOINTS

1. The **tibiofibular joint** is a synovial joint between the lateral condyle of the tibia and the head of the fibula. Note this joint.
2. Note that the tibia and fibula are joined by the **interosseous membrane**. *Clean the surfaces of this membrane.*
3. *Next examine the* **tibiofibular syndesmosis**. *Clean the* **anterior** *and* **posterior tibiofibular ligaments** *and examine them.*

ANKLE JOINT

Review the tendons in relation to this joint and define the capsule which is thin in front and behind. Note on the medial side the attachment of the **medial (deltoid) ligament** which fans out from the medial malleolus of the tibia to the navicular bone, plantar calcaneonavicular ligament, neck of talus, sustentaculum tali of the calcaneus and to the body of the talus. *Identify on the lateral side the* **anterior talofibular**, **calcaneofibular** and **posterior talofibular ligaments**. *Cut through the capsule and ligaments, separate the foot from the leg and examine the articular surfaces. Observe* that the superior **(trochlear)** articular area of the talus is wider in front. This helps to lock the ankle joint in dorsiflexion. *Examine* the tibiofibular mortise and see the **interosseous ligament of the inferior tibiofibular joint**.

ARCHES OF THE FOOT

Identify the **medial** *and* **lateral longitudinal arches** *of the foot*, bearing in mind that the differences in the heights of the medial and lateral arches are a reflection of their functional differences. *Observe* that the calcaneus forms the posterior pillar while the heads of the metatarsals form the anterior pillar. The **transverse arch** is obvious across the bases of the metatarsal bones. This forms only half an arch. Try to understand the part played by the following in the maintenance of the arches:

(a) bony configuration;
(b) ligaments, particularly the plantar ligaments;
(c) long tendons and the intrinsic muscles of the foot;
(d) plantar aponeurosis (the central part).

JOINTS OF THE FOOT

1. *Clean and define the various* **dorsal** *and* **plantar ligaments** *by removing the muscles and tendons of the foot.* Note that the ligaments on the dorsum of the foot are weak while those on the plantar surface are thick and strong.
2. *On the plantar surface examine the* **long plantar ligament** stretching between the calcaneal tuberosity, the ridge on the cuboid bone and the adjacent bases of the metatarsal bones thus bridging the fibularis longus tendon. *Cut this ligament and define the* **plantar calcaneocuboid ligament** which lies deep to the long plantar ligament.

Subtalar Joint

Clean the capsule and the **medial** *and* **lateral talocalcanean ligaments** of the **talocalcanean joint** on the medial and lateral sides of the foot, respectively. *Cut the ligaments.*

Talocalcaneonavicular Joint

1. *On the plantar surface clean the important* **plantar calcaneonavicular** (spring) **ligament** of the **talocalcaneonavicular joint**. Note that this ligament stretches between the **sustentaculum tali of the calcaneus** and the plantar surface of the navicular. *Cut the ligament and verify* that it contains a cartilaginous facet articulating with the head of the talus.
2. *Open the joint on the dorsum and medial side and examine* the strong **interosseous talocalcanean ligament** which extends between the **neck of the talus** and the anterior upper part of the calcaneus. This ligament is important in inversion and eversion of the foot. *Cut the ligament* in order to free the talus.

Calcaneocuboid Joint

Note the capsule. *Open the joint on its dorsum and observe* the corresponding articular surfaces. What strong ligaments lie beneath this joint?

Transverse Tarsal Joint

1. Note that the transverse tarsal joint is formed by the **talocalcaneonavicular** and **calcaneocuboid joints** which lie in the same transverse plane. What movements are possible at these joints?
2. Note the presence of **plantar, dorsal** and **interosseous ligaments** in relation to the *other smaller joints of the foot.*

Metatarsophalangeal and Interphalangeal Joints

1. *Examine the capsule and the thickened* **plantar** *and* **collateral ligaments** *at the* **metatarsophalangeal** *and* **interphalangeal joints**. *Cut the capsules on the dorsal surface and examine the articular surfaces.*
2. *Examine the four* **deep transverse metatarsal ligaments** which unite the plantar ligaments of the adjoining metatarsophalangeal joints. These ligaments hold the metatarsal heads together. Dorsal to the ligaments are the interosseous muscles, whereas the lumbricals and digital nerves and vessels are on the plantar surface.

Summary

The ankle joint is a hinge joint in which the range of plantar flexion is greater than dorsiflexion. In addition, there is some degree of side-to-side movement possible in the plantar flexed position.

Since the line of weight falls in front of the ankle joint there is a tendency for the tibiofibular mortise to slide forward on the trochlear surface of the talus. This is resisted by the strong posterior parts of the medial and lateral ligaments which are directed *downwards and backwards.* During dorsiflexion, the widest anterior part of the trochlea comes in contact with the narrowest, posterior part of the tibiofibular mortise. As a result, no side-to-side movement is possible.

It must be appreciated that the foot serves as a propulsive organ during locomotion and as a supporting pedestal during weight bearing. Consequently, the foot is constructed to meet these demands. The foot possesses longitudinal and transverse arches. The **medial longitudinal arch** is higher and more suited for propulsive efforts, whereas the **lateral arch** is flattened and suited for weight bearing. The **transverse arch** runs across the distal parts of the tarsals and bases of the metatarsals. Each foot forms only half of the transverse arch, the other half being completed by the opposite foot. The transverse arch helps both in propulsion and weight transmission. The moiety of the bones contribute to the formation of the arches of the foot while the maintenance of these arches depends on: (a) intersegmental ties, i.e. ligaments extending between adjacent bones, as well as ties between anterior and posterior pillars; (b) tendons passing under the highest point of the arch and supporting it from below; (c) tendons which suspend the arches from above. In addition, the muscles of the sole act as extensile ligaments.

Since the foot is also an organ which can adapt itself while walking along uneven surfaces, some degree of mobility must be permitted between the bones of the foot without, however, weakening its main functions of support and propulsion. In this connection the amount of movement, i.e. inversion and eversion, permitted at the subtalar and midtarsal joints must be comprehended. It must also be noted that inversion is maximal during plantar flexion and eversion during dorsiflexion of the foot. The association of eversion with dorsiflexion of the foot is perhaps due to the fact that the evertors were originally a part of the extensor group. This also explains their common nerve supply.

Objectives for Dissection Schedule 12

Topic: Ankle joint

General objective

Comprehend the essential features of the osteoligamentous structures.

Specific objectives

1. Define the articulating surfaces of the ankle joint in the skeleton.
2. Describe the attachments of the ligaments of the ankle joint.
3. Demonstrate the tendons in relation to the joint in the living.
4. Demonstrate the possible movements of the joint and the muscles involved.
5. Analyse the reasons for the side-to-side movement of the joint that occurs in the plantar flexed position.
6. Interpret the different radiographic views of the joint.

Topic: Joints of the foot

General objective

Comprehend the movements of the various joints of the foot.

Specific objectives

1. Demonstrate the movements taking place at the subtalar and midtarsal joints.
2. Demonstrate the muscles involved in inversion and eversion.
3. Analyse the above movements in terms of supination and pronation of the hand.
4. Analyse the formation and maintenance of the arches of the foot.

Additional Objectives for Lower Limb

Topic: Review of the lower limb

General objective 1

Comprehend the arrangement and distribution of the blood vessels and lymphatics of the lower limb.

Specific objectives

1. Define the course of the femoral, popliteal, anterior and posterior tibial and dorsalis pedis arteries. Illustrate the surface markings of the first two arteries.
2. Review the distribution of the profunda femoris artery and discuss its role in collateral circulation.
3. Demonstrate the peripheral pulses in the lower limb, the points of arterial compression, and measurement of blood pressure.
4. Identify the great and small saphenous veins, and enumerate the sites of the perforating veins.
5. Demonstrate the deep veins of the lower limb.
6. Describe the venous drainage and apply this knowledge to the occurrence of:
   (a) varicose veins;
   (b) calf vein thrombosis.
7. Enumerate the locations of the superficial and deep lymph nodes and compare the lymphatic drainage to that of the upper limb.
8. Interpret arteriograms, venograms and lymphangiograms.

General objective 2

Comprehend the nerve supply of the lower limb.

Specific objectives

1. Illustrate the surface markings of the sciatic, tibial, common fibular, femoral and saphenous nerves.

2. Explain the motor and sensory deficits in lesions of the femoral, sciatic, tibial and common fibular nerves.
3. Demonstrate the segmental innervation of the joints, muscles and skin.

General objective 3

Comprehend the anatomical basis of the maintenance of the erect posture and walking.

Specific objectives

1. Analyse the maintenance of the erect posture by discussing some important muscular and ligamentous supports in the hip, knee and ankle joints.
2. Demonstrate the walking cycle with the muscles involved in each phase.

Section 3

THORAX

Introduction

The thorax constitutes the upper part of the trunk. It is like a truncated cone which is flattened from before backwards. In the adult the shape of the thorax in transverse section is reniform whereas it is more rounded in the infant. Thus, the human thorax contrasts sharply from that of ordinary mammals in that it is more or less spindle-shaped in transverse section. The shape of the human chest is the outcome of man's arboreal ancestry.

The bony thoracic cage is made up of 12 **thoracic vertebrae**, 12 pairs of **ribs** and their **costal cartilages**, and the **sternum**. The sternum has three parts: (1) the **manubrium** lying opposite the third and fourth thoracic vertebrae; (2) the **body** of the sternum opposite the fifth, sixth, seventh and eighth thoracic vertebrae; and (3) the **xiphoid process**. The junction between the manubrium and the body of the sternum is the **sternal angle**, a palpable landmark at the level of the second **sternocostal joint**. This corresponds to the lower border of the body of the fourth thoracic vertebra. The manubrium and the body of the sternum are joined together by fibrocartilage to form a secondary cartilaginous joint which permits only a restricted amount of movement during respiration. However, the **sternocostal joints** with the exception of the first are of the synovial type in which a greater freedom of movement is possible.

The thorax has an inlet and an outlet. The **superior aperture of the thorax** is formed by the upper end of the manubrium sterni, the first pair of ribs and the first thoracic vertebra. Through this inlet various structures pass from the neck into the thorax and vice versa. The **inferior aperture of the thorax** is formed by the twelfth thoracic vertebra, the lower six costal cartilages and the xiphisternal joint. It is closed by a fibromuscular partition, the **diaphragm**, which is an important muscle involved in respiration.

The cavity of the thorax has three subdivisions — a single midportion called the **mediastinum** containing the heart, the large vessels, the trachea, the oesophagus and nerves, while the two lateral portions — one on either side — contain the lungs with their coverings.

Overview of Schedule 13

Before you begin dissection note:

THORACIC WALL AND LUNGS

Relevant skeletal features:

thoracic cage — sternum; costal cartilages; ribs; thoracic vertebrae; inlet; outlet;
sternum — manubrium; body; xiphoid process; jugular notch; sternal angle;
rib — head; neck; tubercle; shaft; angle; costal groove.
typical intercostal space

Subcutaneous structures:

anterior and lateral cutaneous branches of intercostal nerves.

Muscles:

intercostals (external, internal, innermost).

Nerves:

thoracic (intercostal), phrenic.

Arteries:

internal thoracic; anterior and posterior intercostal.

Veins:

internal thoracic; anterior and posterior intercostal.

Pleurae and lungs:

pleural reflection; surfaces and borders of lungs; root of lungs; fissures; lobes; bronchopulmonary segments.

Surface anatomy:

surface marking of pleura, lungs and fissures.

Clinical anatomy:

auscultation of breath sounds; plain X-ray of chest; bronchogram; bronchoscopy; paracentesis thoracis; bronchopulmonary segments.

Dissection Schedule 13

THORACIC WALL AND LUNGS

1. *With the body on its back remove any remaining fascia and the remnants of the pectoral, serratus anterior and latissimus dorsi muscles.* Note the lateral cutaneous branches of the intercostal nerves in the **midaxillary line** as you remove the tissues. After noting the upper three slips of origin of the **obliquus externus abdominis** from ribs 5, 6, 7 *detach them* so that the *superficial layer* of intercostal muscles, namely the **external intercostals**, can be viewed in the upper six spaces. *Observe* that the fibres of these muscles run downwards and forwards. Note that each external intercostal muscle is replaced anteriorly by the **external intercostal membrane** medial to the **costochondral junction**.

2. *Remove the external intercostal muscles of the upper two or three* intercostal spaces. *Define* the *intermediate layer* formed by **internal intercostal muscles** running downwards and backwards, i.e. in a direction opposite to that of the external intercostals. The internal intercostals are replaced posteriorly by the **internal intercostal membranes** medial to the **angles of the ribs**.

3. *Remove the internal intercostal muscles of the upper two or three* intercostal spaces and *examine* the *innermost layer* of intercostal muscles which do not form a continuous sheet. They consist of three parts:
   (a) **transversus thoracis** passing between the lower third of the posterior surface of the sternum and the deep surfaces of the costal cartilages 2–6.
   (b) **intercostalis intimi** occupying the middle two-fourths of the intercostal spaces; and
   (c) **subcostals** covering the lower intercostal spaces close to the vertebral bodies. Only the intercostalis intimi and part of the transversus thoracis can be seen at this stage.

4. *Find the* **internal thoracic artery** running 1–2 cm lateral to the margin of the **sternum** in front of the transversus thoracis muscle. Note that the artery divides into the **superior epigastric** and **musculophrenic** branches in the sixth intercostal space. *Find the* **anterior intercostal arteries** arising

from the internal thoracic artery and anastomosing with the **posterior intercostal arteries**.

5. *In the upper part of the intercostal space search for the nerve and vessels lying in the* **costal groove** *close to the lower margin of the rib and the* **pleura** which lies deep to the innermost intercostals. *Secure the main* **thoracic (intercostal) nerve** and note that it has **lateral cutaneous, anterior cutaneous, muscular** and **collateral branches**. The collateral branch runs along the upper border of the rib below. All the intercostal as well as the innermost layer of muscles are supplied by the adjacent thoracic nerves.

6. Note that the **posterior intercostal vein,** the posterior intercostal artery and the thoracic nerve lie in that order from above downwards in the costal groove. The posterior intercostal arteries anastomose anteriorly with the anterior intercostal arteries from the internal thoracic artery. Note that the **neurovascular plane** lies between the internal and innermost layers of intercostal muscles.

7. *Next remove the anterior part of the thoracic cage. With a small saw cut transversely through the middle of the manubrium sterni. Then with a scalpel cut backwards along the first intercostal space as far as the* **posterior axillary line,** *all the time taking care not to cut through the parietal pleura which is adherent to the innermost layer of thoracic muscles and ribs. Next, with a pair of shears, cut through ribs 2, 3, 4, 5, 6, 7, 8 vertically along the posterior axillary line. Finally make an oblique cut forwards and upwards to the xiphisternal junction which is then cut transversely using the scalpel and bone shears as necessary. As far as possible try not to damage the parietal pleura. Now remove the anterior part of the thoracic cage.*

8. *Next examine the internal aspect of the part of the thoracic cage that has been removed. Identify* the transversus thoracis and the internal thoracic artery and look for one or two thoracic nerves.

Whenever necessary replace this part of the thoracic cage for reference.

9. Before you examine the **pleura** note that each lung is invested by a double-layered serous membrane. The outer part of the membrane, the **parietal pleura**, lines the inner surface of the corresponding half of the chest wall, a large part of the upper surface of the **diaphragm** and the **mediastinum** (the structures occupying the middle part of the thorax). The inner part of the membrane, the **visceral (pulmonary) pleura**, covers the surface of the lung and lines the fissures between the lobes.

Different regions of the parietal pleura have distinctive names: the part ascending into the neck over the summit of the lung is the **cervical pleura**; the part lining the internal aspect of the thoracic cage and the sides of the vertebral bodies is the **costal pleura**; that covering the thoracic surface of the diaphragm is the **diaphragmatic pleura**; and that applied to the mediastinum is the **mediastinal pleura**.

10. *Make a cruciform incision in the parietal pleura and reflect the flaps to expose the lungs covered by the* **visceral pleura**. You are now in the **pleural cavity** which is between the two layers of the pleura. *Pass your hand over the lungs and locate its* **apex, base (diaphragmatic surface), mediastinal** *and* **costal surfaces**. *On the mediastinal surface palpate the* **root of the lung** *and the* **pulmonary ligament**. The latter is a fold of pleura immediately below the root of the lung. *Explore the* **costodiaphragmatic recess** *by passing your hand between the diaphragm and thoracic cage.* This recess allows for expansion of the lungs during inspiration.

11. *Examine the levels of reflection of the parietal pleurae on the two sides.* Note that the cervical parietal pleura on both sides extends into the root of the neck for about 1–2 cm above the *medial third* of the clavicle. *From here trace the parietal pleurae downwards* until they *almost meet* each other in the midline behind the sternum at the level of the **sternal angle**. The two layers then continue to lie near the midline till they reach the level of the fourth costal cartilage where the *left layer diverges* so that it is about 1 cm away from the lateral margin of the sternum at the level of the sixth costal cartilage. Here it curves laterally as the inferior margin reaching the eighth rib at the **midclavicular line**, the tenth rib at the **midaxillary line** and the twelfth rib at the **paravertebral line**. The levels of reflection

of the *right parietal pleura* are the same as those of the left except that the right layer continues to run close to the midline behind the sternum down to the sixth costal cartilage.

12. *Now examine the limits of the lungs.* The *lower limits* of the lungs are *two ribs above those of the parietal pleura* at the midclavicular, midaxillary and paravertebral lines, i.e. at the level of the sixth, eighth and tenth ribs, respectively. The upper limits of the lungs follow more or less the outline of the pleurae.

13. *Identify the* **phrenic nerves** covered by mediastinal pleura and lying on either side of the **pericardium** and *in front of the root of each lung. Trace these nerves to the diaphragm.*

14. *Remove the lungs by dividing the roots and pulmonary ligaments.* Note that the *root of each* lung contains a **bronchus, pulmonary artery** and **superior** and **inferior pulmonary veins**. These structures enter and leave the **hilum of the lung**.

15. *Examine each lung in turn and identify its* **apex, base, costal surface** and **medial surface**, *and its* **anterior**, **posterior** *and* **inferior borders**. Note that the anterior and inferior margins are sharp while the posterior border is rounded.

16. **Left Lung**: *Identify the* **cardiac notch** along the lower part of the anterior border of the lung. This notch corresponds to the area where the left pleura recedes away from the midline between the fourth and sixth costal cartilages. *Observe* the **oblique fissure** passing from the posterior border to the inferior margin thus dividing this lung into **superior** and **inferior lobes**. Note the tongue-shaped process of the superior lobe situated between the cardiac notch and the oblique fissure. This is known as the **lingula**.

    Observe the following impressions on the **medial (mediastinal) surface**: (a) **cardiac impression** in front of and below the hilum; (b) groove for the **thoracic aorta** behind the hilum and in front of the posterior border; (c) groove for the **arch of aorta** situated above the hilum; (d) grooves for the **left subclavian** and **common carotid arteries** passing upwards from the groove for the arch of the aorta; the impression for the common carotid artery is in front of that for the subclavian artery.

Note the arrangement of structures passing through the hilus: *from before backwards* these are the **superior pulmonary vein, pulmonary artery** and **bronchus.**

17. **Right Lung**: *Identify the* **oblique fissure**. From about the middle of the oblique fissure, observe the **horizontal fissure** passing forwards to the anterior border. These two fissures divide the right lung into **superior, middle** and **inferior lobes.**

    Now identify the impressions seen on the **medial surface**: (a) cardiac impression in front of and below the hilum; (b) groove for the **azygos vein** in front of the posterior border and arching forwards above the hilum; (c) groove for the **superior vena cava** passing upwards from the anterior end of the groove for the azygos vein; (d) groove for the **inferior vena cava** in front of the pulmonary ligament; (e) groove for the **oesophagus** behind the hilum and in front of the groove for the azygos vein.

    Note the arrangement of structures passing through the hilum: *from before backwards* these are the **superior pulmonary vein, pulmonary artery** and **bronchus**. The bronchus *above* the pulmonary artery is known as the *eparterial bronchus.*

18. *Observe* that the **trachea** divides into two **main bronchi** which in turn subdivide into **lobar bronchi** — two on the left and three on the right. Note the presence of **bronchopulmonary lymph nodes** in relation to the lobar bronchi at the hilum. Note that **bronchial arteries** accompany the lobar bronchi of the lungs. These arteries arise from the thoracic aorta or from the upper posterior intercostal arteries. *Trace the lobar bronchi further into the lungs* and note their subdivision into **segmental bronchi**; each segmental bronchus supplies a pyramidal-shaped area of the lung termed the **bronchopulmonary segment**. Note that each segmental bronchus is accompanied by a branch of the pulmonary artery whereas the corresponding vein runs in between segments and therefore drains adjacent bronchopulmonary segments. *Examine museum specimens and your atlas* showing *ten* bronchopulmonary segments in the right and left lung.

Summary

The intercostal nerves are the ventral rami of the thoracic spinal nerves. They supply the adjacent intercostal muscles and skin. The lower six nerves pass into the abdominal wall after leaving the intercostal spaces. The intercostal nerve is a segmental nerve and also supplies the adjacent parietal pleura which is sensitive to pain. However, the visceral pleura is devoid of such innervation and is consequently insensitive to pain.

The lungs which occupy the lateral portions of the thoracic cavity are lateral outgrowths from the foregut. Each lung invaginates the pleural cavity from its medial side. As a result, the roots of the lungs and pulmonary ligaments are found on the mediastinal surface of the lung. During respiration, the roots of the lungs move downwards, forwards and outwards so that there is room for expansion of the posterior parts of the lungs. In addition, there is possibly differential expansion between the lobes of the lungs during respiration and this may be assisted by the fissures which allow freedom of movement between the lobes. The right lung is shorter and heavier than the left lung and its inferior surface is pushed upwards by the right lobe of the liver and overlying cupola of the diaphragm. Each lung is divisible into ten bronchopulmonary segments. This enables the surgical removal of a diseased segment of the lung.

The levels of reflection of pleura and lungs must be comprehended. For example, you should know that the cervical pleura is about 1–2 cm above the medial third of the clavicle. This is due to the fact that the first rib slopes downwards and forwards from its vertebral towards its sternal end. As a result, an accidental puncture through this region could produce a **pneumothorax**. This will also explain why sounds of breathing from the apex of the lungs are better heard over the supraclavicular region than from behind. Moreover, it must be known that the pleural cavity overlaps the upper abdominal organs, so that an injury through the lower part of the pleural cavity could involve the organs occupying the upper part of the abdomen.

Objectives of Dissection Schedule 13

Topic: Pleurae and lungs

General objective

Comprehend the disposition of the pleurae and lungs and the clinical importance of this knowledge.

Specific objectives

1. Identify the cervical, costal, mediastinal and diaphragmatic pleurae.
2. Demonstrate the reflection of the visceral pleura at the hila and thc fissures of the lungs and the formation of the pulmonary ligament.
3. Orientate the right and left lungs.
4. Surface mark the pleura and lungs including the lung fissures and cardiac notch.
5. Identify the main pleural recess.
6. Discuss the anatomical principles involved in the selection of sites for paracentesis thoracis in cases of pleural and pericardial effusion.
7. Discuss the significance of the innervation of the parietal pleura.
8. Explain the importance of the bronchopulmonary segments in surgery and physiotherapy.

Overview of Schedule 14

Before you begin dissection note:

SUPERIOR AND MIDDLE MEDIASTINUM

Superior mediastinum and contents:

thymus; brachiocephalic veins; phrenic and vagus nerves; arch of aorta and branches; trachea; oesophagus.

Middle mediastinum and contents:

pericardium — fibrous; serous (parietal, visceral); transverse sinus; oblique sinus;
heart — surfaces and borders; coronary arteries; coronary sinus; cardiac veins; atria; ventricles; innervation;
great vessels — ascending aorta; pulmonary trunks; superior and inferior venae cavae.
main bronchi

Surface anatomy:

surface marking of heart.

Clinical anatomy:

apex beat; percussion of borders; auscultation of heart sounds; X-ray of chest (pulmonary conus, aortic knuckle); E.C.G.

Dissection Schedule 14

SUPERIOR AND MIDDLE MEDIASTINUM

1. *Again remove the cut portion of the sternum along with the attached* **costal cartilages** and **ribs**. Preserve the removed portion of the sternum and costal cartilages for later study.

2. *Examine the* **mediastinum** which is the space between the two pleural sacs. The mediastinum is subdivided into a **superior** and an **inferior mediastinum**. That part which lies above a plane passing from the **sternal angle** to the junction between the vertebrae T4 and T5 is the superior mediastinum and the part below the plane is the inferior mediastinum. The inferior mediastinum is further subdivided into an **anterior mediastinum** situated in front of the heart, and a **posterior mediastinum** lying behind the heart and the upper posterior surface of the diaphragm while the heart and the roots of the great vessels lie in the **middle mediastinum**.

3. *Identify the bilobed* **thymus gland**, if present, occupying the superior mediastinum and the upper part of the anterior mediastinum. Observe that it overlaps not only the great vessels but also the upper portion of the pericardium. The gland receives its blood supply from the internal thoracic artery.

4. *Remove the thymus.* The **fibrous pericardium** covering the heart as well as the large vessels lying cranial to the pericardium can now be viewed. *Displace the remainder of the manubrium forwards* along with the first rib in order to *clean* the **left brachiocephalic vein** which lies under cover of the upper half of the manubrium. This vein commences behind the left sternoclavicular joint and passes superficial to the **arch of the aorta** to join the **right brachiocephalic vein** at the lower border of the right first costal cartilage to form the **superior vena cava**. *Next clean the right brachiocephalic vein.*

5. *Clean the vessels arising from the arch of the aorta.* These are from right to left: the **brachiocephalic trunk, left common carotid artery** and **left subclavian artery**. Note a small artery, the **thyroidea ima**, which if present

arises from the brachiocephalic trunk and ascends into the neck to supply the **thyroid gland**. *Identify* the **trachea** and **oesophagus** which lie behind the arch of the aorta.

6. *Replace the cut portion of the sternum and ribs* and note that the arch of the aorta lies behind the lower half of the manubrium, i.e. entirely in the superior mediastinum.

7. *Trace the* **phrenic nerves** *cranially*. Note that the right nerve lies lateral to the right brachiocephalic vein and superior vena cava while the left nerve descends between the left common carotid and left subclavian arteries to cross the arch of the aorta. In the interval between these two arteries, *find the* **left vagus nerve** which lies posterior to the left phrenic nerve. *Trace the left vagus nerve* as it descends in front of the arch of the aorta where it gives off the **left recurrent laryngeal nerve**. *Secure this nerve as it hooks under the aortic arch* and the **ligamentum arteriosum**. The ligamentum arteriosum is a fibrous band passing from the left pulmonary artery to the aortic arch. It is a remnant of the **ductus arteriosus**. *Clean the* **superficial part of the cardiac plexus** lying in the concavity of the aortic arch and superficial to the ligamentum arteriosum. Sympathetic branches from the superior cervical, middle cervical, cervicothoracic and second, third, fourth and fifth thoracic ganglia as well as branches from the right and left vagus nerves contribute to the **cardiac plexus**.

8. *Find the* **left superior intercostal vein** passing between the left phrenic and vagus nerves to drain into the left brachiocephalic vein. It drains the second and third intercostal spaces.

9. *Now identify* the **right vagus nerve** as it passes *behind* the root of the right lung and trace it upwards and note how it enters the thoracic inlet by passing superficial to the right subclavian artery.

10. *Next examine the attachments of the* **fibrous pericardium** *to the central tendon of the diaphragm and to the walls of the great vessels.* The sternopericardial ligaments attaching it to the back of the sternum have already been cut. *Expose the heart by a cruciform incision through the front of the fibrous pericardium.* Note that the inner surface of the fibrous pericardium is smooth as it is lined by the **parietal layer of the serous pericardium**. The serous layer of pericardium which is intimately adherent

to the heart is the **visceral layer**. Observe that this layer is reflected along the great vessels where it becomes continuous with the parietal layer.

11. *Identify the* **right** *and* **left auricles** *of the* **atria**, *the* **ventricles**, *the* **ascending aorta** *and* **pulmonary trunk**. Note that the **coronary sulcus** separates the atria from the ventricles while the **anterior** and **posterior interventricular grooves** lie between the ventricles. *Trace the superior and inferior venae cavae towards the right atrium.*

12. Note the orientation of the heart. Observe that the **base of the heart** is situated above and posteriorly while the **apex** is directed antero-inferiorly and to the left. *Verify* that the major part of the *base of the heart is formed by the* **left atrium** which lies opposite the middle four thoracic vertebrae. Note that the right atrium lies mostly in front of the left atrium while the **diaphragmatic surface** of the heart lies against the diaphragm.

13. *Pass your index finger behind* the **ascending aorta** *and* **pulmonary trunk** *and in front of the superior vena cava to explore the* **transverse sinus of the pericardium**. *Note that your finger is above the left atrium* as it lies within the transverse sinus.

    Lift the apex of the heart and pass your finger along the posterior surface of the heart and note the **oblique sinus of the pericardium** which lies between the inferior vena cava and right pulmonary veins on the right and the left pulmonary veins on the left. Note that the oblique and transverse sinuses are separated from each other by reflections of the visceral pericardium along the superior border of the left atrium.

14. *Clean the superior vena cava and observe* that its upper half is extrapericardial and the lower half intrapericardial. Note that the **vena azygos** joins it posteriorly at the lower end of the extrapericardial portion.

15. *Now remove the heart. First divide the inferior vena cava and pulmonary veins close to the heart. Lift the heart upwards* and review the reflections of the serous pericardium and the boundaries of the oblique sinus. Note the opening of the inferior vena cava in the central tendon of the diaphragm. This corresponds to the level of the eighth thoracic vertebra. *Cut the*

reflections of the visceral pericardium along the superior border of the left atrium. Next divide the ascending aorta, the pulmonary trunk and the superior vena cava. Lift out the freed heart.

The heart

1. Now that the heart is freed *identify and trace the* **left coronary artery** as it runs between the pulmonary trunk and the left auricle to enter the **coronary sulcus**, where it divides into the **anterior interventricular** and **circumflex** branches. *Trace the anterior interventricular branch* along the **anterior interventricular groove** towards the apex of the heart. *Follow the circumflex branch* which runs in the coronary sulcus. *Secure the small* **left marginal branch** arising from the circumflex artery.

2. *Next identify the origin of the* **right coronary artery** from the right side of the ascending aorta and *trace it* first between the pulmonary trunk and right auricle and subsequently along the coronary sulcus where it gives off its **right marginal branch**. *Trace the right coronary artery* further along the posterior surface where it divides into a large **posterior interventricular** branch and a smaller terminal branch which anastomoses with the terminal part of the circumflex branch of the left coronary artery. *Trace the posterior interventricular branch* which runs in the **posterior interventricular groove** towards the apex along the diaphragmatic surface of the heart.

3. *Identify*: (a) the **great cardiac vein** lying in the anterior interventricular groove along with the anterior interventricular branch of the left coronary artery; (b) the **middle cardiac vein** running along the posterior interventricular groove, and accompanying the posterior interventricular branch of the right coronary artery; (c) the **left** and **right marginal veins** along the corresponding margins of the heart; (d) the **small cardiac vein** occupying the right extremity of the coronary sulcus and receiving the right marginal vein. *Trace these veins towards the* **coronary sinus**. The major part of the coronary sinus lies between the left atrium and left ventricle. *Follow the coronary sinus to its entry into the right atrium.*

4. *Now open the four chambers of the heart in the following manner:*

The right atrium

Pass the blade of a long knife through the superior vena caval opening down into the right atrium and out through the inferior vena caval opening. Cut laterally to open the right atrium. Then use scissors to make a second cut through the anterior wall of the right atrium at right angles to the first cut. Extend this into the apex of the right auricle. Remove any clots from the atrial cavity and thoroughly wash out the atrium so that its internal features are clearly displayed.

The right ventricle

Pass a long-bladed knife through the right atrioventricular opening between the anterior and septal cusps until it emerges through the apex of the right ventricle. When the knife is in this position, open the ventricle by cutting antero-laterally to the left. Next pass the knife from the lower end of the ventricular incision upwards through the pulmonary valve and out of the cut end of the pulmonary trunk. Now cut anteriorly, thus increasing the exposure of the interior of the right ventricle and at the same time opening the pulmonary trunk. Remove any clots and wash out the ventricle.

The left atrium

Make a vertical cut through the wall of the atrium to join the two right pulmonary openings. Do the same with the two left pulmonary veins. Make a transverse cut to join these two small vertical incisions and extend this cut as far as the apex of the left auricle and so open the left atrium posteriorly. Wash out the interior of this chamber.

The left ventricle

First pass the knife through the left atrioventricular opening until it emerges through the apex of the left ventricle. When the knife is in this position, open the left ventricle by cutting laterally to the left. Next pass the knife from the lower end of this incision upwards between the anterior cusp of the mitral valve and the interventricular septum through the aortic valve and out through the cut end of the aorta. Now cut posteriorly to expose the interior of the left ventricle and the ascending aorta. Clean out any clots that may still be present.

5. *Observe the following features in the* **right atrium**:
   (a) **crista terminalis**, a ridge running between the anterior margins of the superior and inferior venae cavae. (The **sinuatrial node** lies near the upper end of the crista terminalis.) Note the muscular ridges, the **musculi pectinati**, running from the crista terminalis into the auricular part of the atrium. Observe that the atrial wall *behind* the crista terminalis is smooth. This posterior portion of the atrium is the **sinus venarum**;
   (b) the **interatrial septum** separating the two atria. In the septum, note the **fossa ovalis** (a depression) and **limbus fossae ovalis** forming a raised margin above and in front of the fossa;
   (c) **orifice of the superior vena cava**;
   (d) **orifice of the inferior vena cava**;
   (e) **right atrioventricular orifice** guarded by the **tricuspid valve** (**anterior**, **posterior** and **septal cusps**);
   (f) **orifice of the coronary sinus** situated between the last two orifices. (Situated above the opening of the coronary sinus and lying in the atrial septum is the **atrioventricular node**.)

6. *Next observe the interior of the* **right ventricle** and note:
   (a) **trabeculae carneae** which are muscular ridges in the wall of the ventricle. This portion of the ventricle is the **inflow tract**;
   (b) three **papillary muscles** which are conical muscular projections from the ventricular wall. Note the positions of these papillary muscles (**anterior**, **posterior** and **septal**);
   (c) **chordae tendineae** which are fibrous cords arising from the papillary muscles to be attached to the **tricuspid valve cusps** a little away from their free margins. Identify these cusps which are termed **anterior**, **posterior** and **septal** according to their positions;
   (d) right atrioventricular orifice which admits three fingers;
   (e) **pulmonary orifice** guarded by the **pulmonary valve** with three cusps. Note that the pulmonary trunk arises from the smooth upper part of the right ventricle known as the **conus arteriosus** (the **outflow tract**);
   (f) note that a band of muscle passed (now torn) from the septum to the anterior wall of the ventricle. This was the **septomarginal trabecula** (moderator band) which conveyed the **right branch of the atrioventricular bundle**.

7. *Now examine the interior of the* **left atrium** and note:
   (a) **openings of the four pulmonary veins** into the smooth portion of the atrium;
   (b) **left atrioventricular orifice** guarded by an anterior and a posterior cusp;
   (c) left auricle forming the anterior part of the atrium and showing the presence of musculi pectinati.

8. *Finally observe the following features in the interior of the* **left ventricle**:
   (a) trabeculae carneae as in the right ventricle (this region is the **inflow tract**);
   (b) left atrioventricular (mitral) orifice guarded by the **mitral valve**. Note that the anterior cusp of the mitral valve intervenes between the mitral and aortic orifices. It is smooth on both surfaces as blood passes to and from the ventricle on either side of this valve cusp;
   (c) **anterior** and **posterior papillary muscles**;
   (d) chordae tendineae arising from the papillary muscles and getting attached to the **anterior** and **posterior cusps** of the **bicuspid (mitral) valve**;
   (e) **aortic vestibule** which is the smooth upper and anterior part of the left ventricle leading into the aorta (this region is the **outflow tract**);
   (f) **aortic orifice** guarded by the **aortic valve** which is composed of three cusps like the pulmonary valve;
   (g) in the cut ascending aorta identify three dilatations (**aortic sinuses**) at the root of the aorta, just above the valve cusps. Observe that the right coronary artery arises from the **right aortic sinus** and the left coronary artery from the **left aortic sinus**.

   Observe that the left ventricular wall is about three times thicker than the right. Why?

9. Note that the **interventricular septum** is placed obliquely so that its right surface which is convex looks forwards and to the right. *Feel the upper membranous and the lower muscular parts of the septum.*

10. *Observe* that the pulmonary trunk lies first to the right, then in front and finally to the left of the aorta. Note that the right pulmonary artery passes behind the aorta.

Summary

In order to understand the orientation of the heart, it must be appreciated that the heart has a **base** placed posteriorly, a **diaphragmatic surface** in relation to the diaphragm and an **anterior surface**. The axis of the heart, i.e. from base to apex runs obliquely downwards, forwards and to the left. Moreover, the heart is rotated in such a way that the right atrium lies almost in front of the left atrium so that the interatrial septum separating the two chambers forms the posterior wall of the right atrium. Similarly, the right ventricle tends to lie in front of the left. As a result, both the interatrial and interventricular septa are inclined at about 45° to the sagittal plane. Thus, the slope of the septa is such that their anterior surfaces are directed forwards and to the right. Moreover, the ventricles lie anterior to the atria so that the blood from the atria flows more or less in a horizontal direction into the ventricles and not vertically downwards, as is usually imagined.

The right and left coronary arteries which supply the heart arise from the ascending aorta opposite the right and left aortic cusps in relation to the corresponding aortic sinuses. The left coronary artery is preponderant in that it supplies more of the heart than the right. However, the right artery usually supplies such important structures as the sinuatrial and atrioventricular nodes, the former being known as the pace maker. Sometimes, these nodes are supplied by the left coronary artery. The pace of the heart is reduced if the sinuatrial node is nonfunctional and the ventricular rhythm is further reduced if the A.V. node is also damaged. Although these nodes possess intrinsic rhythmic activity, this can be modified by the nerves supplying the nodes. These nerves are derived from the **superficial** and **deep parts of the cardiac plexus**, the branches of which run along the right coronary artery to supply the S.A. and A.V. nodes.

The branches of the two coronary arteries anastomose both in the coronary sulcus and in the interventricular grooves. These anastomoses are insufficient to maintain a collateral circulation when one of the main arteries or one of its larger branches is blocked suddenly. However, the collateral circulation can sometimes maintain the viability of the heart if the blockage has been gradual. When one of the main branches of the left or right coronary artery is blocked suddenly by a blood clot, i.e. **coronary thrombosis**, it results in death (**infarction**) of the cardiac muscle supplied by the vessel. Pain resulting from ischaemia (reduced blood supply) or infarction is felt retrosternally and sometimes referred along the medial side of the left upper limb.

Objectives for Dissection Schedule 14

Topic: The heart

General objective

Comprehend the morphology of the heart and pericardium.

Specific objectives

1. Demonstrate the attachments of the fibrous pericardium.
2. Demonstrate the reflections of the serous pericardium and the formation of the oblique and transverse sinuses.
3. Identify the ascending aorta, pulmonary trunk and venae cavae giving embryological reasons for their anatomical disposition.
4. Identify the chambers of the heart on its external surface.
5. Orientate the borders and surfaces of the heart and indicate the chambers contributing to these borders and surfaces.
6. Outline the origin, course and distribution of the coronary arteries.
7. Demonstrate the internal features of the right atrium.
8. Demonstrate the internal features of the right ventricle.
9. Demonstrate the internal features of the left atrium.
10. Demonstrate the internal features of the left ventricle.
11. Illustrate the surface marking of the heart.
12. Indicate the areas for auscultation of heart sounds.

Overview of Schedule 15

Before you begin dissection note:

SUPERIOR AND POSTERIOR MEDIASTINUM AND JOINTS OF THORAX

Superior and posterior mediastinum and contents:

aorta — ascending; arch; thoracic; branches;
venae cavae — superior; inferior;
trachea — thoracic part; main bronchi;
oesophagus — thoracic part; constrictions;
nerves — vagus; sympathetic trunk; splanchnic nerves;
nerve plexuses — cardiac; pulmonary; oesophageal;
veins — posterior intercostal; hemiazygos; accessory hemiazygos; azygos;
thoracic duct — course.

Surface anatomy:

arch of aorta; superior vena cava; inferior vena cava; azygos vein; openings in the diaphragm.

Clinical anatomy:

barium swallow; oesophagoscopy.

Joints of thorax:

manubriosternal — secondary cartilaginous type;
sternocostal — synovial type except the first sternocostal joint which is a primary cartilaginous joint;
interchondral — synovial type except that between the ninth and tenth costal cartilages which is fibrous;
costovertebral — synovial type with double synovial cavities; radiate ligament; intraarticular ligament;

costotransverse — synovial type; superior costotransverse ligament; costotransverse ligament; lateral costotransverse ligament; *no costotransverse joints for the eleventh and twelfth ribs.*

Clinical anatomy:

movements of the thoracic cage during respiration.

Dissection Schedule 15

SUPERIOR AND POSTERIOR MEDIASTINUM AND JOINTS OF THORAX

SUPERIOR AND POSTERIOR MEDIASTINUM

1. *Re-examine the large vessels arising from the arch of the aorta and trace them towards the root of the neck.* Note the division of the brachiocephalic trunk into the **right subclavian** and **right common carotid arteries** lying behind the **right sternoclavicular joint**.

2. *Replace the heart* and note that the **oesophagus** lies immediately behind the left atrium.

3. *Now, remove the pulmonary arteries and the remains of the pericardium and clean the trachea* which lies partly above and partly behind the arch of the aorta. Note that it bifurcates into the right and left main bronchi opposite the lower border of the fourth thoracic vertebral body. Observe the presence of **tracheobronchial lymph nodes** which lie in front of the lower part of the trachea. *Examine the two main bronchi* and note that the right main bronchus is almost vertical, i.e. in line with the direction of the trachea, whereas the left one is more horizontal.

4. *Identify the* **deep part of the cardiac plexus** which lies on the anterior aspect of the tracheal bifurcation. The cardiac plexus receives branches from the right and left vagus nerves, all the cervical sympathetic and the upper five thoracic ganglia and supplies the heart. It also sends branches to the bronchi.

5. *Trace the thoracic part of the* oesophagus which lies posterior to the trachea and note the *constrictions* where the arch of aorta and left bronchus cross it. *Follow the oesophagus down to the* **oesophageal opening** in the diaphragm, which is opposite the level of the tenth thoracic vertebra. *Secure the* **left recurrent laryngeal nerve** *at the aortic arch and trace it upwards* as it lies in the groove between the trachea and oesophagus.

6. *Follow the* **right** *and* **left vagus nerves** *distally*. Observe that the main part of each vagus nerve passes behind the root of the lungs to form the **posterior pulmonary plexus**. Note the contributions from the second, third, fourth and fifth thoracic sympathetic ganglia to this plexus. *Trace*

each vagus nerve from the lower end of this plexus towards the oesophagus where the left and right nerves form the **oesophageal plexus.**

7. *Trace the oesophageal plexus downwards* towards the diaphragm where it gives rise to the **anterior** and **posterior vagal trunks** which follow the oesophagus through the **oesophageal opening of the diaphragm** opposite the tenth thoracic vertebra. Each trunk carries both right and left vagus nerve fibres.

8. *Clean* the **sympathetic trunks** and their ganglia which lie on either side of the thoracic vertebral bodies. There are usually eleven ganglia. *Locate* the **cervicothoracic ganglion** opposite the neck of the first rib. Note that **grey** and **white rami communicans** connect the ganglia with the thoracic nerves. *Secure* the **greater splanchnic nerve** arising from the fifth to the ninth ganglia and the **lesser splanchnic nerve** from the ninth and tenth ganglia. These ganglia are found close to the sides of the respective thoracic vertebral bodies. *Trace these splanchnic nerves downwards towards the* **crura of the diaphragm** which they pierce before entering the abdomen. Note that the greater splanchnic nerves provide branches to the oesophageal plexus.

9. *Clean the descending* **thoracic aorta** *and trace it towards the diaphragm* where it passes through the **aortic orifice** of the diaphragm opposite the twelfth thoracic vertebra. *Trace the* **posterior intercostal arteries** *from the aorta to the lower nine intercostal spaces.* These arteries anastomose with the **anterior intercostal arteries**. Note that the aorta also has **bronchial, oesophageal, phrenic** and **mediastinal branches** all of which are small arteries.

10. *Identify* the **superior intercostal artery**, a branch of the **costocervical trunk** which is a branch of the subclavian artery in the root of the neck. Note that it supplies the first two intercostal spaces. Observe the following structures which lie opposite the neck of the first rib: the cervicothoracic sympathetic ganglion, superior intercostal artery and the **ventral ramus of the first thoracic nerve**. *Trace the ventral ramus of the first thoracic nerve which ascends over the first rib to join the brachial plexus.*

11. Observe that the first intercostal space of both sides is drained by the **first posterior intercostal vein** which drains into the corresponding

brachiocephalic vein. Note that the **left superior intercostal vein** drains the second and third intercostal spaces. Its termination into the left brachiocephalic vein has already been seen.

12. *Identify* the **thoracic duct** and **azygos vein** passing through the aortic opening of the diaphragm. *Trace the azygos vein upwards* where it arches over the root of the right lung to enter the superior vena cava just outside the pericardium. *Secure the following tributaries of the azygos vein*:
    (a) **right superior intercostal vein** draining the second and third intercostal spaces;
    (b) **right posterior intercostal veins** of the lower eight spaces;
    (c) **accessory hemiazygos vein** receiving the fourth to eighth posterior intercostal veins and the **hemiazygos vein** draining the lower posterior intercostal veins of the left side of the thorax. They pass behind the aorta and thoracic duct to join the azygos vein opposite the seventh and eighth thoracic vertebral bodies. Note that the **oesophageal veins** drain into the azygos veins.
13. *Trace the thoracic duct upwards* in front of the thoracic vertebral bodies up to the fifth thoracic vertebra where it inclines towards the left. It then ascends upwards into the neck on the left side of the oesophagus.
14. Medial to the angle of the lower ribs *identify* the **subcostales muscles**, which are part of the innermost intercostals.

JOINTS OF THORAX

1. *These joints should be studied on your cadaver and on a skeleton.*
2. In the portion of sternum and costal cartilages that has been preserved *study the following joints*: (a) **manubriosternal joint**. Note that a fibrocartilaginous disc intervenes between the manubrium and the body of the sternum. This is an example of a secondary cartilaginous joint; (b) **sternocostal joints**. Note that the first sternocostal joint is a primary cartilaginous joint and that the union between the second and seventh costal cartilages and the sternum is by synovial joints.
3. *Clean one or two costovertebral joints.* Note that the capsule is strengthened anteriorly by **radiate ligaments** which pass to the two vertebrae related to

the rib and to the **intervertebral disc**. The head of most ribs has two demifacets which articulate with the bodies of two adjacent vertebrae by synovial joints. In these cases an intervening **intraarticular ligament** extends from the rib to the intervertebral disc, thus dividing the synovial cavity into two.

4. Note that there is a synovial joint between the articular part of the **tubercle of the rib** and the corresponding **transverse process** of the vertebra (**costotransverse joint**). The capsule of the joint is strengthened by the **superior costotransverse, costotransverse** and **lateral costotransverse ligaments**.

5. Note that there are synovial joints between the sixth, seventh, eighth and ninth cartilages (**interchondral joints**).

Summary

The oesophagus extends from the lower end of the **pharynx** to the **cardiac orifice of the stomach**. It is constricted at its commencement, where the left bronchus and the arch of the aorta cross in front of it and where it pierces the diaphragm. These have to be borne in mind during **oesophagoscopy**. The oesophagus runs *behind* the left atrium. Thus any enlargement of the left atrium, for example in **mitral stenosis**, can cause symptoms of **dysphagia**. The oesophagus deviates a little to the right of the midline as it lies behind the heart and consequently produces a visible impression on the mediastinal surface of the right lung in front of the groove for the azygos vein.

The other structures of interest in this region are the trachea and thoracic duct. The fact that the right main bronchus, which is one of the terminal divisions of the trachea, runs vertically carries with it the danger of foreign bodies entering it more frequently than into the left main bronchus. The tracheobronchial lymph nodes are closely related to the left recurrent laryngeal nerve which may sometimes be compressed by these nodes leading to hoarseness of the voice.

The thoracic duct commences from the upper end of a sac known as the **cisterna chyli** which is situated in front of the upper two lumbar vertebrae in the abdomen. The thoracic duct is a thin-walled vessel draining lymph from almost the entire body except the right upper limb, the right half of the thorax and the right side of the head and neck. It is provided with a number of valves. It terminates by opening into the junction of the left subclavian and internal jugular veins.

Movements of the Thoracic Cage during Respiration

In normal respiration there is simultaneous movement of the thoracic cage and diaphragm. During inspiration the volume of the thorax is increased by an increase in one or more of its diameters (anteroposterior, transverse, or vertical) as a result of which air is sucked into the lungs.

In *inspiration* the increase in the anteroposterior diameter is brought about by rotation of the second to the seventh ribs around an axis traversing their heads and tubercles. This rotation results in an elevation of their costal cartilages and the sternum resulting in the so-called 'pump handle' type of movement. In addition, there is a limited amount of movement occurring around an anteroposterior axis passing through the costotransverse and sternocostal joints — the so-called 'bucket-handle' type of movement. This increases the transverse diameter of the thorax which is especially marked in the region of the fifth to seventh ribs. In the region of the eighth, ninth and tenth ribs, there is a splaying out of the costal margin due to diaphragmatic contraction. During *forced inspiration* the first rib also moves upwards and forwards along with the manubrium, thereby increasing the anteroposterior diameter of the thoracic inlet. The last two ribs are not actively involved in movements of the thoracic cage as they are usually fixed by the muscles of the posterior abdominal wall. This fixation enables a more efficient contraction of the diaphragm.

Objectives for Dissection Schedule 15

Topic: Superior and posterior mediastinum

General objective 1

Comprehend the principles of the arrangement of the structures in the superior and posterior mediastinum.

Specific objectives

1. Define the limits of the superior mediastinum and enumerate the structures contained within it from before backwards.
2. Demonstrate the surface markings of the arch of the aorta and its branches.
3. Demonstrate the course of the thoracic part of the oesophagus and its sites of constriction.
4. Define the extent and course of the descending thoracic aorta.
5. Summarise the formation and termination of the first intercostal, superior intercostal, accessory hemiazygos, hemiazygos and azygos veins.
6. Outline the origin, course and relations of the thoracic duct.
7. Illustrate the areas drained by the thoracic and right lymphatic ducts.

General objective 2

Comprehend the anatomical principles in normal respiration.

Specific objectives

1. Define the articulating areas on: (a) the heads of the ribs and (b) the vertebrae.
2. Define the slope of the thoracic inlet.
3. Understand the significance of the downward slope of the ribs.
4. Explain the possible roles of the primary respiratory muscles — the diaphragm in abdominal respiration and the intercostals in thoracic respiration.
5. Define the axes of the 'bucket handle' and 'pump handle' types of movement of the ribs during respiration.

6. Explain how an increase in the three diameters of the thorax facilitates entry of air, venous blood and lymph into the thorax.

7. Enumerate the accessory muscles of respiration and indicate their role in: (a) forced inspiration; (b) forced expiration (bronchospasm).

Additional Objectives for Thorax

Topic: Chest wall

General objective

Comprehend the important anatomical features of the chest wall.

Specific objectives

1. Define the term 'typical intercostal space'.
2. Describe the disposition of the three layers of the intercostal muscles.
3. Indicate the 'neurovascular plane' and the order of structures in the costal groove.
4. Describe the formation, course and distribution of a thoracic mixed spinal nerve.
5. Illustrate how the thoracic wall retains the primitive segmental pattern of innervation.
6. Explain the anatomical principles and hazards involved in paracentesis thoracis.
7. Demonstrate the technique of percussion by which the borders of the heart and lungs can be defined.
8. Indicate the positions of the apex beat and the cardiac valves on the chest wall.
9. Describe the manoeuvres by which cardiac sounds in different areas can be accentuated.
10. Identify the features of the thoracic cage and diaphragm in radiographs of the chest during full inspiration and expiration.

Topic: Thoracic viscera

General objective

Comprehend the clinical importance of the basic anatomical features of the thoracic viscera.

Specific objectives

1. Demonstrate the position of the trachea at the thoracic inlet by palpation.
2. Demonstrate the relations of the trachea and extrapulmonary bronchi.
3. Define the subdivisions of the thoracic cavity.
4. Explain how a sound knowledge of the orientation of the heart, ventricular septum, and the conducting system is necessary for the understanding of the electrocardiograph.
5. Interpret anteroposterior and lateral views of: (a) plain radiographs of the chest; (b) radiographs of the chest after a barium swallow.
6. Explain the anatomical principles involved in oesophagoscopy and bronchoscopy.
7. Explain the anatomical basis of the following signs and symptoms of disease: (a) occurrence of dysphagia in left atrial enlargement; (b) 'tracheal tug' in aortic aneurism; (c) hoarseness of the voice due to mediastinal lymphadenitis; (d) symmetrical 'notching' of the ribs in coarctation of the aorta.

Section 4

ABDOMEN

Introduction

The **abdomen** is that part of the trunk which lies below the thorax. Like the thorax, the abdomen has a cavity which is enclosed by walls. The walls of the abdomen can be conveniently divided into three parts — an upper part formed by the lower portions of the thoracic cage, an intermediate portion comprising the anterolateral and posterior abdominal walls, and a lower portion formed by the bony pelvis with its muscular and ligamentous attachments. The cavity of the abdomen is limited superiorly by the **diaphragm** and inferiorly by another sheet of muscle placed across the bony pelvis, the **pelvic diaphragm**. The **inlet of the pelvis (pelvic brim)** or **linea terminalis** is used as a landmark to divide the cavity of the abdomen into an upper abdomen proper and a lower **pelvic cavity**. It must be remembered that these two cavities are functionally and developmentally one unit.

The serous membrane lining the inner aspect of the abdominal wall is called the **parietal peritoneum** while that covering the viscera is known as the **visceral peritoneum**. The space between these two layers is known as the **peritoneal cavity** which is a capillary interval containing a film of lubricating fluid. The peritoneal cavity acts as one enormous bursa which permits varying degrees of freedom of movement for the abdominal and pelvic organs.

The disposition of the abdominal viscera can be understood more easily if one visualises the arrangement of these viscera in the early embryo. In the embryo, the most ventral structure filling the abdominal cavity is the **liver**, which lies ventral to the gut. Dorsolateral to the gut are those structures which developed from the intermediate mesoderm such as the **kidneys** and **suprarenals**. Dorsal to the gut are the large vessels, i.e. **aorta** and **inferior vena cava**.

In the adult, the arrangement is similar to that in the embryo except that the space occupied by the liver is smaller, with the result that the intestines have come ventrally to abut against the anterior abdominal wall. This disposition of the intestines is also facilitated by the presence of long folds of peritoneum — **mesenteries** — which allow them greater freedom of movement. Those structures which are not provided with a fold of peritoneum and which lie against the posterior abdominal wall behind the peritoneum are said to be retroperitoneal.

Finally, it must be remembered that the mobile diaphragm causes the abdominal viscera to move with respiration. This is most marked in the organs lying directly under the diaphragm and is of clinical importance.

Overview of Schedule 16

Before you begin dissection note:

ANTERIOR ABDOMINAL WALL AND EXTERNAL GENITALIA

Relevant skeletal features:

thoracic cage — lower part;
vertebral column — lumbar region;
hip bones — pubic symphysis; pubic crest; pubic tubercle; pectineal line; anterior superior iliac spine; iliac crest.

Relevant landmarks:

linea alba; umbilicus; linea semilunaris; midaxillary line; posterior axillary line.

Planes of abdomen:

vertical; transpyloric; transtubercular.

Regions of abdomen:

epigastric; umbilical; pubic; right and left hypochondriac; right and left lateral; right and left inguinal.

Subcutaneous structures:

anterior and lateral cutaneous branches of lower thoracic (intercostal) nerves; subcostal nerve; iliohypogastric nerve; ilioinguinal nerve; fatty and membranous layers of the superficial fascia.

Muscles:

obliquus externus abdominis; obliquus internus abdominis; cremaster muscle; transversus abdominis; rectus abdominis; pyramidalis; rectus sheath.

Inguinal region:

Superficial inguinal ring; deep inguinal ring; inguinal canal.

Nerves:

muscular branches of lower thoracic ; subcostal; iliohypogastric; ilioinguinal; genitofemoral.

Arteries:

lower posterior intercostal; subcostal; lumbar; superior epigastric; inferior epigastric.

Veins:

veins accompanying the above arteries.

External genitalia:

male — testis and its coverings; spermatic cord and its contents; scrotum; penis;
female — round ligaments; clitoris; vulva.

Surface anatomy:

superficial inguinal ring; deep inguinal ring; inguinal canal.

Clinical anatomy:

surgical incisions on the anterior abdominal wall; vasectomy; inguinal hernia; hydrocele; undescended testis.

Dissection Schedule 16

ANTERIOR ABDOMINAL WALL AND EXTERNAL GENITALIA

Surface Anatomy of the Anterior Abdominal Wall

1. With the body lying on its back and with a skeleton available for reference, *begin the study of the abdomen by examining the surface of the abdominal wall on the cadaver.* At a convenient moment revise what you learn on your own body.

2. *The regions of the abdomen*:

   The abdomen is divided into regions. *With the point of your scalpel lightly draw a line transversely across the body* through a point midway between the **jugular notch of the sternum** and the upper border of the **pubic symphysis**. This line represents the **transpyloric plane**, which passes through the lower border of the first lumbar vertebra. *Draw a further horizontal line across the body* at the level of the **tubercles of the iliac crests**. This is known as the **transtubercular plane**. *Draw a vertical line upwards on each side*, commencing from a point midway between the pubic symphysis and the **anterior superior iliac spine**. In this way the abdomen is divided into nine regions. These are, from above downwards: the **epigastric**, **umbilical**, **pubic** in the middle, flanked on either side by the **hypochondriac**, **lateral** and **inguinal regions**.

   The *transpyloric plane* marks the position of the **pylorus**, which lies 1–2 cm to the right of the midline; the blind end, or **fundus**, of the **gall bladder**; the hila of the **kidneys**; and the lowest limit of the **spinal cord**.

   In a young healthy adult the navel, or **umbilicus**, lies at the level of the intervertebral disc between the third and fourth lumbar vertebrae. As age advances and fat is deposited, the umbilicus tends to lie below this level.

Superficial Anterior Abdominal Wall

3. *Make the following incisions*:
   (a) *a vertical incision along the midline from the* **xiphoid process** *to the upper margin of the pubic symphysis encircling the umbilicus*;

(b) *from the pubic symphysis laterally to the* **pubic tubercle** *and thence a curved incision along the fold of the groin to the anterior superior iliac spine*; (*if not already made*);

(c) *from the anterior superior iliac spine along the iliac crest as far as the level of the* **posterior axillary line**.

Reflect the skin flap.

4. (a) *Next make a vertical incision through the* **superficial fascia** *in the ventral midline of the body extending from the xiphoid process to the symphysis pubis.*

   (b) *Make a horizontal incision extending from the anterior superior iliac spine to the ventral midline of the body.* The superficial fascia below the horizontal incision has a superficial fatty and a deeper membranous layer.

   (c) *Insert a finger deep to the membranous layer and in front of the underlying aponeurotic portion of the external oblique muscle. Separate* the membranous layer from the muscle inferiorly.

   (d) *Identify the* **spermatic cord** (in the male) *or* **round ligament of the uterus** (in the female) above and lateral to the pubic tubercle. Note that *the finger can be passed medial to the cord into the* **perineum**. However, the finger cannot enter the thigh laterally because of the fusion of the membranous layer to the deep fascia of the thigh, the **fascia lata**.

5. *Reflect the fascia of the abdominal wall laterally*. Note that the anterior cutaneous branches of the lower five thoracic, subcostal (T12) and iliohypogastric (L1) nerves become cutaneous about 3–4 cm from the midline. The seventh thoracic nerve supplies the skin over the xiphoid while the tenth thoracic nerve supplies the skin around the umbilicus.

6. Note the lateral cutaneous branches of the lower five thoracic nerves and the lateral cutaneous branches of the subcostal and iliohypogastric nerves along the **midaxillary line**. The latter two nerves cross the iliac crest to pass into the gluteal region.

Muscles of the Anterior Abdominal Wall

7. *Remove the remains of the superficial fascia and clean the first muscle layer* which is the **obliquus externus abdominis**. Note the absence of deep fascia over the muscle. Why is deep fascia absent over the anterior abdominal wall?

8. The *origin* of the external oblique muscle is from the outer surfaces of the lower eight ribs where its slips of origin interdigitate with those of the **serratus anterior** and **latissimus dorsi muscles**. Observe that the muscle fibres slope downwards, forwards and medially. Note the *insertion* of the posterior part of the muscle into the *anterior half* of the outer lip of the **iliac crest**. *Trace the anterior aponeurotic portion to its insertion* into the **linea alba, pubic crest, pubic tubercle** and **anterior superior iliac spine**. Note that the linea alba is a bloodless, thickened fibrous band between the symphysis pubis and xiphoid while the "rolled in" aponeurotic part of the muscle between the pubic tubercle and anterior superior iliac spine is the **inguinal ligament**.

9. *Detach the external oblique muscle from the ribs and iliac crest. Make a horizontal incision through the muscle from the anterior superior iliac spine to the* **linea semilunaris**. *Reflect the upper part of the external oblique medially and examine the* **obliquus internus abdominis muscle** whose fibres run upwards, forwards and medially, i.e. in a direction opposite to that of the external oblique. The internal oblique *originates* from the *lateral two thirds* of the inguinal ligament, the *anterior two thirds* of the middle lip of the iliac crest and the **thoracolumbar fascia**. Note its aponeurotic *insertion* into the lower four costal cartilages, xiphoid process, linea alba and the pubic crest. *Observe that the part of the aponeurosis passing towards the upper two thirds of the linea alba splits* to enclose the paramedian muscle called the **rectus abdominis**.

10. *Taking care make a vertical incision in the internal oblique muscle from the costal margin to the anterior superior iliac spine. From here extend the incision horizontally to the linea semilunaris. As you reflect the muscle forwards observe* the main nerves and vessels of the abdominal wall lying on the horizontally running fibres of the **transversus abdominis muscle**. This is the neurovascular plane.

Now verify the *origin* of the transversus abdominis muscle from the *lateral half* of the inguinal ligament, the *anterior two thirds* of the inner lip of the iliac crest, thoracolumbar fascia and the inner surfaces of the lower six costal cartilages. Note its *insertion* into the xiphoid process, linea alba, pubic crest and pectineal line.

The Rectus Sheath

11. *Open the aponeurotic covering of the rectus muscle called the* **rectus sheath** *by a vertical paramedian incision from the lower rib margin to the pubic crest. Identify* the **rectus abdominis muscle** which has vertically disposed fibres and exhibits transverse **tendinous intersections** on its anterior surface. *Verify the attachments* of the rectus muscle to the pubic crest and symphysis pubis inferiorly and to the outer surface of the xiphoid and seventh, sixth and fifth costal cartilages superiorly. Near the lower end of the rectus observe the slender **pyramidalis muscle** lying anteriorly and running from the pubic crest and symphysis to be inserted into the linea alba above.

Note that all the muscles of the anterior abdominal wall are supplied by the lower six thoracic and L1 nerves, except rectus abdominis (lower six thoracic nerves) and pyramidalis (subcostal nerve).

12. *Divide the rectus muscle transversely in the middle and reflect the two halves*. Note the thoracic and subcostal nerves entering the sheath and piercing the rectus to become subcutaneous and the anastomosis between the **superior** and **inferior epigastric arteries**, as well as those between their accompanying veins on the deep surface of the muscle. What is the significance of these arterial and venous anastomoses?
13. *Examine the anterior and posterior walls of the rectus sheath at the following levels*:
    (a) at the level of the xiphoid, the anterior wall of the sheath is formed by the external oblique aponeurosis while posteriorly the muscle rests directly on the costal cartilages. Note that the superior epigastric artery enters the deep surface of the rectus by passing between the sternal and costal origins of the **diaphragm**;

(b) from the xiphoid to a level midway between the umbilicus and symphysis pubis, the anterior wall is formed by the external oblique aponeurosis and the **anterior lamella of the internal oblique** while the posterior wall is formed by the **posterior lamella of the internal oblique** and aponeurosis of the transversus abdominis;

(c) below a level midway between the umbilicus and symphysis pubis, the aponeurosis of all the three muscles pass in front of the rectus muscle, while the posterior wall is deficient and, thus, the rectus lies directly on the **fascia transversalis**.

Note that the posterior wall ends inferiorly in a sharp border called the **arcuate line**. The inferior epigastric artery enters the rectus sheath by ascending in front of the margin.

The Inguinal Canal

14. *Now turn your attention to the inguinal region and the dissection of the* **inguinal canal**.

The inguinal canal is an oblique intermuscular passage 5 cm long, situated above the medial half of the inguinal ligament. It transmits the **spermatic cord** in the male and the **round ligament of the uterus** in the female. The inguinal canal is directed medially, downwards and forwards and extends from the **deep inguinal ring** in the fascia transversalis to the **superficial inguinal ring** in the external oblique muscle. The deep inguinal ring is situated 1.5 cm above the **midinguinal point** — a point half way between the anterior superior iliac spine and the symphysis pubis. The superficial inguinal ring is situated above the pubic tubercle. Note that the external oblique aponeurosis forms the anterior wall of the inguinal canal.

Identify the superficial inguinal ring above the pubic tubercle and note that the spermatic cord or the round ligament of the uterus emerges through it.

15. *From the lateral end of the horizontal incision already made in the external oblique aponeurosis, make a cut running downwards, forwards and medially, parallel to and a finger's breadth above the inguinal ligament. Cut towards the pubic symphysis, passing above the superficial inguinal ring. Reflect the superior and inferior portions of the cut external oblique aponeurosis and carefully examine the concave upper surface of the*

inguinal ligament. Follow the inguinal ligament medially to the pubic tubercle. Note the extension of the ligament backwards to the **pecten of pubis**. This is called the **lacunar ligament**. *Observe* that it is triangular with its sharp base facing laterally.

16. Note the triple relationship of the lower fibres of the internal oblique to the spermatic cord or round ligament of the uterus. The fibres of the internal oblique arising from the inguinal ligament first *pass in front* of the cord or round ligament, then *above* it and finally *behind* the cord or round ligament where the muscle contributes to a part of the **conjoint tendon**. Thus, the fibres of this muscle contribute to the anterior wall, roof, and to the posterior wall of the inguinal canal in that order. You may find the fibres of the **cremaster muscle** passing on to the spermatic cord from the lower edge of the internal oblique and transversus abdominis muscles.

17. *Detach the fibres of the intenal oblique arising from the inguinal ligament and turn this part of the muscle medially. Now identify the lower margin of the transversus abdominis muscle and follow its fibres* as they arch medially where they will be found to join those of the internal oblique to form the conjoint tendon. *Examine the attachment of this tendon* to the pubic crest and pecten pubis. The conjoint tendon is formed by those fibres of the internal oblique and transversus abdominis muscles that originate from the inguinal ligament. Note that the conjoint tendon lies immediately posterior to the superficial inguinal ring, thus contributing to the posterior wall of the inguinal canal.

18. *Observe* that the fascia transversalis forms the posterior wall of the inguinal canal in this region.

19. *Exert traction* on the spermatic cord or the round ligament of the uterus and *identify* the deep inguinal ring, a deficiency in the fascia transversalis 1.5 cm above the midinguinal point. *Confirm that the deep ring lies lateral to the inferior epigastric vessels. Follow the spermatic cord or round ligament medially* and note how it lies on the lacunar ligament and upper grooved surface of the inguinal ligament which therfore constitute the floor of the inguinal canal. Now review the boundaries of the inguinal canal:

— the *anterior* wall is formed by the external olique aponeurosis in its entirety and by the internal oblique in its lateral half behind the aponeurosis;

— the *posterior* wall is formed by the conjoint tendon in the medial half of the canal and behind it by the fascia transversalis in all the length of the canal;

— the *roof* is formed by the lower arching fibres of the internal oblique and transversus abdominis muscles, and

— the *floor* is formed by the inguinal ligament and most medially by the lacunar ligament.

20. *Secure the ilioinguinal nerve* which reaches the inguinal canal by passing deep to the internal oblique or by piercing it close to the deep inguinal ring.

21. Next note the coverings of the **spermatic cord**. These coverings are generally fused and cannot be separated. They are the **external spermatic fascia** (continuation of external oblique), cremaster muscle and its fascia (continuation of internal oblique and transversus abdominis) and **internal spermatic fascia** (continuation of fascia transversalis) from superficial to deep.

    Try to identify some of the contents of the spermatic cord: **ductus deferens, testicular vessels, pampiniform plexus of veins,** lymph vessels, autonomic nerve plexuses and **genital branch of the genitofemoral nerve**. All these structures enter the deep inguinal ring and traverse the entire length of the canal. The ilioinguinal nerve traverses only the medial part of the canal. Note the easy access to the ductus deferens *by a small incision on the upper lateral scrotal skin.*

Male External Genitalia

1. *Begin by examining* the **external urethral opening** at the tip of the terminal enlarged part of the penis known as the **glans penis**. At the junction of the glans and the shaft *observe* the double fold of skin over the glans known as the **prepuce** or foreskin. The prepuce is attached to the glans on the ventral surface by the **frenulum**, along which runs the artery to the prepuce. Note the midline raphe running along the inferior aspect of the shaft of the penis and continuing as a ridge in the midline round the scrotum.

2. *Incise the skin of the dorsum of the penis longitudinally proximal to the glans and reflect it. Identify* the **dorsal vein, artery** and **nerve of the penis** on the dorsum. *Examine the continuity of the membranous layer of the superficial fascia of the lower abdomen over the pubes into this region.* In the midline it surrounds the penis, lines the scrotum subcutaneously as the **dortos muscle**, and then spreads laterally to be attached to the ischiopubic rami. Posteriorly, this layer extends between the **ischial tuberosities** to fuse with the thickened layer of deep fascia which also stretches between the ischiopubic rami known as the **perineal membrane**.

3. *Incise the scrotal skin on the lateral side, withdraw the* **testis** *and trace the continuity of the coverings of the spermatic cord over the testis. Remove these coverings and identify the* **tunica vaginalis** which is a serous sac consisting of visceral and parietal layers continuous with each other at the posterior margin of the testis and surrounding it in front and at the sides.

4. *Now follow the ductus deferens* and note that it leads to the **epididymis**. This part of the epididymis is the **tail** and is followed by the **body**, and then by the **head** which surmounts the upper pole of the testis like a helmet. The epididymis is fixed to the back of the testis by areolar tissue, but note that the body of the epididymis is separated from the testis by an infolding of the tunica vaginalis called the **sinus of the epididymis**. The opening of the sinus faces posterolaterally.

5. *Make a transverse section through the testis* and examine its structure. Under the visceral layer of the tunica vaginalis note the tough fibrous coat of the testis, the **tunica albuginea**. *Observe* a thickening of the tunica albuginea at the back of the testis called the **mediastinum testis**. Note that the testis is subdivided into a number of **testicular lobules** by incomplete fibrous **testicular septa** radiating from the mediastinum to the tunica albuginea. Each of these compartments contains two or more highly coiled **convoluted seminiferous tubules** which open into the **rete testis** situated inside the mediastinum. Fifteen to 20 delicate **efferent ducts** emerge from the upper part of the rete testis and pass into the head of the epididymis.

6. *Now make a transverse section through the shaft of the penis* and note that it consists of the two dorsal **corpora cavernosa** and a ventral **corpus spongiosum**, each containing vascular erectile tissue. *Identify* the terminal

part of the urethra, the **spongy urethra**, in the middle of the corpus spongiosum.

Female External Genitalia

1. *Observe* the prominence above the pubes due to accumulation of fat in the superficial fascia. This is the **mons pubis**. Below it is the **pudendal cleft** (or **vulva**) through which the genitourinary system opens to the exterior. The vulval orifice is guarded on either side by two rounded folds of skin the **labia majora** which are devoid of hair medially and are kept moist by the secretion of sebaceous glands. Between these folds are the **labia minora**.
2. *When traced forwards* the labia minora become prominent as they approach the **clitoris**, the homologue of the penis. They then split to enclose the clitoris. Their anterior folds form the **prepuce of the clitoris**, while the posterior folds form the **frenulum**. *Draw back the prepuce* and note the **glans of the clitoris**. Note that the **dorsal vein, artery** and **nerve of the clitoris** are situated on the dorsum of the clitoris. Do not search for them. The clitoris is composed of erectile tissue.
3. *When the labia minora are separated*, the **vaginal orifice** is seen. In a virgin it will be covered by a membrane called the **hymen** which is perforated in the middle. Between the hymen and the posterior parts of the labia minora are the openings of a pair of glands called the **greater vestibular glands** (of Bartholin). *Anterior to the vaginal orifice note* the puckered **external opening of the urethra**.

Summary

In the study of the anterior abdominal wall you must comprehend the formation of the rectus sheath and the inguinal canal as both of them are of clinical importance. In addition, the development of the anterior abdominal wall must be understood since a failure of normal development of this region can result in **ectopia vesicae**, a condition in which the mucosa of the urinary bladder is exposed to the exterior through a cleft in the lower abdominal wall. Furthermore, the region of the umbilicus is also a site at which various anomalies can occur:

(a) **congenital umbilical hernia** in which there is a prolapse of the midgut loop through the region of the umbilicus; normally the midgut loop is withdrawn into the abdomen during early fetal life;

(b) retention of a **vitellointestinal duct**, i.e. the connection between the yolk sac and midgut; this duct may remain patent and when the umbilical cord is cut after delivery of the fetus, the contents of the gut can escape through the patent duct to the exterior;

(c) retention of a patent **urachus** (median umbilical ligament) will allow the escape of urine to the exterior through the region of the umbilicus.

The testis descends through the inguinal region which is a part of the anterior abdominal wall. Thus, the abdominal wall provides the coverings for the testis and spermatic cord. Owing to the descent of the testis, the inguinal region is made weak. The site of weakness is at the region of the deep and superficial inguinal rings. These sites are usually well protected. For example, the area behind the superficial inguinal ring is reinforced by the conjoint tendon. The deep inguinal ring is protected anteriorly by the shutter action of the lower fibres of the internal oblique muscle. There are other mechanisms which also operate to provide strength to the region of the deep inguinal ring. These must also be studied.

The essential similarity of the external genitalia in the two sexes is readily comprehended if their development is briefly reviewed. Mesenchymal cells of the primitive streak region migrate around the **cloacal membrane** to form a pair of elevated folds. These **cloacal folds**, one on either side of the midline, unite anteriorly to form the **genital tubercle**. Further growth separates the cloacal folds into anteriorly placed **urethral folds** and posterior **anal folds**. Subsequently, a pair of **genital swellings** appear lateral to these urethral folds. *In the male*, these swellings enlarge and grow towards each other to fuse in the midline and give rise to the scrotum. At the same time the genital tubercle rapidly undergoes lengthening giving rise to the penis. This lengthening causes the urethral folds to keep pace and form a **urethral groove** the lips of which subsequently fuse to form the spongy urethra. *In the female*, the genital tubercle is a smaller structure and constitutes the clitoris which is a miniature penis. The genital swellings remain separate as the labia majora while the urethral folds also do not fuse and give rise to the more medially and deeply placed labia minora.

Objectives for Dissection Schedule 16

Topic: Anterior abdominal wall

General objective

Comprehend the arrangement of the structures in the region.

Specific objectives

1. Define the nine regions of the abdomen.
2. Define the attachments of the external oblique, internal oblique, transversus and rectus abdominis muscles.
3. Analyse the actions of these muscles both alone and in combination.
4. Illustrate the constitution of the rectus sheath just above the level of: (a) the symphysis pubis; (b) umbilicus; and (c) the costal margin.
5. Enumerate the contents of the rectus sheath.
6. Indicate the significance of the anastomoses between superior and inferior epigastric arteries and veins.
7. Illustrate the dermatomic pattern of the anterior abdominal wall.

Topic: Inguinal canal

General objective

Comprehend the clinical importance of the arrangement of the structures in the region.

Specific objectives

1. Orientate the pelvic girdle and show the correct disposition of the inguinal and lacunar ligaments in the anatomical position.
2. Indicate the surface marking of the superficial and deep inguinal rings.
3. Describe the length and direction of the inguinal canal.
4. Describe the walls, roof and floor of the canal.
5. Describe the contents of the canal in both sexes.

6. Discuss the protective mechanisms of the canal.
7. Analyse the methods of differentiating indirect from direct inguinal hernias.

Topic: External genitalia

General objective

Comprehend the arrangement of the external genitalia in both sexes.

Specific objectives

1. Describe the development of the gonads and the descent of the testis.
2. Describe the manner of the formation of the coverings of the testis, including the tunica vaginalis.
3. Illustrate the transverse sections of the testis and penis.
4. Describe the blood supply and lymphatic drainage of the testis.
5. Describe the different parts of the epididymis and the origin and course of the ductus deferens.
6. Describe the male external genitalia.
7. Describe the female external genitalia.

Overview of Schedule 17

Before you begin dissection note:

ABDOMINAL CAVITY, STOMACH AND INTESTINES

Peritoneum:

parietal; visceral; greater sac; omental bursa; omental foramen; median umbilical fold; medial umbilical fold; falciform ligament; left triangular ligament; lesser omentum; greater omentum; gastrosplenic ligament; lienorenal ligament; mesentery; mesoappendix; transverse mesocolon.

Viscera:

liver	— lower margin; fissure for the ligamentum teres; fissure for the ligamentum venosum; porta hepatis; caudate lobe;
gall bladder	— fundus;
stomach	— fundus; body; pyloric part; greater and lesser curvatures; incisura angularis; sulcus intermedius; stomach bed; interior of the stomach; arterial supply; venous drainage; lymphatic drainage; nerve supply;
jejunum and ileum	— extent; differences; arterial supply; venous drainage; lymphatic drainage; nerve supply;
appendix	— position; arterial supply;
caecum	— posterior relations;
colon	— ascending; transverse; descending; sigmoid; arterial supply; venous drainage; lymphatic drainage; nerve supply.

Portal vein:

formation; location, hepatoportal-systemic anastomoses.

Surface anatomy:

fundus of gall bladder; cardiac and pyloric orifices of the stomach; caecum and appendix.

Clinical anatomy:

referred pain over the umbilical region and pain over the right iliac fossa in appendicitis.

Dissection Schedule 17

ABDOMINAL CAVITY , STOMACH AND INTESTINES

1. *Open the abdomen by means of the following cruciate incision:*
   (a) *a vertical incision through the linea alba (keeping to the left of the midline and the umbilicus), from the xiphoid process above to the pubic symphysis below;*
   (b) *a transverse incision just below the level of the umbilicus, extending on either side to the posterior axillary line.*

   Reflect the four triangular flaps.

2. *Examine the inner aspect of the* **peritoneum**. This consists of a **parietal layer** which lines the walls of the abdominal cavity and a **visceral layer** which covers the abdominal organs to a variable extent. A film of fluid between these two layers facilitates the movement of the organs. The potential space between the two layers is called the **peritoneal cavity**.

   The part of the peritoneal cavity seen now is the **greater sac**. There is a small pocket of the peritoneal cavity which is called the **omental bursa**. This will be seen later.

3. *Identify the peritoneal folds running from the umbilicus. Observe* the sagittal sickle-shaped fold of peritoneum passing from the umbilicus along the anterior abdominal wall towards the liver. This is the **falciform ligament**. *Palpate* its inferior margin and *identify* the cord-like **ligamentum teres** contained within it. This is the remnant of the **left umbilical vein** of the fetus. Running downwards in the midline from the umbilicus to the apex of the urinary bladder is the **median umbilical fold**, raised by the remnant of the **urachus**. On either side of this fold, identify the **medial umbilical folds** which run downwards and laterally to the pelvic brim. These folds contain the obliterated umbilical arteries. Further laterally note the **lateral umbilical folds** raised by the inferior epigastric arteries.

4. *Now study the abdominal viscera in situ. Examine the* **liver** which occupies the right hypochondrium and epigastrium up to the left lateral line. Its lower edge *does not normally project* below the right costal margin. The **fundus of the gall bladder** is at the level of the right ninth costal cartilage in the transpyloric plane.

5. *Identify* the **stomach** occupying the left hypochondrium and epigastrium. Observe that the fold of the peritoneum extending downwards from the **greater curvature of the stomach** is the **greater omentum** and that which extends upwards from the **lesser curvature** to the visceral surface of the liver is the **lesser omentum**. *Pass your hand upwards* along the greater curvature and *feel* the **fundus of the stomach** which lies below the left dome of the diaphragm. *Now palpate* the **spleen** which lies to the left of the fundus in the left hypochondrium. *Palpate* the thickened part of the stomach which lies close to the right margins of the greater and lesser omenta. This is the **pyloric sphincter**. Distal to this is the **duodenum** most of which lies behind the peritoneum against the posterior abdominal wall. *Verify* that the duodenum continues into the **jejunum** and the latter into the **ileum**. The duodenum, jejunum and ileum together form the **small intestine**. Note that the ileum enters the medial side of the **caecum**.

6. The caecum which is situated in the **right iliac fossa** is the blind commencement of the **large intestine** below the **ileocaecal junction.** *Identify* the **vermiform appendix** which is a worm-like prolongation from the medial side of the caecum. *Observe* that the **ascending colon** extends upwards from the upper end of the caecum as far as the **right colic flexure** situated just below the liver where the **transverse colon** begins. The transverse colon ends at the **left colic flexure** opposite the spleen. From here the large intestine continues downwards into the **descending colon**. The descending colon continues into the **sigmoid colon** below the pelvic brim. The next part is the **rectum** which begins at the level of the third sacral vertebra where the sigmoid colon ends.

7. *Now identify the following features of the* **stomach**:
   (a) note that its **fundus** lies above the level of the **cardiac orifice** (where the **oesophagus** enters) and fits into the curvature of the left dome of the diaphragm; this is succeeded by the **body of the stomach**;
   (b) *identify* a notch on the lesser curvature called the **angular notch**. The pyloric part is distal to this notch. The pyloric part is subdivided into the **pyloric antrum** and **pyloric canal** by an indistinct indentation on the greater curvature.

8. *Examine* the **greater omentum** which is attached to the greater curvature. The greater omentum has four layers of peritoneum. The anterior two

layers pass down from the greater curvature of the stomach, recurve and travel upwards to become the posterior two layers. In the fetus, the posterior two layers lie in front of the **transverse mesocolon** as two distinct layers, but fuse subsequently with the transverse mesocolon. Thus, in the adult, the posterior two layers of the greater omentum and the transverse mesocolon *appear* to be continuous. *Verify this.*

9. *Next remove the left lobe of the liver* in order to study the attachments of the lesser omentum and the **abdominal part of the oesophagus**. *Pass your hand to the left of the falciform ligament over the superior surface of the liver and observe that it is reflected on to the diaphragm as the* **left triangular ligament**. *Divide this ligament and remove the left lobe of the liver by cutting through it to the left of the falciform ligament and to the left of the attachment of the lesser omentum. Preserve this part of the liver for later study. Now follow* the lower attachment of the lesser omentum to the abdominal oesophagus, the lesser curvature of the stomach and the first 2–3 cm of the duodenum. Superiorly, note its attachment to the lips of the **porta hepatis** in front and to the **fissure for the ligamentum venosum** and diaphragm behind. *Observe* that the two layers of the lesser omentum become continuous with each other at the right margin of the porta hepatis.

10. *Now examine the right free border of the lesser omentum* which descends from the porta hepatis. *Pass your finger behind this free border where it will enter the* **omental foramen**. This foramen leads into a pocket of the peritoneal cavity known as the **omental bursa**.

    Study the boundaries of the omental foramen. These are: *anteriorly*, the free border of the lesser omentum containing within its layers the **bile duct** in front and to the right, the **hepatic artery** in front and to the left, and the **portal vein** behind; *posteriorly*, the peritoneum covering the **inferior vena cave**; *superiorly*, the **caudate process of the caudate lobe of the liver**; and *inferiorly*, the first part of the duodenum.

    Note that from above downwards the omental bursa lies behind: (a) the caudate lobe of the liver; (b) the lesser omentum; (c) the stomach; (d) the two anterior layers of the greater omentum. *Incise the anterior two layers of the greater omentum about 4 cm below the greater curvature and explore the inside and the extent of the omental bursa. Pass your hand to the left of that portion of the omental bursa lying behind the fundus of the stomach. Your fingers will now encounter the spleen.*

Pass your hand to the left of the fundus and feel the **gastrosplenic ligament** which is a fold of peritoneum that extends from the fundus of the stomach to the **hilum of the spleen**. *Now pass your hand round the* **diaphragmatic surface of the spleen** *to palpate the* **lienorenal ligament** extending from the hilum of the spleen to the left **kidney** which lies against the posterior abdominal wall.

11. *Peel off the anterior layer of the lesser omentum and clean the* **right** *and* **left gastric arteries** lying close to the lesser curvature. *Similarly dissect the* **right** and **left gastroepiploic arteries** lying within the greater omentum a little away from the greater curvature. *Trace the right gastric artery to its origin from the* **common hepatic artery**. *Now clean the* hepatic artery, bile duct and the portal vein in the free margin of the lesser omentum up to the porta hepatis. Observe the presence of lymph nodes around the upper end of the bile duct. *Trace the common hepatic artery downwards towards the upper border of the first part of the duodenum* where it gives off the **gastroduodenal artery** which is retroduodenal. The artery divides into the right gastroepiploic and **superior pancreaticoduodenal arteries**.

12. *Now divide the stomach immediately to the right of the pylorus. Divide the right gastric and the right gastroepiploic vessels and turn the stomach upwards and to the left* to expose the peritoneum on the posterior abdominal wall. *Identify* the **coeliac trunk** arising from the **abdominal aorta** opposite the twelfth thoracic vertebra just above the level of the upper border of the **pancreas**.

    Clean and examine the three branches of the coeliac trunk: (a) **common hepatic**; (b) the **left gastric artery** which courses upwards towards the cardiac orifice where it arches forward to enter the lesser omentum; *identify* its oesophageal branches; and (c) the **splenic artery** as it pursues a tortuous course to the left along the upper border of the pancreas. *Trace this artery* across the front of the left kidney and into the lienorenal ligament. *Identify* its **short gastric** and left gastroepiploic branches, both of which travel in the gastrosplenic ligament to reach the stomach.

    Note that the *common hepatic artery* becomes the *hepatic artery* after giving off the gastrodudenal artery.

13. Note that the **right** and **left gastric veins** enter the portal vein directly. The right **gastroepiploic vein** enters the **superior mesenteric vein** while the left drains into the **splenic vein**.

14. *Observe* the presence of lymph nodes along the course of the main vessels supplying the stomach. Especially important are the **hepatic, subpyloric** and **pancreaticosplenic nodes**.

15. *Carefully strip off the peritoneum from the oesophagus and the anterior and posterior surfaces of the cardiac end of the stomach to examine the* **anterior** *and* **posterior vagal trunks** supplying the stomach. These nerves can be identified by gentle traction on the vagal trunks from the thoracic side of the diaphragm. Note that the *anterior vagal trunk supplies* the anterior surface of the stomach and that its **hepatic branch** runs upwards in the lesser omentum to supply the liver after which it descends again to supply the first part of the duodenum and the pylorus. The *posterior vagal trunk supplies* the posterior surface of the stomach. It also gives off the **coeliac branch** to the **coeliac plexus** of nerves situated over the front and sides of the upper part of the aorta and the coeliac trunk.

16. *Next remove the stomach by cutting across its cardiac end. Examine the posterior relations of the stomach,* i.e. the 'stomach bed'. These are: the diaphragm, left suprarenal gland, spleen, upper part of the left kidney, pancreas and the transverse colon and its mesocolon. *Now open the stomach lengthwise and examine its interior.* Note that its mucous membrane is thrown into folds. *Examine the musculature of the stomach* and note that it has an **outer longitudinal**, a **middle circular** and an **inner oblique layer**.

The Small Intestine

17. The **small intestine**, without the duodenum, is approximately 6 m long. Its upper two-fifths is **jejunum** and its lower three-fifths is **ileum**. The small intestine occupies a central position in the abdominal cavity, below the liver and the stomach, and behind the transverse mesocolon, the transverse colon and the greater omentum. The lowest coils of the intestine lie in the pelvic cavity.

Lift up the coils of the small intestine and examine the attachment of the **mesentery** *to the posterior abdominal wall.* This is the **root of the mesentery** which extends obliquely downwards from the **duodenojejunal flexure** to the **ileocaecal junction** a length of about 15 cm. Within its layers, the mesentery contains the superior mesenteric vessels, nerves and lymphatics of the small intestine, as well as lymph nodes. *Strip off a layer of mesentery and clean the* **jejunal** *and* **ileal branches** arising from the convex side of the **superior mesenteric artery**. *Observe* that these branches subdivide repeatedly to form arterial arcades before sinking into the wall of the gut. These arcades are fewer in the jejunum. Note that the mesentery of the jejunum also contains less fat, hence when the jejunal mesentery is viewed against the light, 'windows' can be seen. The ileum has a longer mesentery and contains more arterial arcades. These probably contribute to its greater mobility.

18. *See if there is a small diverticulum* known as (Meckel's) **diverticulum ilei** arising from the antimesenteric border of the wall of the ileum about 1 m proximal to the ileocaecal junction. It represents the stump of the **vitellointestinal** duct of the fetus.

19. Note that the veins of the small intestines drain into the **superior mesenteric vein**. This vein joins the splenic vein to form the portal vein behind the **neck of the pancreas**. The root of the mesentery is studded with small lymph nodes into which drain the lymph channels running along with the vessels in the mesentery. The efferents from these lymph nodes at the root of the mesentery unite to form the **intestinal lymph trunk** which will ultimately enter a lymph sac called the **cisterna chyli** which is situated in front of the upper two lumbar vertebral bodies. This will be seen later.

20. *Re-examine the jejunal and ileal branches of the superior mesenteric artery, and trace them to their origin.*

21. *Next cut the small intestine at the duodenjejunal flexure and again 10 cm proximal to the ileocaecal junction. Remove the intestine by cutting through the mesentery near the gut. Now cut two 20-cm segments, one from the jejunum and another from the ileum.*

Note that the wall of the jejunum is *palpably thicker*. It is also possible to *feel* the folds of the mucosa.

Next open the two intestinal segments longitudinally with a pair of scissors and wash them. Confirm the presence of the folds of the mucosa called **circular folds**. These folds help to increase the secreting and absorbing surface of the small intestine, and are more prominent in the jejunum. *Observe* that the **intestinal villi** are larger and also more numerous in the jejunum, probably to increase the absorbing surface. In the wall of the ileum note the presence of small solitary lymph nodules as well as large pale oval aggregations of lymphoid tissue called **aggregated lymphatic follicles** (Peyer's patches) along the antimesenteric border.

The Large Intestine

22. Note that the **large intestine** is about 1.5 m long. *Observe* that it is widest at its commencement, the caecum, and becomes progressively narrower towards the anal canal. The component parts are the **caecum, vermiform appendix, ascending colon, transverse colon, descending colon, sigmoid colon, rectum** and **anal canal**. *Identify the following features of the large intestine*: (a) **teniae coli** which consist of three thick bands of longitudinal musculature; (b) **haustrations** or sacculations; (c) **appendices epiploicae** which are small masses of fat enclosed in peritoneum. These features are absent in the appendix and rectum.

23. *Examine the caecum* and note that it is broader than long. *Exert traction* on the caecum and note its mobility due to its complete peritoneal covering. *Observe* the structures on which it lies. These are the **iliopsoas muscles,** the **femoral nerve,** the **lateral femoral cutaneous nerve** and the **external iliac artery**. *Cut through the anterior wall of the caecum and clean its interior to examine the* **ileocaecal orifice**. Note the upper and lower folds of the valve as they protrude into the caecum. The surrounding muscle is thickened around it to form a sphincter. *Next identify the orifice of the vermiform appendix* about 2 cm below the ileocaecal orifice. The appendix is very variable in its position but its opening into the caecum is relatively constant. *Now trace the* **anterior tenia coli** *and see how it leads towards the root of the appendix.* What is the position of the appendix in your cadaver? Usually it is *retrocaecal* or *retrocolic*. *Observe* that the appendix

has its own mesentery by which it is connected to the terminal ileum. This is the **mesoappendix** along which the **appendicular artery** runs.

24. *Now study the relations of the ascending colon.* It is covered with peritoneum on its front and sides. Note the **right paracolic gutter** situated between it and the flank. This gutter can be traced upward over the kidney and behind the right lobe of the liver. *Strip the peritoneum off and observe* that the ascending colon lies on the **iliacus, quadratus lumborum** and **transversus abdominis muscles** separated by the **ilioinguinal** and **iliohypogastric nerves** and the **lumbar arteries**. Note that it also lies *across* the lower part of the right kidney. Its anterior relations are coils of the small intestine and part of the greater omentum.

25. *Trace the transverse colon* as it runs across the upper abdomen from right to left from the **right colic** to the **left colic flexure**. *Observe* its well defined mesentery, the transverse mesocolon, which makes it mobile and hence variable in its position. Note that the proximal end of the transverse mesocolon lies on the duodenum and the head of the pancreas while the distal end lies in front of the left kidney. *Observe* that the major part of the transverse mesocolon is attached to the **body of the pancreas** in a horizontal line lying approximately in the transpyloric plane. *Verify* that the left colic flexure lies opposite the ninth and tenth ribs while the right colic flexure is on a lower level at the tenth and eleventh ribs.

26. *Trace the descending colon down to the pelvic brim* where it becomes the sigmoid colon. *Observe* that its posterior relations are similar to those of the caecum and ascending colon.

27. *Observe* that the sigmoid colon first passes from the left pelvic brim backwards towards the right side of the pelvis and finally turns towards the left to reach the midline where it continues as the rectum. It has a **sigmoid mesocolon** whose attachment forms an inverted "V" with the apex of the "V" lying opposite the bifurcation of the **left common iliac artery** which is here crossed by the **left ureter**. *Verify this.*

28. *Remove the remainder of the peritoneum from the posterior abdominal wall from the level of the pancreas downwards and trace and clean the branches of the superior and inferior mesenteric arteries.*

29. Turn first to the **superior mesenteric artery**. *Identify its origin from the aorta* just below the origin of the coeliac trunk and note how it first passes behind the pancreas and then crosses the **uncinate process of the pancreas** and the third part of the duodenum. You have already seen its jejunal and ileal branches. *Now trace the distribution of its remaining branches*:
    (a) the **middle colic artery** arises at the lower border of the pancreas and enters the transverse mesocolon immediately to supply the proximal two-thirds of the transverse colon. This artery anastomoses with the branches of the **left colic artery** which is a branch of the **inferior mesenteric artery**;
    (b) the **inferior pancreaticoduodenal artery** is a small branch which is given off before the superior mesenteric artery reaches the duodenum. This artery passes to the right between the head of the pancreas and the third part of the duodenum to anastomose with the **superior pancreaticoduodenal artery** which is a branch of the **gastroduodenal artery**; the inferior pancreaticoduodenal artery supplies the pancreas and the duodenum distal to the opening of the bile duct;
    (c) the **right colic artery** runs retroperitoneally across the posterior abdominal wall below the duodenum and divides into the ascending and descending branches which supply the ascending colon and right colic flexure; this artery anastomoses with the middle colic superiorly and ileocolic inferiorly;
    (d) the **ileocolic artery** also runs retroperitoneally and divides into descending and ascending branches to supply the terminal part of the ileum, caecum, appendix and a small part of the ascending colon.

30. *Next trace the* **superior mesenteric vein** which lies to the right of the superior mesenteric artery. Its tributaries correspond to the arterial branches. It also receives the **right gastroepiploic vein**. The superior mesenteric vein joins the splenic vein behind the neck of the pancreas to form the portal vein at the level of the first lumbar vertebra.

31. *Now turn to the* **inferior mesenteric artery** which originates from the aorta about 4 cm above its termination. *Clean its origin and trace its branches*:
    (a) the **left colic artery** runs to the left retroperitoneally in front of the ureter and below the duodenum; it divides into ascending and

descending branches which supply the distal part of the transverse colon and the entire descending colon;

(b) the **sigmoid arteries** give branches to the sigmoid colon after having passed through the lateral limb of the sigmoid mesocolon; these arteries anastomose with the descending branch of the superior left colic above and a branch of the superior rectal below;

(c) the **superior rectal artery** is the continuation of the inferior mesenteric artery at the pelvic brim. It will be seen during the dissection of the pelvis.

Note that the branches of the superior and inferior mesenteric arteries radiate towards the wall of the large gut and anastomose in such a way that they form a continuous circumferential vascular channel extending along the mesenteric border from the caecum to the sigmoid colon. This is called the **marginal artery** and is of clinical importance.

32. *Trace the* **inferior mesenteric vein** which lies to the left of the inferior mesenteric artery. Its tributaries correspond to the arterial branches. The inferior mesenteric vein ascends medial to the left ureter to enter the splenic vein lying behind the pancreas.

33. The lymphatics of the colon follow the vessels and end in the lymph nodes distributed along the course of the vessels. Nearer to the gut are the **colic nodes** and more distal to the gut are **paracolic nodes** from which the lymph is returned to the nodes lying at the root of the mesentery (**preaortic lymph nodes**) before finally passing into the **intestinal lymph trunk**. *Try to identify the preaortic nodes.*

34. Note that the arteries are accompanied by **autonomic nerves** from the **superior** and **inferior mesenteric plexuses**. These plexuses should be noted in relation to the origins of these vessels from the abdominal aorta.

35. *Next carefully remove the large intestine from the caecum downwards to the junction of the descending and sigmoid colon at the pelvic brim. Free the ascending colon from the posterior abdominal wall, cut through the transverse mesocolon close to the colon, free the descending colon from its posterior relations and cut through the colon at the junction of the*

descending and sigmoid colon at the level of the brim of the pelvis. Now remove the freed colon from the abdominal cavity.

Summary

An understanding of the disposition of the peritoneal reflections often presents considerable difficulty to the student. However, this can be overcome if the student comprehends that the gut is suspended by a **dorsal mesentery** along its entire length while the **ventral mesentery** exists only for the stomach and proximal duodenum. Into the ventral mesentery grows the liver. Consequently, the lesser omentum, the coronary and triangular ligaments as well as the falciform ligament are derivatives of the ventral mesentery. Thus, the ventral mesentery passes from the abdominal oesophagus, stomach and proximal duodenum to the diaphragm (in front of the oesophageal orifice), the liver and anterior abdominal wall.

The dorsal mesentery is altered from its embryonic condition so that parts of the gut retain this mesentery while others lose it altogether. For example, the duodenum (except the proximal 2 cm), and the ascending and descending colon lose their mesenteries altogether while the stomach, jejunum, ileum, transverse and sigmoid colon retain their mesenteries. As the omental bursa develops within the mesentery of the stomach, i.e. within the dorsal mesogastrium, the latter enlarges and comes into relationship with the transverse mesocolon with which it later fuses. Moreover, the attachments of the dorsal mesogastrium to the *midline* posterior abdominal wall gets altered with the development of the omental bursa. As a result, the dorsal mesogastrium in the adult is attached the diaphragm, kidney and pancreas. Thus, in the adult these attachments are represented by the gastrosplenic, lienorenal and greater omental folds of peritoneum.

Since the midgut loop in the embryo lies within the umbilical cord and undergoes rotation during its return, malrotation of the gut or even an arrest of withdrawal of the gut into the abdomen may take place.

The position of the appendix is described as being extremely variable. This is entirely due to differential growth rates of the walls of the caecum which makes the appendix occupy different positions depending on which wall of the caecum grows faster and which part grows slower.

The arterial supply of the gut is based on its development. The gut is divisible into fore-, mid- and hindgut and each of these portions has a blood supply of its own. Thus, the foregut is supplied by the *coeliac trunk*. The abdominal part of the foregut includes the lower end of the oesophagus, stomach and proximal duodenum up to the entry of the bile duct. In addition, the liver and part of the pancreas which are outgrowths from the foregut region also receive their blood supply via branches of the coeliac trunk. Furthermore, the spleen which develops inside the dorsal mesogastrium is also supplied by the coeliac trunk. The midgut, which is supplied by the *superior mesenteric artery*, extends from the site of the opening of the bile duct into the duodenum to the junction of the proximal two-thirds and the distal third of the transverse colon. Distal to this is the hindgut which is supplied by the *inferior mesenteric artery*.

Objectives For Dissection Schedule 17

Topic: Abdominal viscera and peritoneum

General objective

Comprehend the basic anatomy of the abdominal viscera and their peritoneal relationships.

Specific Objectives

1. Indicate the positions of the stomach, liver, spleen, small intestine, caecum and appendix.
2. Explain the development of the greater sac and omental bursa of the peritoneum and their disposition in the adult.
3. Illustrate the subdivisions, borders, surfaces and gross features of the stomach.
4. Describe the posterior relations of the stomach.
5. Describe the peritoneal relations of the stomach with special reference to the omenta, the gastrophrenic, gastrosplenic and lienorenal ligaments.
6. Describe the blood supply, nerve supply and lymphatic drainage of the stomach.
7. Indicate the subdivisions of the small and large intestines.
8. Explain the macroscopic differences between:
   (a) the jejunum and ileum; and
   (b) the small and large intestines.
9. Describe the distribution of the coeliac, superior, and inferior mesenteric arteries.
10. Describe the portal vein and its main tributaries; where do the major hepatoportal-systemic anastomoses occur?
11. Indicate the clinical importance of:
    (a) the paracolic gutter;
    (b) positions of the appendix;
    (c) the diverticulum ilei;

(d) the length of the sigmoid mesocolon and volvulus; and
(e) portal obstruction.

12. Interpret radiographs of:
    (a) plain films of the abdomen; and
    (b) the abdomen after a barium meal and after an enema.
13. Interpret an ultrasound of the abdomen.

Overview of Schedule 18

Before you begin dissection note:

LIVER, PANCREAS, DUODENUM AND SPLEEN

Liver:

surfaces and margins; lobes; relations; structures passing through the porta hepatis; bare area; common hepatic duct.

Gall bladder:

subdivisions; relations; arterial supply.

Pancreas:

subdivisions; relations; arterial supply; venous drainage; openings of the pancreatic ducts.

Duodenum:

subdivisions; relations; arterial supply; venous drainage; lymphatic drainage; opening of the bile duct and pancreatic duct.

Spleen:

position; relations.

Portal vein:

formation and its tributaries; hepatoportal-systemic anastomoses.

Surface anatomy:

liver; gall bladder; bile duct; duodenum; spleen.

Clinical anatomy:

portal obstruction; biliary colic.

Dissection schedule 18

LIVER, PANCREAS, DUODENUM AND SPLEEN

1. *Replace the cut portion of the left lobe of the liver in order to study the organ in situ. Observe* the pyramidal shape of the hardened liver. *Verify once again* that it occupies the right hypochondriac and epigastric regions. Note that it has a **diaphragmatic surface** composed of *right, anterior, superior* and *posterior surfaces* and a **visceral surface**. *Observe* that all surfaces except the visceral are related to the diaphragm, which separates the liver from the pleura and lungs. *Study the surface marking of the liver.*
2. *Trace the* **hepatic artery** *into the* **porta hepatis** and note its **right** and **left branches**. *Identify the* **cystic artery** which is given off by the right branch to supply the **gall bladder**. *Turn your attention* to the triangular interval outlined by the **common hepatic duct** on the left, the **cystic duct** on the right and the liver above. This area is of clinical importance. *Trace the* **bile duct** *and observe its formation by the union of the cystic duct with the common hepatic duct.* Note that the common hepatic duct is formed by the union of the **right** and **left hepatic ducts**. *Trace* the **portal vein** to the porta hepatis and note its division into **right** and **left portal branches**.
3. *Now trace the falciform ligament* and note that its two layers diverge. The left layer covers the left surface of the liver and is reflected on to the inferior aspect of the diaphragm as the **left triangular ligament**. *Next follow the right layer* which similarly continues as the **coronary** and **right triangular ligaments** before passing on to the diaphragm. *Divide all these ligaments.*
4. *Divide the structures passing through the porta hepatis as close to the liver as possible. Strip off the peritoneum on the posterior abdominal wall* immediately behind these structures to reveal the **inferior vena cava**. *Follow the inferior vena cava upwards* and note that it lies in a deep groove on the posterior aspect of the liver. *Divide the inferior vena cava above and below the level of the liver avoiding damage to the diaphragm. The liver is now free to be removed for study. Examine its surfaces.*
5. *Observe the features of the posterior surface of the liver which is triangular in shape.* These are from left to right:

(a) a groove or impression for the abdominal part of the oesophagus;
(b) the **ligamentum venosum** lying in a fissure;
(c) the **caudate lobe**;
(d) the inferior vena cava lying in a deep groove and receiving the three main **hepatic veins**; and
(e) the rough triangular surface lying between the **superior** and **inferior layers of the coronary ligament**. This is called the **bare area** as it is not covered by peritoneum. *Observe* the continuity of the left layer of the falciform ligament with the left triangular and the right layer with the coronary ligament.

6. *Now examine the visceral impressions on the inferior surface produced by*:
   (a) the fundus and body of the stomach;
   (b) the pylorus;
   (c) the duodenum;
   (d) the gall bladder;
   (e) the right flexure of the colon;
   (f) the upper part of the right kidney; and
   (g) the right suprarenal gland.

7. Note that the falciform ligament in front and the **fissures for the ligamentum teres** and **venosum** on the inferior and posterior aspects divide the liver into anatomical **left** and **right lobes**. The surgical subdivision, however, is defined by the **fossa for the gall bladder** and the groove for the inferior vena cava. To the left of the fossa, note the **quadrate lobe** in front of the porta hepatis and the caudate lobe behind the porta. *Review the position of structures within the porta hepatis and the attachment of the lesser omentum* to the lips of the porta and to the fissure for the ligamentum venosum.

8. *Examine the gall bladder* and note its blind end, the **fundus**, which projects beyond the inferior margin of the liver. This continues into the **body** which narrows to form a **neck** leading into the **cystic duct.** The cystic duct joins the common hepatic duct to form the bile duct.

9. *Now examine the* **spleen**. Note that it has a **diaphragmatic surface** related to the ninth, tenth and eleventh ribs and a **visceral surface** related to the

stomach, kidney, left flexure of the colon and pancreas. Note the impressions made by these viscera. *Observe* that the **superior border** of the spleen presents characteristic notches.

10. *Next clean and examine the duodenum and pancreas*. The **duodenum** is divided into four parts for convenience of description. *Trace* the first, the **superior part**, which passes upwards, backwards and to the right towards the neck of the gall bladder. Note that the bile duct, portal vein, gastroduodenal artery, with the inferior vena cava still further back are the posterior relations of this part. *Follow* the second, the **vertical part**, as it descends over the medial part of the kidney, being itself overlapped by the head of the pancreas.

    Trace the *third*, the **horizontal part**, as it passes from right to left and note that it crosses the right ureter, right gonadal vessels, inferior vena cava, aorta and right psoas major muscle. *Observe* the *fourth*, the **ascending part**, as it ascends closely applied to the left side of the aorta to terminate in the **duodenojejunal flexure** 2–3cm to the left of the midline at the level of the second lumbar vertebra. Note that a fibromuscular band fixes this flexure to the posterior abdominal wall and also attaches it to the right crus of the diaphragm.

11. *Now study the* **pancreas** which can be divided into a **head** (occupying the "C" of the duodenum), a **neck**, a **body** and a **tail** ending at the **hilus of the spleen**. Behind the neck lies the **portal vein** formed by the union of the **superior mesenteric** and **splenic veins**. A small tongue-like extension of the pancreas called the **uncinate process** lies behind the superior mesenteric vessels. Note that the body is placed behind the omental bursa and has **anterior**, **inferior** and **posterior surfaces** as it is triangular in section. The demarcating margin between the anterior and inferior surfaces is a raised edge, where the fused greater omentum and transverse mesocolon are attached. *Next study the posterior relations of the gland*: the head is related to the inferior vena cava, right renal vein and bile duct; the neck to the portal vein; and the body to the left renal vessels and left kidney. The tail lies in the lienorenal ligament and is related to the splenic hilus. Note that the splenic artery pursues a tortuous course along the upper margin of the gland.

12. *Clean the bile duct downwards to its opening into the duodenum.* Note that its upper or *supraduodenal part* runs in the free border of the lesser omentum. The second or *retroduodenal part* descends behind the first part of the duodenum to the right of the gastroduodenal artery with the portal vein behind while the inferior vena cava is situated still further posteriorly. The third or *pancreatic part* passes downwards and to the right lying in a groove on the posterior surface of the head of the pancreas, sometimes completely embedded in it. The inferior vena cava will be found to be a direct posterior relation of this part of the bile duct.

13. *Remove the pancreatic tissue piecemeal and identify the main* **pancreatic duct** which runs along the length of the gland to join the bile duct and form the **hepatopancreatic ampulla**. *Make a vertical cut in the anterior wall of the second part of the duodenum and examine its interior. Look for an elevation* on the posterior wall called the **greater duodenal papilla**, at the summit of which is the opening of the hepatopancreatic ampulla. *See if there is an opening of the* **accessory pancreatic duct** about 2 cm above the level of the papilla. *Dissect the terminal ends of the bile and pancreatic ducts and observe* the thickening of circular muscle around their ends forming their sphincters.

14. *Now clean the portal vein* formed by the union of the splenic and superior mesenteric veins. *Review* the main tributaries of the portal vein.

15. *Review the course of the inferior mesenteric vein* as it ascends lateral to the inferior mesenteric artery behind the peritoneum and in front of the left psoas major muscle. *Observe* how it crosses the gonadal and renal vessels and passes behind the duodenojujunal flexure to enter the splenic vein which lies behind the pancreas and below the splenic artery.

Summary

Variations in the origin of the hepatic arteries are of considerable importance in surgery and so are the variations in the origin and course of the cystic artery and bile duct. The *gall bladder* is often the site of formation of gall stones, and pain due to gall bladder inflammation is felt in the part of the abdomen overlying its fundus. This is situated at the transpyloric plane where this plane cuts the lateral margin of the right rectus abdominis. Biliary calculi can occur not only in the gall bladder but also along the bile duct where stones coming down from the gall bladder can be impacted. This causes an obstruction to the flow of bile into the duodenum with resultant jaundice.

The *portal vein*, which receives blood from the gut, spleen, pancreas and gall bladder, breaks up into capillaries in the liver which finally drain into the hepatic veins. This circulation is referred to as the **hepatoportal system**. There can be an obstruction to the portal circulation resulting in portal hypertension. Such a condition leads to the formation of dilated veins in the lower oesophagus and lower end of the rectum where there are communications between portal and systemic veins. Oesophageal varices can rupture and give rise to severe haematemesis whereas obstruction at the region of the rectum results in the formation of haemorrhoids. Another site of such portosystemic communication is in the region of the umbilicus where veins around the umbilicus get enlarged in cases of portal obstruction to give rise to the 'caput medusae'.

The *splenic artery* reaches the spleen through the lienorenal ligament. In this ligament lies also the tail of the pancreas. This fact has to be borne in mind during ligature of the splenic artery prior to removal of the spleen. Any damage to the tail of the pancreas results in the escape of pancreatic secretions into the peritoneal cavity causing acute peritonitis.

Objectives For Dissection Schedule 18

Topic: Liver, pancreas, duodenum and spleen

General objective 1

Comprehend the structures of the liver and biliary apparatus.

Specific objectives

1. Indicate the surfaces, borders, as well as the surgical and anatomical subdivisions of the liver.
2. Surface mark the liver, gall bladder and bile duct.
3. Describe the reflection of the falciform, coronary and triangular ligaments and the lesser omentum.
4. Illustrate the relations of the posterior and visceral surfaces of the liver.
5. Indicate the relations of the three parts of the bile duct.
6. Interpret the cholecystograms and liver angiograms.

General objective 2

Comprehend the basic anatomical features of the duodenum, pancreas, spleen and the portal vein.

Specific objectives

1. Identify the duodenum, its subdivisions, general topography and internal and external features.
2. Describe the relations of the four parts of the duodenum in turn.
3. Identify the subdivisions, surfaces and borders of the pancreas.
4. Describe the relations of the different parts of the pancreas.
5. Describe the duct system of the pancreas and its development.
6. Indicate surfaces, borders, notches and surface marking of the spleen.
7. Describe the relations of the diaphragmatic and visceral surfaces of the spleen.

8. Illustrate the tributaries, mode of formation and termination of the portal vein.

9. Discuss the clinical importance of:
   (a) the sites of hepatoportosystemic anastomoses;
   (b) the relationship of the head of the pancreas to the bile duct;
   (c) the relationship of the lymph nodes in the porta hepatis to the bile duct;
   (d) the sphincter mechanism of the bile and pancreatic ducts.

Overview of Schedule 19

Before you begin dissection note:

KIDNEY, SUPRARENAL AND POSTERIOR ABDOMINAL WALL

Kidney:

coverings; relations; arterial supply; venous drainage; hilum.

Ureter:

course; constrictions; arterial supply; nerve supply.

Suprarenal:

relations; arterial supply; venous drainage.

Posterior Abdominal Wall

Muscles:

diaphragm; psoas; quadratus lumborum; transversus abdominis; iliacus.

Nerves:

subcostal; lumbar plexus and branches; sympathetic trunk; coeliac, renal, superior mesenteric, intermesenteric, inferior mesenteric, and hypogastric plexuses.

Arteries:

aorta and branches.

Veins:

subcostal; inferior vena cava and tributaries; azygos.

Lymphatics:

cisterna chyli; right and left lumbar trunks; intestinal lymph trunk.

Surface anatomy:

kidney; ureter; spleen; aorta; inferior vena cava.

Clinical anatomy:

inferior vena caval obstruction; renal infarction; polycystic kidneys; ureteric colic.

Dissection Schedule 19

KIDNEY, SUPRARENAL AND POSTERIOR ABDOMINAL WALL

1. *Observe the general disposition of the two kidneys* which are placed *retroperitoneally. Study the anterior relations* of the **left kidney** which are the left suprarenal gland, spleen, stomach, pancreas, left colic flexure, the coils of small intestine and the superior left colic vessels. Similarly note that the **right kidney** is related anteriorly to the right suprarenal, the liver, duodenum, right colic flexure and coils of small intestine.

2. *Remove the duodenum, pancreas and spleen together in one block after dividing the branches of the coeliac and superior mesenteric arteries as well as the superior mesenteric, inferior mesenteric and portal veins.*

3. From the thoracic region *trace the* **greater** *and* **lesser splanchnic nerves** into the **coeliac ganglia** and the **least splanchnic nerves** into the **renal ganglia**. Note that the coeliac ganglia lie one on either side of the coeliac trunk while the renal ganglia are found in relation to the origin of the renal arteries from the aorta. *Identify and clean the* **lumbar sympathetic trunks** running in front of the vertebral bodies medial to the psoas major muscle. Observe that the right trunk is overlapped by the inferior vena cava while the left one lies to the left of the abdominal aorta. Each trunk has **four ganglia**. Note that the upper two **lumbar splanchnic nerves** from these ganglia join the **coeliac, renal** and **intermesenteric plexuses**. The intermesenteric plexus is found in front of the aorta in between the origins of the superior and inferior mesenteric arteries. *Next identify the* **superior hypogastric plexus** in front of the bifurcation of the aorta. The plexus is reinforced by lumbar splanchnic nerves from the third and fourth lumbar sympathetic ganglia. The plexus then runs down into the pelvis as the **right** and **left inferior hypogastric plexuses**.

4. *Pull the kidney with its fascia forwards and remove the* **pararenal fatty body** which lies posteriorly on the posterior abdominal wall. *Observe* the **renal fascia** enveloping the kidney. *Remove this fascia and expose the kidney and suprarenal gland.* Note that each **suprarenal gland** caps the corresponding kidney. *Trace the three* **suprarenal arteries — superior, middle** and **inferior** — which supply this gland. These arise respectively

from the **inferior phrenic, aorta** and **renal arteries**. Note that each gland is drained by a single vein; the **right suprarenal vein** drains into the **inferior vena cava** and the **left suprarenal vein** into the **left renal vein**.

5. *Lift each kidney forwards and clean its bed. Observe its posterior relations.* These are in its upper third the **diaphragm** and in its lower two-thirds from medial to lateral the **psoas major, quadratus lumborum** and **transversus abdominis muscles**; and from above downwards the **subcostal, iliohypogastric** and **ilioinguinal** nerves and accompanying blood vessels. *Note that the diaphragm separates the kidneys from the pleura and costodiaphragmatic recess.*

6. *Replace the kidneys and observe* that in the region of each hilum the structures encountered from front to back are the **renal vein, renal artery** and **renal pelvis**. Note that each kidney is supplied by a branch from the abdominal aorta. *Observe* that the *left renal vein crosses in front of the aorta* passing just below the pancreas. Above it lies the superior mesenteric artery.

7. *Make a coronal section of the kidney on one side and examine the* **cortex** *and the* **medulla** *with its* **renal pyramids**. The renal pyramids open into 8–16 **minor calyces** which subsequently enter into the two **major calyces**. The major calyces unite to form the **renal pelvis** which continues downwards as the **ureter**. In some cases, the kidney may be lobulated (**fetal lobulation**) or the two kidneys may be fused across the aorta to give rise to the **horseshoe kidney**.

8. *Now clean the ureter* which is closely adherent to the peritoneum. Note that the ureter commences in the renal pelvis and runs half of its course in the abdomen and the other half in the pelvis. *Observe* that it generally runs in front of the **transverse processes of the lumbar vertebrae**. Note its rich arterial supply. In the abdominal part of its course it receives branches from the renal, gonadal and common iliac arteries. The ureter has *three constrictions*: at the pelvic-ureteric junction, at the pelvic brim and where it enters the bladder.

9. *Study the* **abdominal aorta**. Note that it enters the abdomen by *passing behind the* **median arcuate ligament** which extends between the two crura

of the diaphragm. *Observe* the inclination of the aorta towards the left as it runs downwards to divide into the two **common iliac arteries** opposite the body of L4 vertebra. *Review* the anterior relations of the aorta and the disposition of the autonomic plexuses in relation to it. *Observe* the **preaortic** and **paraaortic (lumbar) lymph nodes** distributed along the length of the aorta.

10. *Next clean and study the branches of the abdominal aorta*:
    (a) *ventral branches* — **coeliac** (T12 vertebra); **superior mesenteric** (L1 vertebra); and **inferior mesenteric** (L3 vertebra). These supply the gastrointestinal tract.
    (b) *lateral branches* — **inferior phrenic, middle suprarenal, renal** and **testicular** or **ovarian**. The inferior phrenic arteries supply the diaphragm as well as the suprarenals. The other vessels supply structures developed from the intermediate mesoderm.
    (c) *dorsal branches* — four **lumbar** and a **median sacral**. These give branches to the body wall.
    (d) *terminal branches* — **right** and **left common iliac**.

11. *Clean* the **inferior vena cava** *and its tributaries. Observe* its formation by the union of the two **common iliac veins** in front of the fifth lumbar vertebra to the right of the midline. *Review its anterior relations*. Its main *posterior relations* are the lumbar vertebrae and psoas major muscle below, the right crus of the diaphragm and the right suprarenal gland above, and the right sympathetic trunk along its length. *Observe* that the right lumbar, renal, suprarenal and inferior phrenic arteries also pass behind it. Its tributaries are the lower **lumbar, renal and inferior phrenic veins** as well as the **right suprarenal** and **right gonadal veins**. Note that the left suprarenal and left gonadal veins join the left renal vein.

12. *Now clean the diaphragm and study it*. Note its origins:
    (a) *vertebral*: by means of *two* **crura** from the front of the lumbar vertebral bodies, the **right crus** from the upper three and the **left crus** from the upper two vertebrae. *Trace the other slips of origin* from the **medial** and **lateral arcuate ligaments**. *Define the attachments* of the medial arcuate ligament from the body of the first lumbar vertebra to its transverse process. *Observe* how it bridges across the psoas muscle.

Similarly study the attachments of the lateral arcuate ligament from the transverse process of the first lumbar vertebra to the twelfth rib. *Observe* how it arches across the quadratus lumborum muscle.

(b) *costal*: by six slips from the lower six costal cartilages. See how these interdigitate with the slips of origin of the transversus abdominis.

(c) *sternal*: by two slender slips from the back of the xiphoid process.

Trace all the fibres as they converge on to the **central tendon**. Work out the actions of the diaphragm and recall that it is innervated by the phrenic nerve. *Now identify the following structures transmitted behind or through the diaphragm*:

(a) the aorta, azygos vein and the thoracic duct pass through the **aortic hiatus** behind the **median arcuate ligament** at the level of T12;

(b) the psoas muscle and the sympathetic trunk behind the medial arcuate ligament;

(c) the quadratus lumborum muscle and the subcostal vessels and nerve behind the lateral arcuate ligament;

(d) the oesophagus, the vagal trunks and the oesophageal branches (or tibutaries) of the left gastric artery (or vein) through the **oesophageal opening** at T10. Note that the fibres of the right crus cross over to the left side to encircle the oesophagus;

(e) the inferior vena cava and **right phrenic nerve** through the **opening for the inferior vena cava** at T8 vertebra;

(f) the superior epigastric artery between the sternal and costal origins of the diaphragm;

(g) the **left phrenic nerve** on the left side.

13. *Review* the subcostal, iliohypogastric and ilioinguinal nerves. *Identify* the **genitofemoral nerve** which will be seen to emerge on the anterior surface of the psoas major muscle at the level of L3 vertebra. *Find the* **femoral nerve** *between the psoas and iliacus muscles and observe the* **obturator nerve** *passing into the pelvis along the medial border of the psoas.*

14. *Now clean and study the attachments of the muscles of the posterior abdominal wall.* These are the **psoas major, iliacus, quadratus lumborum** and occasionally the **psoas minor**.

The *psoas major muscle arises* from: (a) the lower part of the body of T12 and from the bodies of the lumbar vertebrae; (b) the intervertebral discs; (c) fibrous arcades arching over the four lumbar arteries; and (d) the anterior surfaces of the transverse processes of the lumbar vertebrae. The muscle is *inserted* into the lesser trochanter of the femur.

The *iliacus muscle arises* from the iliac fossa of the hip bone and is also *inserted* into the lesser trochanter of the femur.

Both these muscles are supplied by L2, 3, 4 nerves.

The *quadratus lumborum muscle arises* from the iliac crest, iliolumbar ligament, and transverse processes of the lower lumbar vertebrae. It is *inserted* partly into the upper lumbar transverse processes and partly into the medial half of the twelfth rib. This muscle is enclosed between the anterior and middle lamellae of the **thoracolumbar fascia** while the psoas is covered by the **psoas fascia** which continues inferiorly as the **iliac fascia** over the iliacus muscle.

The *psoas minor originates* from the bodies of T12 and L1 vertebrae and its *insertion* is into the **pecten of the pubis**. This muscle is not always present.

15. *Trace the* femoral, genitofemoral, **lateral femoral cutaneous**, and obturator nerves proximally into the substance of the psoas and *expose the* **lumbar plexus** *on one side by removing the psoas piecemeal.* Note the origins of the following nerves:
    (a) the lateral femoral cutaneous nerve from L2, 3;
    (b) the femoral nerve from L2, 3, 4 dorsal divisions; and
    (c) the obturator nerve from L2, 3, 4 ventral divisions.

    Trace the **lumbosacral trunk** formed from the descending branches of L4 and ventral ramus of L5. This trunk descends over the **ala of the sacrum** into the pelvis.

16. *Next follow the common iliac arteries* as they pass laterally towards the **sacroiliac joints** where they divide into the **external** and **internal iliac arteries**. The internal iliac artery descends backwards into the pelvis where it will be followed later. *Trace the external iliac artery* as it lies on the psoas and then as it runs round the **pelvic brim** to pass under the **inguinal ligament** at the **midinguinal point** to become the **femoral artery**. At this

point the **external iliac vein** which is a continuation of the **femoral vein** lies medial to the artery . *Now follow the vein proximally* to the sacroiliac joint where the **internal iliac vein** joins it to form the **common iliac vein.** Note that the left common iliac vein is medial to the corresponding artery, while the right is posterolateral to its artery. The left common iliac vein receives the **median sacral vein**. Note the formation of the **inferior vena cava** by the union of the two common iliac veins opposite L5 vertebra.

17. Having examined the lumbar plexus and the iliac vessels *complete the examination of the posterior abdominal wall by studying the cisterna chyli and azygos vein.*

18. The **cisterna chyli**, a dilated sac about 6 cm long and 6 mm wide, is a reservoir for lymph from the abdomen and lower limbs. *Observe that the cisterna lies between the right crus of the diaphragm and the aorta in front of the vertebral bodies of L1 and L2.* It receives the **intestinal** and **lumbar lymph trunks**. The latter drain the lower limbs, pelvis, kidneys, suprarenals and gonads.

    Observe that the upper end of the cisterna chyli continues as the **thoracic duct** and enters the thorax through the aortic hiatus of the diaphragm.

19. Note that the **azygos vein** arises either from the inferior vena cava or as an upward continuation of the ascending lumbar vein. *Trace it upwards as it leaves the abdomen through the aortic hiatus to the right of the thoracic duct.*

Summary

The *kidneys* and *ureters* are some of the important structures placed against the posterior abdominal wall and you must know their positions. In the living, this can be revealed by injecting an iodine-containing dye intravenously. The dye, which is radio-opaque, is subsequently excreted by the kidney and an X-ray will then reveal the position of the kidneys and ureters. This method of obtaining the outline of the urinary apparatus is known as *intravenous pyelography*. Another method of obtaining the outline of the kidneys and ureters is by injecting the dye via the ureters, i.e. *retrograde pyelography*. In this way, ureteric calculi, dilatation of the pelvis of the ureter (*hydronephrosis*), tumours, as well as anomalies of the kidneys and ureters can be diagnosed.

Each kidney is supplied by a renal artery which divides into an anterior and a posterior branch which then divide into five **segmental arteries**, each of which is an end artery. Since the anastomosis between these segmental arteries is poor, an occlusion of one of the segmental vessels could lead to an infarct, i.e. death of the segment supplied by the corresponding artery. Moreover, the superior and inferior segmental arteries may arise independently and this can give rise to aberrant renal arteries.

The *ureters* which are closely adherent to the peritoneum have three sites of constriction. At these sites a stone (*ureteric calculus*) can get impacted. As the ureter tries to get rid of the calculus by contraction of its musculature there is resultant colic (*renal colic*) in which the pain radiates from the loin towards the groin. This radiation of pain depends on the segmental innervation of the ureter from T10-L2 spinal segments.

The *lumbar sympathetic trunks* provide most of the postganglionic fibres to the lower limb arteries. Consequently, lumbar sympathectomy often provides an improvement in the blood supply to the lower limbs when there is a spasm or narrowing of the lower limb arteries. However, the results may be unsatisfactory if there are intermediate ganglia in relation to the rami communicans of the lumbar nerves. Such ganglia escape when the lumbar sympathetic trunks are removed. As they are able to provide an alternative route of postganglionic fibres to the lower limb, the spasm of the vessels continues to persist.

Objectives for Dissection Schedule 19

Topic: Kidneys, ureters and suprarenal glands

General objective

Comprehend the basic structural features of the kidneys, ureters and suprarenal glands.

Specific objectives

1. Indicate the surfaces, poles, hilum and surface projection of each kidney and enumerate the structures at the hilum from front to back.
2. Describe the fascial and anterior relations of the kidneys and suprarenal glands.
3. Describe the 'bed' of the kidneys.
4. Describe the vascular supply of: (a) the suprarenals, and (b) the kidneys with special reference to vascular segmentation.
5. Illustrate the transverse and coronal sections of the suprarenals and kidneys.
6. Identify the renal pyramids, minor and major calyces, and the ureter.
7. Describe the course, relations, constrictions and blood supply of the ureters and surface mark them.
8. Interpret intravenous and retrograde pyelograms in health and disease.
9. Interpret an ultrasound of the kidneys.

Topic: Vessels and nerves of the abdomen

General objective

Comprehend the arrangement of the nerves, blood supply and lymphatics of the abdomen.

Specific objectives

1. Indicate the surface marking of the aorta and inferior vena cava.
2. Describe the territory of supply of the dorsal and lateral branches of the aorta.

3. Describe the formation, tributaries, course and relations of the inferior vena cava and the vena azygos.
4. Indicate the position of the cisterna chyli and describe its tributaries, viz. lumbar and intestinal lymph trunks.
5. Describe the course of the superior and inferior mesenteric veins and their territory of venous drainage.
6. Outline the course of the lumbar sympathetic trunk.
7. Describe the termination of the splanchnic nerves and the location and area of distribution of the coeliac, mesenteric and hypogastric plexuses.

Topic: Diaphragm, muscles of the posterior abdominal wall and lumbar plexus

General objective

Comprehend the functional anatomy of the muscles of the region and the arrangement of the lumbar plexus.

Specific objectives

1. Describe the vertebral, costal and sternal origins of the diaphragm and the formation of its central tendon.
2. Describe the attachments of the psoas major, quadratus lumborum and iliacus.
3. Analyse the parts played by the diaphragm and quadratus lumborum in respiration.
4. Discuss the actions of the psoas and iliacus.
5. Illustrate the principles of the formation and distribution of the lumbar plexus.
6. Illustrate the constitution of the posterior abdominal wall.

Overview of Schedule 20

Before you begin dissection note:

PELVIC VISCERA

Relevant skeletal features:

hip bones — ilium; ischium; pubis;
sacrum — ala; anterior sacral foramina; sacral promontory; sacroiliac joint;
coccyx — coccygeal vertebrae; sacrococcygeal articulation;
bony pelvis — greater pelvis; lesser pelvis; inlet; outlet; diameters; ligaments.

Peritoneum:

male — sigmoid mesocolon; rectovesical pouch;
female — sigmoid mesocolon; rectouterine pouch; vesicouterine pouch; broad ligament of uterus; mesosalpinx; mesovarium; suspensory ligament of the ovary; uterosacral folds.

Rectum:

flexures; ampulla; relations; arterial supply; venous drainage; lymphatic drainage; nerve supply.

Uterus:

position; subdivisions; cavity; arterial supply; venous and lymphatic drainage; support; pubocervical ligament; transverse cervical ligament; uterosacral ligament; round ligament.

Uterine tubes:

intramural part; isthmus; ampulla; infundibulum; fimbriae; abdominal ostium.

Ovary:

attachments; relations; arterial supply; venous drainage; nerve supply; ligament of ovary.

Vagina:

fornices; relations.

Urinary bladder:

shape; surfaces; internal architecture; relations in both sexes; arterial supply; venous drainage; nerve supply.

Ureter:

pelvic part — course; termination; arterial supply in both sexes.

Ductus deferens:

course; termination.

Seminal vesicle:

shape; position; duct.

Prostate:

shape; size; position; subdivisions; capsules; prostatic venous plexus; prostatic urethra; openings of ducts.

Surface anatomy:

fundus of urinary bladder; fundus of uterus.

Clinical anatomy:

prolapse of uterus; prolapse of rectum; enlargement of prostate; spread of cancer from pelvic viscera.

Dissection Schedule 20

PELVIC VISCERA

1. Before beginning the dissection of the pelvis *you should follow the reflection of the peritoneum in the pelvis* and then *examine* the pelvic viscera *in situ. In both male and female cadavers trace the peritoneum* over the **urinary bladder** which lies just behind the **symphysis pubis** and observe how the peritoneum is carried over its superior surface as a *loose fold* and is then reflected down over the upper part of its posterior surface. *Now trace the peritoneum separately in both sexes.*

In the male

2. Note the peritoneal reflection from the back of the bladder onto the anterior surface of the *middle third* of the **rectum**. The pouch of peritoneum between the two viscera is called the **rectovesical pouch**. *Now identify* the **ductus deferens** which raises a fold of peritoneum as it runs downwards and medially from the **deep inguinal ring** towards the back of the bladder. Posteriorly, *observe* the fold of peritoneum raised by the **ureter** as it runs down across the **ala of the sacrum**, and then inclines anteriorly and medially towards the superolateral angle of the bladder.

In the female

3. Note that the **uterus** lies between the bladder and **rectum**. The peritoneum passes from the bladder on to the anterior surface of the body of the uterus forming the **vesicouterine pouch**. It then passes over the uterus to its posterior surface where it descends down to cover the upper part of the **vagina**. From here it is reflected onto the anterior surface of the *middle third* of the rectum giving rise to the **rectouterine pouch**.

   Now identify the double fold of peritoneum which lies on either side of the uterus. This is the **broad ligament** which extends to the side walls of the pelvis. Within the broad ligament are the **uterine tubes** and **ovaries**. That part of the broad ligament extending from the lateral end of the uterine tube and ovary to the pelvic wall is called the **suspensory ligament of the**

ovary. The ovarian vessels and nerves traverse this ligament on their way to supply the ovary. The uterine tubes lie along the free border of the ligament subtended by the **mesosalpinx** (part of the broad ligament), while the ovaries are situated below the tubes. Each ovary is intimately attached to the posterior layer of the broad ligament which provides it with a short mesentery known as the **mesovarium**. *Inside the broad ligament identify the* **round ligament of the uterus** *and the* **ligament of the ovary**. The round ligament begins at the junction of the uterine tube with the uterus and runs forwards and laterally in the broad ligament and then crosses the brim of the pelvis to enter the inguinal canal through the deep inguinal ring. The ligament of the ovary can be seen stretching from the medial side of the ovary to the side of the uterus. Note the folds of peritoneum raised by the round ligament and the ligament of the ovary.

Now observe two other folds of peritoneum which lie on either side of the rectouterine pouch. These extend from the lower part of the posterior surface of the uterus to the sacrum and are known as the **rectouterine folds**. *Within these folds feel the condensations of extraperitoneal tissue called* **uterosacral ligaments**.

Posteriorly, *observe* also the fold of the peritoneum raised by the **ureter** as it runs down across the **ala of the sacrum**, and then inclines anteriorly and medially to pass under the broad ligament to the superolateral angle of the bladder.

In the male and female pelves

4. *Now examine median sagittal sections of prosected male and female pelves or of models* and note that the pelvic organs rest on a muscular diaphragm called the **pelvic diaphragm**. This is formed chiefly by the **levator ani muscles** and fascia which are attached to the anterior and lateral walls of the pelvis and which meet in the midline. The pelvic diaphragm *marks the lowest limit of the abdominal cavity below which is the* **perineum**. *Examine* the terminal parts of the alimentary and genitourinary systems which pass through the pelvic diaphragm in the midline to enter the perineum. From behind forwards these are the **anal canal, vagina** and **urethra** in the female and the anal canal and urethra in the male.

5. *Next identify the* **sigmoid mesocolon** *once again and trace its medial limb downwards towards the rectum. Open the medial limb of the sigmoid mesocolon and trace the* **inferior mesenteric artery** which continues as the **superior rectal artery**. *Cut through the sigmoid mesocolon and remove the sigmoid colon between ligatures.* Note that the rectum does not have a mesentery, taeniae coli, sacculations or appendices epiploicae. *Peel the peritoneum off the rectum and observe* that the rectum has anteroposterior and lateral flexures.

6. *Strip the peritoneum carefully from the lateral walls of the pelvis, preserving the ureters which are adherent to it. Remove the parietal peritoneum from the anterior surface of the sacrum* and note the continuation of the **superior hypogastric plexus** into the pelvis as the **right** and **left inferior hypogastric plexuses** lying on either side of the rectum.

7. *Trace the* **internal iliac artery** *downwards and backwards* from where it begins in front of the sacroiliac joint. *Observe* that the internal iliac vein lies above and posterior to the artery while the ureter is below and in front of the artery. *Try to trace* the middle rectal arteries arising from the internal iliac arteries and passing medially to the sides of the rectum. *Observe* that these branches lie in a condensation of pelvic fascia which also contains branches of the inferior hypogastric plexuses.

8. *Dissect away the fascia to mobilise the rectum. Now identify the lower dilated part of the rectum*, the **ampulla**. The ampulla will be seen to be anchored to the sacral hollow by dense pelvic fascia. *Lever the ampulla away from the sacrum and identify* the **median sacral artery** and its branches supplying the ampulla. *Now observe* the other posterior relations of the rectum which are the sacrum, coccyx, piriformis muscles and the sacral plexuses.

9. *Those of you who are dissecting a female pelvis proceed to* No. 10 and *those who are dissecting a male pelvis proceed to* No. 26. However, whichever body you are dissecting, you must also study that of the opposite sex. Therefore, arrange as conveniently as is possible to work on two cadavers.

Dissection of the pelvic organs in the female

10. *Begin by examining the uterus and its adnexae in your cadaver. During the course make constant reference to a median sagittal section of a prosected or model female pelvis so as to confirm your findings.*

    Note that the **uterus** is normally bent forwards at right angles to the vagina and to the plane of the pelvic brim (**anteverted position**). The uterus is also usually flexed forwards on itself (**anteflexed position**) at the junction of the cervix and body. *Next identify the different parts of the uterus.* That part above the openings of the uterine tubes is the **fundus** while the main part below the fundus is the **body**. The narrow terminal cylindrical part of the uterus is the **cervix**. In **nulliparae** the junction between the body and the cervix is indicated by the presence of a broad groove known as the **isthmus**.

    Observe that the vagina encircles the lower part of the cervix to form the **vaginal fornix (anterior, lateral** and **posterior fornices**). The part of the uterine cervix lying above the vagina is called the **supravaginal portion of the cervix** and the part lying within the vagina is called the **vaginal portion of the cervix**. *Observe* that the cervix passes through the *anterior wall of the vagina*, and consequently the posterior fornix is deeper.

11. *Now clean the uterine tubes and ovaries. Observe the different parts of the uterine tube.* The narrow proximal portion embedded in the uterine wall is the **intramural part**. This is followed by a constricted part called the **isthmus** which is continued laterally as the wider **ampulla of the uterine tube** which subsequently becomes the funnel-shaped **infundibulum**. The infundibulum opens into the peritoneal cavity via the **abdominal ostium**. Hence, the peritoneal cavity is open to the exterior in the female. Note the finger-like processes called the **fimbriae** projecting from the infundibulum.

12. *Next examine the* **ovary** which lies in the superior (posterior) leaf of the broad ligament. Its uterine end is attached to the uterus by the ligament of the ovary. Note that the ovary is separated only by peritoneum from the **superior vesical artery, obturator nerve** and **vessels** and the **obturator internus muscle** which lie on the lateral pelvic wall. *Identify the mesovarium and trace the branches of the ovarian vessels into the organ*

entering it through the **ovarian hilum**. Note that the **ovarian artery** arises from the abdominal aorta and that its terminal branches end by anastomosing with branches of the **uterine artery** (see below). Note that the **right ovarian vein** drains into the inferior vena cava and the **left** drains into the left renal vein.

13. *Return to the* **ureter** *and clean and trace it downwards* from the front of the bifurcation of the **common iliac artery**; *strip away the connective tissue around it* and note its rich vascular supply from the vesical arteries. *Trace it to the level of the* **ischial spine** where it passes beneath the root of the broad ligament. *Proceed very carefully and clean the uterine artery which will be seen crossing from lateral to medial above the ureter as the ureter lies close to the lateral fornix of the vagina. Trace the ureter to its termination into the bladder.*

14. *Then trace the uterine artery proximally to its origin* from the **internal iliac artery**. *Remove the broad ligament and trace the artery distally* to the side of the uterus which it supplies. Note that some ascending branches end by anastomosing with the ovarian artery. *As you trace the uterine artery near the lower part of the uterus observe* the thickened condensations of fibrous tissue and muscle fibres around it. Note that this band connects the supravaginal part of the cervix and the dome of the vagina to the side wall of the pelvis. This is the **transverse cervical ligament** which plays an important role in steadying the vagina and uterus.

15. *Identify the attachments of the* **uterosacral ligaments** which pass backwards from the cervix and vagina to the front of the sacrum. And note that the **pubocervical ligaments** pass forwards from the cervix and vagina to the neck of the bladder and on to the back of the pubes.

16. *Trace the superior vesical artery* arising from the patent portion of the **umbilical artery** and supplying the upper part of the bladder.

17. *Now examine the* **urinary bladder** *and observe* that it is roughly pyramidal in shape, having a **superior surface**, two **inferolateral surfaces**, a **fundus (base)**, an **apex** and a **neck**. The fundus is the posterior surface which is related to the lower part of the uterus and upper part of the vagina. The neck rests on the pelvic diaphragm and is continuous inferiorly with the

urethra. *Observe* that the fascia round the neck of the bladder is condensed to form the **pubovesical** and pubocervical ligaments which makes it the most fixed part.

18. Having studied the rectum, uterus with its uterine tubes and urinary bladder *in situ, you next proceed to remove these organs in one piece for further study.*

19. *First, carefully release the rectum from its adjacent lateral structures. Then divide the round ligaments close to the deep inguinal ring and the uterine and vaginal arteries close to their origins. Cut the ureter and the ovarian artery at the pelvic brim. Strip off the suspensory ligament of the ovary from the pelvic wall. Pull the uterus laterally and separate the attachments of the broad ligament from the pelvic floor on both sides.*

    Next, using a curved pair of scissors or a scalpel, cut through the lower end of the rectum just above the pelvic floor. Cut across the pelvic part of the vagina and finally cut the urethra below the neck of the bladder also at the level of the floor of the pelvis. Try not to damage the pelvic floor. In this operation, due to the narrow confines, you may at times have to cut from before backwards or from behind forwards. Now remove the rectum, uterus and bladder in one piece from the pelvic cavity for further study.

20. *Carefully separate the rectum from the vagina using a scalpel and forceps. Open the rectum and clean out its interior in order to study it.* Note that the mucous membrane has a variable number of horizontal folds, but the most constant of these are usually present on the concave sides of the lateral flexures.

21. *Next carefully separate the uterus from the bladder using a scalpel and forceps. Clean the uterus.*

22. *Then make a coronal section through the uterus* and note that its cavity inside the body is triangular. The **cavity of the uterus** continues into the fusiform **cervical canal of the uterus**. At the upper end of the cervical canal is the **internal os of the uterus,** while at the lower end of the canal which opens into the lumen of the vagina is the **external os of the uterus**.

23. *Now follow the* **vagina** *downwards* and note its relations: *anteriorly*, to the bladder above and urethra below; *posteriorly*, to the rectum above and

anal canal below; *laterally,* from above downwards to the uterine artery, transverse cervical ligament, ureter and levator ani muscle. Note that the **vaginal artery** arises from the internal iliac artery and supplies the vagina and lower part of the bladder (this artery replaces the **inferior vesical** of the male).

24. *Next, using a cruciate incision, open the urinary bladder in order to examine the interior. Make a sagittal midline cut through the superior surface of the bladder and the anterior junction of the two inferolateral surfaces. Then make a horizontal incision through the junction of the superior and inferolateral surfaces. Reflect the four flaps.*

    Examine the interior of the bladder. Observe the folds in the mucous membrane. On the posterior surface *identify* the **internal opening of the urethra** and the two **openings of the ureters**. Note that the triangular area of mucosa between these three orifices is smooth and constitutes the sensitive **trigone of the bladder**. The thickened ridge connecting the two ureteric orifices is the **interureteric fold**.

25. *Once more review* the midline pelvic effluent canals leaving the pelvis between the medial edges of the **levator ani muscles**, the **urogenital hiatus**. These are from before backwards the **urethra**, the **vagina**, and the **anal canal** behind the **perineal body**.

    This completes the examination of the female pelvic viscera. *Now examine the contents of the male pelvis* (No. 26).

Dissection of the pelvic organs in the male

26. *During the course of your pelvic dissection make constant reference to a median sagittal section of a prosected or model male pelvis.* Note that below the neck of the bladder is a firm pyramidal organ, with its base applied to the neck of the bladder and its apex to the pelvic diaphragm. This is called the **prostate**.

27. *Identify* the **ureter** in the abdomen once again. *Trace it down to the front of the bifurcation of the common iliac artery and on into the pelvis. Strip the peritoneum and connective tissue off the ureter* and note its rich vascular supply from the vesical arteries. *Follow it in front of the* **internal iliac artery** *and then medially to its termination* in the superolateral angle of the bladder. (See No. 31.)

28. *Trace the* **ductus deferens** *from the* **deep inguinal ring** *across the anterior aspect of the lateral pelvic wall and follow it to the back of the urinary bladder.* Note that in its terminal course the ductus deferens crosses the ureter from lateral to medial. Next *identify* the lobulated **seminal vesicles** on the posterior aspect of the bladder.

29. *Trace the* **superior vesical artery** arising from the patent portion of the **umbilical artery** and supplying the upper part of the bladder. Note that the **inferior vesical artery** arises from the internal iliac artery and supplies the lower part of the bladder, the seminal vesicles and the prostate.

30. *Now examine the* **urinary bladder**. *Observe* that it is roughly pyramidal in shape having a **superior** and two **inferolateral surfaces**, a **fundus (base),** an **apex** and a **neck**. The fundus is the posterior surface and is related to the seminal vesicles and the terminal part of the ductus deferens. The neck of the bladder rests on the prostate and is continued into the urethra. *Observe* that the fascia around the neck of the bladder is condensed to form ligaments which makes the neck the most fixed part of the bladder. These are the **puboprostatic ligaments** which are attached to the back of the pubis.

31. *Next remove, in one piece, the rectum, the urinary bladder, seminal vesicles, the two ductus deferens, the prostate and the remains of the two ureters. First, carefully release the rectum from its adjacent lateral structures. Then cut the ductus deferens at the deep inguinal ring on both sides; cut the ureters at the pelvic brim, and then cut the vessels that supply the pelvic organs.*

    Next, using a curved pair of scissors or a scalpel, carefully remove the rectum, bladder and prostate by cutting across the lower end of the rectum and the urethra below the prostate but above the pelvic floor. Try not to damage the pelvic diaphragm. In this operation, due to the narrow confines, you may at times have to cut from before backwards or from behind forwards. Now remove the rectum, bladder and prostate in one piece from the pelvic cavity for further study.

32. *Carefully separate the rectum from the bladder using a scalpel and forceps. Open the rectum and clean out its interior in order to study it.* Note that

the mucous membrane has a variable number of horizontal folds, but the most constant of these are usually present on the concave sides of the lateral flexures.

33. *Then clean the posterior surface of the bladder* and observe that the ductus deferens comes to lie medial to the seminal vesicle whose duct joins it to form the **ejaculatory duct**. *Trace the ejaculatory duct* inferiorly behind the neck of the bladder into the **prostate**. *Clean the fascia surrounding the prostate* and note that the fascia is continuous with the fascia around the bladder neck. *As you clean this fascia note* the plexus of veins around the neck of the bladder and **base of the prostate**. This is the **prostatic venous plexus**. Note that the **apex of the prostate** rests on the pelvic diaphragm. The neck of the bladder leads into the urethra whose proximal part is thus surrounded by the prostate and is hence called the **prostatic urethra**.

34. *Next using a cruciate incision, open the urinary bladder and prostate, in order to examine their interior. First, gently push one limb of a blunt pair of forceps up the prostatic urethra and into the bladder. Then make a sagittal midline cut through the superior surface of the bladder and the anterior junction of the two inferolateral surfaces, and continue the cut vertically downwards through the anterior part of the prostate on to the limb of the forceps. Next make a horizontal incision through the junction of the superior and inferolateral surfaces. Reflect the four flaps.*

35. *Examine the interior of the bladder. Observe* the folds in the mucous membrane. *On the posterior surface identify* the **internal opening of the urethra** *and the two* **openings of the ureters**. Note that the triangular area of mucosa between these three orifices is smooth and constitutes the sensitive **trigone of the bladder**. The thickened ridge connecting the two ureteric orifices is the **interureteric fold**. In most cadavers a bulge caused by the middle lobe of the prostate, the **uvula vesicae**, can also be seen on the posterior wall just above the neck of the bladder.

36. *Now separate the cut edges of the prostate and examine the interior of the* **prostatic urethra**. *Observe* the **urethral crest** which is a midline ridge on its posterior wall. On this crest *look for* the **colliculus seminalis**, a midline eminence. In the centre of this is a small opening leading into a

blind diverticulum called the **prostatic utricle**, the counterpart of the uterus and vagina. On either side of the mouth of the utricle is a slit-like opening of the ejaculatory duct which you may not be able to see. Lateral to the urethral crest *identify* the **prostatic sinus**. This is a curved groove into which many small ductules of the prostate open. That part of the prostate lying between the ejaculatory ducts posteriorly and the prostatic urethra anteriorly is called the **middle lobe of the prostate**.

Finally, note that the prostate has a true histological capsule in addition to the fascial capsule. The prostatic venous plexus lies between the fascial and histological capsules.

37. Once more *review* the midline pelvic effluent canals leaving the pelvis between the medial edges of the **levator ani muscles**, the **urogenital hiatus**. These are from before backwards the **urethra** and the **anal canal** which is behind the **perineal body**.

38. This completes the examination the male pelvic viscera. *Now examine the contents of the female pelvis* (No.10).

Summary

The arrangement of the pelvic viscera is best comprehended by briefly recalling the subdivision of the **primitive cloaca** by the **urorectal septum**. The *anteriorly* placed **urogenital sinus** develops into a cranial dilation, the urinary bladder and a narrower urethra caudally. Tubular evaginations of the wall of the proximal part of this urethra gives rise to the prostate which therefore surrounds this part called the prostatic part of the urethra in the male. The *posteriorly* placed **anorectal canal** develops into the terminal parts of the alimentary canal indicated by their names. The genital ducts and their derivatives, viz. seminal vesicles in the male, the uterus and its adnexae in the female, grow in between the bladder in front and the rectum behind maintaining an intermediate position. Another feature of interest is that though the urinary bladder is developed mostly from the endoderm of the cloaca its trigone is mesodermal in origin. The sympathetic innervation of the bladder is predominantly to the trigone. This is very sensitive to pain, e.g. from calculi or cancer.

The relationship of the rectouterine pouch to the vagina and its accessibility through the posterior fornix of the vagina, as well as the laxity of the reflection of the peritoneum on to the superior surface of the bladder, have important clinical applications.

The pelvic fascia though described as parietal and visceral entities is essentially one continuous layer. Its disposition as loosely arranged and ill defined layers over the distensible viscera such as the bladder, rectum and uterus, and as dense well defined layers where support is needed such as in the ligaments of the uterus, rectum and around non-distensible organs such as the prostate must be appreciated. For example, when the levator ani muscles and the ligaments in relation to the uterus and rectum become weak, there is a tendency for the occurrence of **prolapse** of the uterus and the rectum.

A common condition affecting the male in his later years is enlargement of the prostate gland. The anatomical basis of the different methods of approaching the prostate (transurethral, perineal, etc.) must be fully comprehended. The reasons for the great respect with which the surgeons regard the prostatic venous plexus during all operations on the prostate, and the importance of the plexus in the spread of prostatic cancer must also be appreciated. The relations, blood supply and the radiographic location of the ureter are also of great importance as the ureter is the site of impaction of calculi and it is also vulnerable to damage during surgical procedures in the lower abdomen and pelvis. Finally, the blood supply, lymphatic drainage and the relations of the rectum must be known, as this is one of the common sites of occurrence of cancer.

You must also be aware that some of the pelvic organs are very variable in their position just like the abdominal viscera. Thus, though the ovary is described as occupying the **ovarian fossa** it must be realised that this is true only in nulliparae. The ovary never returns to the fossa after the first pregnancy and its subsequent position is extremely variable. Another pelvic organ which shows variability is the sigmoid colon. It can even extend up to the umbilical region or even higher particularly when it has a long mesentery which predisposes it to become twisted on its pedicle causing a condition called **volvulus**.

Objectives for Dissection Schedule 20

Topic: Pelvic viscera

General Objective

Comprehend the arrangement of the pelvic viscera and their peritoneal relationships.

Specific objectives

1. Describe the reflection of pelvic peritoneum with special reference to the formation of the vesicouterine, rectouterine and rectovesical fossae.
2. Describe the reflections and contents of the broad ligaments of the uterus.
3. Describe the position, surfaces, apex, base and neck of the urinary bladder.
4. Describe the relations of the surfaces of the bladder and its internal appearance.
5. Indicate the developmental parts of the bladder and analyse the innervation of these parts.
6. Describe the prostate, its capsules and lobes.
7. Illustrate the formation and termination of the ejaculatory duct and the parts of the male urethra.
8. Indicate the position and peritoneal relationships of the ovaries, uterus, uterine tubes and vagina.
9. Identify the component parts of the uterus and uterine tubes.
10. Discuss the supports of the uterus and the causes of uterovaginal prolapse.
11. Describe the walls, fornices and relations of the vagina.
12. Describe the blood supply and lymphatic drainage of the ovary, uterus and vagina.
13. Interpret hysterosalpingograms.
14. Interpret an ultrasound of:
    (a) the pelvic viscera of a female;
    (b) the pelvic viscera of a male.

Overview of Schedule 21

Before you begin dissection note:

BLOOD VESSELS, NERVES AND MUSCLES OF THE PELVIS

Arteries:

internal iliac, divisions and branches; median sacral.

Veins:

internal iliac and tributaries; venous plexuses.

Nerves:

sacral plexus; coccygeal plexus; autonomic plexuses.

Muscles:

piriformis; obturator internus; levator ani and its subdivisions. *Pelvic diaphragm, perineal body.*

Clinical anatomy:

pelvic diaphragm and mechanics of labour.

Dissection Schedule 21

BLOOD VESSELS, NERVES AND MUSCLES OF THE PELVIS

1. *Clean the* **internal iliac artery** *and its branches. To get a clear view of these branches remove the accompanying veins.* Note the branches of the **pelvic autonomic plexuses** that you may encounter and the positions of the **pelvic lymph nodes** at the origins of most of the arterial branches.

2. Note that the internal iliac artery divides into an **anterior** and a **posterior division**. The posterior division gives only parietal branches whereas the anterior division gives both parietal and visceral branches.

3. *From the posterior division trace the following parietal branches*:
   (a) the **iliolumbar artery** which passes *upwards* beneath the psoas, this artery gives off iliac and lumbar branches;
   (b) two **lateral sacral arteries** which pass through the **anterior sacral foramina**;
   (c) the **superior gluteal artery** which passes between the **lumbosacral trunk** and the **first sacral nerve** to emerge through the **greater sciatic foramen** above the **piriformis muscle**.

4. *Next trace the parietal branches of the anterior division* which are:
   (a) the **obturator artery**, which runs forwards along the lateral pelvic wall *below the obturator nerve* to leave the pelvis through the **obturator foramen** to enter the medial aspect of the thigh;
   (b) the **internal pudendal artery**; and
   (c) the **inferior gluteal artery** — these latter two arteries are the terminal branches of the anterior division. *Trace their exit from the pelvis below the piriformis muscle and through the greater sciatic foramen.*

   The *visceral branches* of the anterior division are:
   in the *male* — **superior vesical, middle rectal** and **inferior vesical arteries**.
   in the *female* — **superior vesical, middle rectal, uterine** and **vaginal arteries**.

5. *Next examine the nerves of the pelvis.* Passing forwards on the lateral wall and accompanying the obturator artery is the **obturator nerve**. *Now trace*

the lumbosacral trunk into the pelvis. Observe that this trunk lies posteromedial to the obturator nerve and runs across the sacroiliac joint to take part in the formation of the **sacral plexus** by joining the anterior primary rami of the upper sacral nerves.

6. Note that the plexus lies: (a) lateral to the **anterior sacral foramina**; (b) on the piriformis muscle; and (c) *external* to the pelvic fascia. Also note that the blood vessels lie *internal* to the fascia. *Identify the first sacral nerve* immediately below the superior gluteal artery.

7. *Now trace the branches of the sacral plexus. First, try to find the nerves arising from the ventral aspect of the sacral nerve roots.* These are the nerves to the obturator internus and quadratus femoris muscles; they leave the pelvis through the greater sciatic foramen. Do not spend time looking for them. *Now lift the plexus and find the nerves arising from the dorsal surface of the plexus.* These are the nerves to the piriformis, perforating branch of S2, 3 and the **posterior femoral cutaneous nerve**. The fourth sacral nerve joins the fifth sacral and coccygeal nerves to from the **coccygeal plexus** on the surface of the coccygeus muscle . *Next identify the* **superior** *and* **inferior gluteal nerves** *and trace them as they leave the pelvis through the greater sciatic foramen, the former above and the latter below the piriformis. Finally, clean the terminal branches of the plexus* which are the **sciatic** and **pudendal** nerves. These nerves exit through the greater sciatic foramen below the piriformis. Identification of all these nerves is clearer on examination of the gluteal region.

8. *Now clean and study the attachments of*: (a) the **piriformis muscle** to the middle three pieces of the sacrum; and (b) the **obturator internus** to the side wall of the lesser pelvis. *Follow their tendons through the greater and lesser sciatic foramina, respectively.* Their insertions on to the femur were (will be) seen in the gluteal region. *Next identify* the **coccygeus muscle** passing from the ischial spine to the last piece of the sacrum and the first piece of the coccyx. *Observe* how it lies edge to edge with the posterior margin of the **levator ani muscle**, helping to form the **pelvic diaphragm**.

9. *Next clean and study the attachments* of the levator ani muscle. *First trace its origins* from the back of the **pubis**, the **ischial spine** and from a fibrous

band between the two. The latter band of origin is called the **tendinous arch of the levator ani muscle**.

From this wide origin *trace the muscle fibres backwards and medially to their insertion* in the midline where they meet the fibres of the opposite side. Note that they form a series of U-shaped loops around the pelvic organs providing them with support as well as contributing to their sphincteric mechanism.

Note that the **pubic** (anterior) **part** of the levator ani muscle is composed of three sets of muscle fibres: a medial set, the **levator prostatae muscle** in the *male* (the corresponding fibres in the *female* are called the **pubovaginalis muscle**); an intermediate set, the **puborectalis muscle**; and a lateral set, the **pubococcygeus muscle**, in both males and females.

In the *male* the **levator prostatae muscle** is *inserted* into the fibromuscular **perineal body**. In the *female* the **pubovaginalis muscle** crosses the side of the **vagina** to *reach* the perineal body. Some of its fibres actually blend with the muscular walls of the vagina and together with fibres from the contralateral muscle form a partial sphincter.

In both sexes the **puborectalis muscle** passes across the side of the rectum to loop around the **anorectal junction** by joining with its fellow of the opposite side. Some of the fibres become continuous with the deeper part of the **external anal sphincter** and the outer longitudinal coat of the rectum. The muscle loop angulates the anorectal junction forwards.

The **pubococcygeus muscle** is mainly *inserted* into the **anococcygeal body**, the coccyx and into the lowest part of the sacrum in both sexes.

Posterior to the pubococcygeus lies the **iliococcygeus** (posterior) part of the levator ani muscle. Its fibres pass medially *below* the pubococcygeus to be *inserted* into the anococcygeal body, coccyx and lower part of the sacrum. The pubococcygeal and iliococcygeal muscles together with their insertion into the anococcygeal body form the **levator ani shelf** which supports the rectum directly and in the *female* the uterus indirectly.

Note that the anterior gap between the pillars of the right and left levator ani is known as the **urogenital hiatus**. This gap transmits the urethra in the *male* and the urethra and vagina in the *female*.

Observe how the levator ani muscle of the two sides slope towards the midline to form a muscular gutter.

The levator ani is supplied by the third and fourth sacral nerves and the pudendal nerves which supply the anterior parts.

10. *Now review the structures passing though the greater and lesser sciatic foramina.* Note that these structures which exit through these foramina, were (will be) encountered when you dissected the gluteal region.

Summary

You must be aware that the **pelvic diaphragm** (pelvic floor) is composed of fascia (**superior fascia of the pelvic diaphragm**), a muscle layer (levator ani and coccygeus) and fascia (**inferior fascia of the pelvic diaphragm**) from above downwards. The muscle layer provides support for the pelvic viscera, particularly when intraabdominal pressure is raised as in micturition, defaecation and parturition, and it reinforces the rectal and urethral sphincters.

The manner of arrangement of structures within the narrow confines of the pelvic cavity shows the maximum utilisation of the available space. In the narrow space outside the **parietal pelvic fascia** are found the lumbrosacral plexus and its branches, which are least distensible, while the most distensible structures which are the pelvic organs such as the bladder, uterus, rectum, etc., are provided with the maximum amount of room in the pelvic cavity.

As to the arrangement of the muscles and nerves that leave the pelvic cavity, it is clear that they can exit only through the greater and lesser sciatic foramina en route to the gluteal region or perineum. In this respect it must be recalled that the piriformis muscle exits through the greater sciatic foramen and has superior gluteal vessels and nerves above it, and the sciatic and pudendal nerves below it during its passage through the foramen.

The important role of the levator ani muscles in the support and integrity of the pelvic organs must be thoroughly understood. Another important feature of these muscles is that they slope towards each other to form a gutter in the midline. The gutter-like arrangement of the two muscles rotates the foetal head into the anteroposterior plane as it descends through the pelvis. This is of paramount importance in the mechanics of normal labour. The levator ani may become partially torn during a difficult childbirth. As a result the support of the pelvic viscera may be diminished, the uterus descends (*prolapse*) and urinary incontinence may occur. The diameters of the bony pelvis at its inlet and outlet are also important for the same reason.

Finally, you must appreciate the role of the **lateral sacral veins** and their communications with the **vertebral venous plexus** in the mechanism of spread of cancer from the pelvic viscera to the axial skeleton.

Objectives for Dissection Schedule 21

Topic: Pelvic blood vessels and nerves

General objectives

Comprehend the arrangement and distribution of the pelvic blood vessels and nerves.

Specific objectives

1. Identify the aortic bifurcation, common iliac, external iliac and internal iliac arteries.
2. Identify the lumbrosacral trunk and enumerate the structures descending across the ala of the sacrum.
3. Enumerate the branches of the two divisions of the internal iliac artery and outline their territories of supply.
4. Describe the location of prostatic, vesical and uterovaginal venous plexuses and their drainage.
5. Indicate the positions of pelvic lymph nodes and their area of drainage.

Topic: Pelvic musculature

General objective

Comprehend the functional anatomy of the pelvic muscles.

Specific objectives

1. Describe the origin and insertion of the levator prostatae (pubovaginalis), puborectalis, pubococcygeus, iliococcygeus and coccygeus portions of the pelvic diaphragm.
2. Analyse the actions of the levator ani muscle with reference to:
   (a) its components — pubovaginalis, puborectalis;
   (b) its role in the support of the pelvic viscera at normal times and during various stresses; and
   (c) its role in the mechanics of labour.

Overview of Schedule 22

Before you begin dissection note:

PERINEUM

Perineum:

boundaries.

Ischioanal fossa boundaries

Rectum and anal canal:

sphincters; relations; mucous membrane; arterial supply; venous drainage; portosystemic anastomosis; nerve supply.

Urogenital region:

subcutaneous perineal pouch; superficial perineal pouch and contents; deep perineal pouch and contents.

Nerves:

pudendal nerve and branches.

Arteries:

internal pudendal artery and branches.

Veins:

internal pudendal vein and tributaries.

Lymphatics:

superficial inguinal lymph nodes.

Surface anatomy:

pudendal canal.

Clinical anatomy:

rectal examination; vaginal examination; pudendal block anaesthesia.

Dissection Schedule 22

PERINEUM

1. The clinical **perineum** is the floor of a groove between the upper parts of the thighs and between the lower parts of the buttocks. This is the region of the external genitalia and anus.

2. The anatomical perineum is the **inferior pelvic aperture** which is a diamond-shaped space bounded by the symphysis pubis, the conjoint rami (inferior ramus of pubis and ramus of ischium) ischial tuberosity, sacrotuberous ligament and the coccyx. *Verify these landmarks on a bony pelvis*. Note that the perineum is situated below the pelvic diaphragm.

   For convenience the perineum is subdivided into two triangles by drawing a line across the inferior pelvic aperture between the centres of the two ischial tuberosities. The triangle behind the line, with the coccyx as its apex, is called the **anal region**. It contains the anal canal and, on each side of the anal canal, an **ischioanal fossa**. The triangle in front of the line, with the pubic symphysis at its apex, is called the **urogenital region**. It contains the urethra and external genitalia.

   Note the position of the two regions: the urogenital region is more or less in a horizontal plane and the anal region is set at about 120° to the urogenital region.

3. *You will first explore the anal region and subsequently the urogenital region in the male and female cadaver. Also examine prosected specimens and models.*

Anal Region

1. *With the male or female body in the prone position and the pelvis elevated make the following incisions*:
   (a) *in the* **male** — *a median incision from the coccyx to the root of the penis encircling the anus and the neck of the scrotum; in the* **female** — *a median incision from the coccyx to the pubis encircling the anus and the labia majora;*
   (b) *a transverse incision from one ischial tuberosity to the other.*

   Reflect the skin flaps and remove the fat and fascia and in the male the scrotum as well.

2. *Examine the muscular sphincter surrounding the anal canal.* This is the **sphincter ani externus**. *Clean it* and note that it has three parts which together surround the length of the anal canal:
   (a) the *subcutaneous part* surrounds the anal orifice;
   (b) the *superficial part* encircles the middle part of the anal canal and extends from the **anococcygeal body** behind the anal canal to the **perineal body** (see below) in front;
   (c) the *deep part* will be found encircling the upper end of the anal canal; this part also has contributing fibres from the puborectalis part of the levator ani muscle.

   The sphincter is supplied by:
   (a) the **inferior rectal nerve** accompanied by vessels passing from the region of the ischial tuberosity towards the anal canal; and
   (b) the perineal branch of S4.

   The upper two-thirds of the anal canal is encircled by the **internal sphincter**, which is in fact a thickening of the inner circular smooth muscle of the gut. Also, observe the U-shaped fibres of the puborectalis part of the levator ani muscle which loop around the upper part of the anal canal to sling the **anorectal junction** forwards.

3. *Next examine the relations of the anal canal* and note that the anococcygeal body is behind it. The perineal body separates the anal canal from the root of the penis in front in the *male* and from the lower end of the vagina in the *female*. *Open the anal canal along its posterior aspect and study its interior.* Observe the longitudinal folds in the lining mucous membrane called the **anal columns**. Connecting the lower ends of these vertical columns are horizontal folds of mucosa known as the **anal valves**. *Identify these valves.*

4. Lateral to the anal canal is the **ischioanal fossa** which is wedge shaped. Note that its *lateral wall* is formed by the ischium and the obturator internus muscle covered by **obturator fascia**. The *medial wall* is formed by the sphincter ani externus and the levator ani muscle with its covering, the **inferior fascia of the pelvic diaphragm**; the *roof* is the meeting place of the levator ani and obturator internus muscles; the *anterior wall* is formed by the **body of the pubis** and fascia, which will be examined later. *Posteriorly* lie the sacrotuberous ligament and the gluteus maximus muscle. The *floor* is formed by the skin and fascia of the buttock.

Carefully remove the fat and demonstrate the ischioanal fossa. Then trace the **inferior rectal nerve** *laterally to its parent trunk, the* **pudendal nerve**, which is found to traverse a fascial tunnel, the **pudendal canal**, on the lower inner surface of the obturator internus. *Trace the pudendal nerve forwards* and note that it divides into the **dorsal nerve of the penis (clitoris)** and the **perineal nerve**. The latter gives off the **posterior scrotal nerves** (or **labial nerves** in the female) in the anterior part of the canal. The perineal nerve and the dorsal nerves of the penis (or clitoris) will then be seen running forwards into the **deep perineal pouch** (see below).

Urogenital Region

Those of you who are dissecting a male perineum proceed to the section dealing with the *Urogenital Region in the Male* and those who are dissecting a female perineum proceed to the section dealing with the *Urogenital Region in the Female*. However, whichever body you are dissecting, you must also study that of the opposite sex. Therefore, arrange as conveniently as is possible to work on two cadavers.

Urogenital Region in the Male

With the body in the supine position and the pelvis elevated:

Subcutaneous perineal pouch

1. Note that the **membranous layer of superficial fascia** which you exposed when you removed the superficial fat from the anterior abdominal wall is attached to the medial margin of the pubic bones anteriorly, to the **pubic arch** laterally, and to the posterior border of the **perineal membrane** posteriorly. The membranous layer also lines the inner aspect of the scrotum (as the **dartos muscle**) and forms a sleeve for the **body of the penis**. Deep to this membranous layer lies the **subcutaneous perineal pouch**, a potential space between the membranous layer below and the **perineal deep fascia** above.
2. *Remove the remains of the membranous layer of superficial fascia by cutting along its attached margins. Clean the region. You will now see the* **perineal deep fascia** which is attached to the posterior margin of the

perineal membrane and at the sides to the ischiopubic rami. *Next carefully remove the perineal deep fascia.* You are now in the **superficial perineal pouch.**

Superficial perineal pouch

3. The **superficial perineal pouch** lies between the perineal deep fascia (below) and the perineal membrane (above). It contains the root of the penis (two **crura** and the **bulb of the penis**) and its associated muscles, and branches of the **internal pudendal vessels** and **pudendal nerves.** The muscles in the pouch are the **ischiocavernosus, bulbospongiosus** and **superficial transverse perineal muscles.**
4. *Explore and clean the superficial perineal pouch and try to find the following:*
   (a) The **ischiocavernosus muscles,** which arise from the corresponding ramus of the ischium to sweep over the **crus of the penis** to gain insertion into it.
   (b) The **bulbospongiosus muscle,** which arises from the perineal body and from a median raphe on the inferior aspect of the **corpus spongiosum (bulb of the penis).** The fibres sweep dorsally to be inserted onto the corpus.
   (c) The **superficial transverse perineal muscles,** which are poorly developed, are two small slips arising from the posterior part of the ramus of the ischium and run transversely to be inserted into the perineal body. They form the posterior boundary of the urogenital region. *Do not waste time looking for these two muscles.*

   All these muscles are supplied by the perineal branch of the pudendal nerve and the internal pudendal vessels.
5. Having studied the superficial perineal pouch and its contents *remove these structures as follows:*
   (a) *Divide the dorsal vein, arteries and nerves of the penis just distal to the* **arcuate ligament of the pubis.**
   (b) *Separate the crura and bulb of the penis, together with their muscles, from their attachments to the perineal membrane and pubic arch, working from behind forwards. As you do so you will have to divide the relevant vessels and nerves.*

(c) *Divide the* **urethra** *where it enters the upper surface of the bulb of the penis.*

(d) *Finally, remove the superficial transverse perineal muscles if you can find them.*

In this way the remainder of the penis is detached entirely and the perineal membrane is exposed completely.

6. Note that the **perineal membrane** is a triangular membrane which extends across the pubic arch and is attached to the ischiopubic rami. Posteriorly, in the midline, it is attached to the perineal body. And in front, between the apex of the membrane and the **arcuate pubic ligament**, the **deep dorsal vein of the penis** passes to the **prostatic plexus of veins**. The membrane is traversed by the urethra and the ducts of the **bulbourethral glands** (which open into the penile portion of the urethra).

7. Note also the perineal body which is a fibromuscular mass located between the anal canal behind and the perineal membrane in front. Here several muscles meet and fuse. These are the bulbospongiosus, external anal sphincter, superficial and deep transverse perineal and levator ani (levator prostatae) muscles. The perineal body is much more important in the female than in the male, since it is an indirect support for the pelvic organs.

Deep perineal pouch

8. The **deep perineal pouch** is a space whose superficial (inferior) covering is the perineal membrane and whose deep (superior) covering is a layer of fascia. This fascia fills the gap between the two ischiopubic rami and laterally, on either side, is coextensive with the fascia covering the obturator internus. Medially its upper surface fuses with the **inferior fascia of the pelvic diaphragm**. The perineal membrane and the obturator fascia extension fuse posteriorly at the posterior border of the urogenital region. Thus the pouch is not an enclosed space but is open above. This space together with its coverings and muscles forms a protective barrier for the urogenital hiatus.

9. The deep perineal pouch is occupied by the **external urethral sphincter muscle**, which surrounds the **intermediate part of the urethra**, the two

deep transverse perineal muscles, the two **bulbourethral glands** and vessels and nerves.

The intermediate part of the urethra is the section of the urethra which lies between the prostate above and the bulb of the penis below.

The deep transverse perineal muscles arise from the ramus of the ischium and are inserted into the perineal body and decussate around the sphincter urethrae to fuse with the fellow of the opposite side. These muscles help to stabilise the urethra in the midline.

Exposure of the inferior surface of the levator ani muscle in the male

10. *Since it is difficult to dissect the deep perineal pouch proceed directly to remove the coverings and contents of the deep perineal pouch,*
    (a) *carefully cut along its lateral attachments to the ischiopubic rami and reflect medially. Then divide the urethra transversely at that level;*
    (b) *clear away the remaining fascia from the inferior surface of the levator ani muscles* (**inferior fascia of the pelvic diaphragm**), *stripping it forwards and medially.*
11. Note that you now have:
    (a) removed part of the anterior wall of the ischioanal fossa;
    (b) exposed the gap between the levator ani muscles, the **urogenital hiatus**, which is filled with fascia, and through which the urethra passes.
12. This completes the examination of the urogenital region of the male. *Now examine the female urogenital region.*

Urogenital Region in the Female

With the body in the supine position and the pelvis elevated:

Subcutaneous perineal pouch

1. Note that the **membranous layer of superficial fascia** which you exposed when you removed the superficial fat from the anterior abdominal wall is attached to the medial margin of the pubic bones anteriorly, to the **pubic arch** laterally, and to the posterior border of the **perineal membrane** posteriorly. Medially, the membranous layer passes through the deeper portions of the **labia majora** and becomes attached to the margins of the

vaginal orifice in the perineal membrane. It also forms a sleeve for the **body of the clitoris**. Deep to this membranous layer lies the **subcutaneous perineal pouch**, a potential space between the membranous layer below and the **perineal deep fascia** above.

Also note the **vestibule of the vagina**, which is a cleft between the **labia minora**. It contains the openings of the **vagina**, the **urethra** and the **ducts of the greater vestibular glands**. The **external urethral orifice** is situated behind the **clitoris** and immediately in front of the **vaginal orifice**.

2. *Remove the remains of the membranous layer of superficial fascia by cutting along its attached margins. Clean the region. You will now see the* **perineal deep fascia** which is attached to the posterior margin of the perineal membrane, at the sides to the ischiopubic rami, and medially to the margins of the vaginal orifice. *Carefully remove the perineal deep fascia*. You are now in the **superficial perineal pouch.**

Superficial perineal pouch

3. The **superficial perineal pouch** lies between the perineal deep fascia (below) and the perineal membrane (above). It contains the root of the clitoris (two **crura** and the **bulb of the vestibule**) and its associated muscles and branches of the **internal pudendal vessels** and the **pudendal nerves,** and the two **greater vestibular glands**. The muscles in the pouch are the **ischiocavernosus, bulbospongiosus** and **superficial transverse perineal muscles.**

4. *Explore and clean the superficial perineal pouch. Try to find*:
   (a) The **ischiocavernosus muscles** which arise from the corresponding ramus of the ischium and embrace the crura of the clitoris.
   (b) The **bulbospongiosus muscle** is split and separated from the contralateral half by the lower part of the vagina. It arises from the perineal body and passes forward around the vaginal orifice to be inserted partly into the side of the pubic arch and partly into the root and the dorsum of the clitoris. In its course it covers the **bulb of the vestibule.** The bulb of the vestibule consists of paired elongated masses of erectile tissue which lie at the side of the vaginal opening.

The **greater vestibular glands** are two small, round bodies located immediately behind the bulb of the vestibule and their ducts open close to the vaginal orifice. They are often atrophied in old age.

(c) The **superficial transverse perineal muscles**, which are poorly developed, are two small slips arising from the posterior part of the ramus of the ischium and run transversely to be inserted into the perineal body. They form the posterior boundary of the urogenital region. *Do not waste time looking for these two muscles.*

All these muscles are supplied by the perineal branch of the pudendal nerve and the internal pudendal vessels.

5. Having studied the superficial perineal pouch and its contents *remove these structures as follows*:
   (a) *Pull the clitoris downwards and divide its vessels and nerves distal to the* **arcuate ligament of the pubis**.
   (b) *Detach the crura and the bulb of the vestibule, together with their muscles, from the pubic arch and the perineal membrane, beginning anteriorly and working backwards. As you do so you will have to divide the relevant vessels and nerves.*
   (c) *Finally remove the superficial transverse perineal muscles if you can find them.*

   In this way the clitoris is detached entirely and the perineal membrane is exposed completely.

6. Note that the **perineal membrane** is a triangular membrane which extends across the pubic arch and is attached to the ischiopubic rami. Posteriorly, in the midline, it is attached to the perineal body. And in front, between the apex of the membrane and the **arcuate pubic ligament**, the **deep dorsal vein of the clitoris** passes to the **vesical plexus of veins**. The perineal membrane is traversed by the urethra anteriorly and the vagina posteriorly.

7. Note also the perineal body which is a fibromuscular mass located between the anal canal behind and the vagina in front. Here several muscles meet and fuse. These are the bulbospongiosus, external anal sphincter, superficial transverse perineal, urogenital and levator ani (pubovaginalis) muscles. The perineal body is an indirect support for the pelvic organs. It may be damaged during **parturition**. To avoid injury, the opening for the passage

of the foetal head may be enlarged by incising the posterior wall of the vagina and the nearby part of the perineum (**episiotomy**) lateral to the perineal body.

Deep perineal pouch

8. The **deep perineal pouch** is a space whose superficial (inferior) covering is the perineal membrane and whose deep (superior) covering is a layer of fascia. This fascia fills the gap between the two ischiopubic rami and laterally, on either side, is coextensive with the fascia covering the obturator internus. Medially its upper surface fuses with the **inferior fascia of the pelvic diaphragm**. The perineal membrane and the obturator fascia extension fuse posteriorly at the posterior border of the urogenital region. Thus the pouch is not an enclosed space but is open above. This space with its coverings and muscles forms a protective barrier for the urogenital hiatus.

9. The deep perineal pouch is occupied by the **urogenital sphincter**, which surrounds the urethra and connects with the vagina, and by vessels and nerves.

   The urogenital sphincter arises from the inferior ramus of the pubis and the perineal body and encircles the vagina and urethra, thereby helping to fix these two structures.

   The female urethra is about 4 cm long and extends from the neck of the bladder to the external urethral orifice in the vestibule of the vagina. It is intimately adherent to the anterior wall of the vagina.

Exposure of the inferior surface of the levator ani muscle in the female

10. *Since it is difficult to dissect the deep perineal pouch proceed directly to remove its coverings and contents*:
    (a) *carefully cut along its lateral attachments to the ischiopubic rami and reflect medially. Then divide the urethra and vagina transversely at that level*;
    (b) *clear away the remaining fascia from the inferior surface of the levator ani muscles* (**inferior fascia of the pelvic diaphragm**), *stripping it forwards and medially*.

11. Note that you now have:
    (a) removed part of the anterior wall of the ischioanal fossa;
    (b) exposed the gap between the two levator ani muscles, the **urogenital hiatus**, which is filled with fascia, and through which the vagina and urethra pass.

12. This completes the examination of the urogenital region of the female. *Now examine the male urogenital region.*

The Nerves and Arteries of the Perineum in Both Sexes

1. The **pudendal nerve (S2,3,4)**
   The pudendal nerve furnishes most of the innervation to the perineum. *Pick up the pudendal nerve in the* **pudendal canal**, which is in the lateral wall of the **ischioanal fossa**, and note that it gives off the following branches:
   (a) the **inferior rectal nerve** which supplies the levator ani and external anal sphincter muscles and the lower half of the anal canal;
   (b) the **perineal branch** (mixed nerve) which supplies the skin of the scrotum (labia) and the muscles in the superficial perineal pouch.
   (c) the **dorsal nerve of the penis** (or **clitoris**); this branch courses along the inner aspect of the ischiopubic ramus and supplies the muscles in the deep perineal pouch. It then runs on the dorsum of the penis (or clitoris) and supplies the skin, prepuce and glans.

2. The **internal pudendal artery**
   The internal pudendal artery is a branch of the **internal iliac artery**. The artery accompanies the pudendal nerve in the pudendal canal. It supplies the structures in the urogenital region. Note the following branches:
   (a) the **deep artery of the penis** (or **clitoris**) which pierces the crus and runs in the substance of the corpus cavernosum;
   (b) the **dorsal artery of the penis** (or **clitoris**) which pierces the perineal membrane and runs along the dorsum of the penis (or clitoris).

Summary

The **ischioanal fossa** is important because of its vulnerability to infection. This vulnerability is due to its close proximity to the anal canal and to the fact that it is filled with fat that is poorly vascularised.

The **anal canal** shows several important features. It is the site of portosystemic anastomoses and hence bleeding from varicose veins may occur in cases of portal hypertension. Straining due to chronic constipation also predisposes to similar varicosity of the rectal veins leading to the common condition of 'piles' or **haemorrhoids**. The anal canal also exhibits a 'mucocutaneous junction'. The skin below the junction is very sensitive to pain as it is innervated by the pudendal nerve, which is a **somatic nerve**, whereas the mucous membrane above, which is innervated by **visceral nerves**, is insensitive to pain. This is of considerable clinical importance. Thus tearing of the anal valves due to a scybalous mass of faeces in chronic constipation gives rise to a linear ulcer extending down into the anal skin which then gives rise to an excruciatingly painful condition called **fissure-in-ano**.

In the *female urogenital space*, attention should be paid to the area between the vagina and the anal canal known as the **perineal body**. Its importance can be gauged by the fact that it is this region between the anus and the posterior wall of the vagina that is referred to as the 'perineum' by gynaecologists. Its overwhelming importance is due to the fact that it supports the pelvic organs, especially the uterus.

Another region of importance is the upper part or dome of the vagina. The close proximity of the uterine artery and the ureter to the lateral fornix, and the accessibility of the rectouterine pouch via the posterior fornix should always be borne in mind as their clinical implications are profound.

It must also be borne in mind that a considerable amount of information regarding the pelvic structures is obtained by introducing an examining finger into the rectum (**rectal examination**) and vagina (**vaginal examination**). Piles, cancer of the rectum, enlarged pelvic lymph nodes, prostatic hypertrophy, uterovaginal prolapse, cancer of the uterine cervix, and prolapsed ovaries are a few of the conditions diagnosed in this way.

Finally, it is important to recall that the **pudendal canal** lies on the lateral wall of the ischioanal fossa above the medial margin of the ischial tuberosity which is an easily palpable landmark. With a finger in the rectum or vagina acting as a guide it is possible to inject a local anaesthetic in order to produce analgesia of the perineum to enable a number of surgical procedures in the region, including forceps delivery.

Objectives for Dissection Schedule 22

Topic: Perineum

General Objective

Comprehend the basic anatomical arrangements of the region.

Specific Objectives

1. Describe the formation and contents of the superficial perineal pouch.
2. Describe the formation and contents of the deep perineal pouch.
3. Indicate the position of the pudendal canal.
4. Indicate the course and branches of the pudendal neurovascular bundle.
5. Define the boundaries of the ischioanal fossa.
6. Describe the sphincters of the anal canal.
7. Describe the structures that are palpable during rectal and vaginal examinations in the living.
8. Discuss the anatomical principles involved in:
   (a) ischioanal abscess;
   (b) fissure and fistulae of anal canal;
   (c) pudendal block anaesthesia;
   (d) Bartholin's abscess;
   (e) haemorrhoids;
   (f) the clinical applications of the pectinate line;
   (g) faecal incontinence resulting from accidental damage to the puborectalis sling.

Additional Objectives for Abdomen

Topic: Peritoneal reflections

General objective

Comprehend the disposition of the peritoneum and its clinical applications.

Specific objectives

1. Illustrate the disposition of the peritoneum:
   (a) in a sagittal section through the abdomen;
   (b) in horizontal sections through the abdomen at the level of the omental foramen.
2. Explain the clinical importance of:
   (a) the right paracolic gutter;
   (b) the relations of the omental foramen;
   (c) the omental bursa;
   (d) the pararectal fossae.

Topic: Abdominal viscera

General objective

Comprehend the clinical importance of the basic anatomical features of the abdominal viscera.

Specific objectives

1. Indicate the features by which the following can be identified during an abdominal operation (laparotomy):
   (a) jejunum; (b) ileum; (c) large intestine; (d) the vermiform appendix; (e) the proximal and distal ends of a loop of small intestine;
2. Discuss the effects of partial or complete obstruction of:
   (a) the bile duct; (b) the pancreatic duct; (c) ureter; (d) uterine tubes; (e) small intestine; (f) large intestine; (g) the portal vein; (h) the inferior vena cava; (i) the aortic bifurcation.

3. Indicate the structures encountered during a surgical approach to the kidney from the back.

4. Discuss the anatomical basis of:
   (a) maldescent and malposition of the testis; (b) torsion of the testis; (c) torsion of the kidney; (d) needle aspiration of the liver; (e) infarcts of the kidney; (f) sigmoidoscopy; (g) urethral catheterisation and cystoscopy; (j) approaches to the prostate gland; (k) portosystemic anastomoses; (l) pelvimetry; (m) cystocoele and rectocoele; (n) hiatus hernias; (o) diaphragmatic hernias.

5. Discuss the clinical importance of the relationship of the liver, spleen and kidneys to the pleura.

6. Describe the anatomical features by which a physician confirms an enlargement of these organs by palpation and percussion:
   (a) liver; (b) spleen; (c) kidneys; (d) caecum; (e) stomach.

7. Correlate the microstructure to the function of the different parts of the alimentary canal from the mouth to the anal canal.

8. Interpret the radiographic appearances of:
   (a) oesophageal varices; (b) normal and altered duodenal 'cap'; (c) normal gas shadows in the gastrointestinal tract; (d) cystograms.

Topic: Nerves of abdomen

General Objective

Comprehend the important principles of the innervation of the abdominal viscera.

Specific objectives

1. Discuss the mechanism of defaecation and faecal incontinence.

2. Discuss the mechanisms of micturition and urinary incontinence.

3. Explain the probable mechanisms of:
   (a) 'colicky' abdominal pain;
   (b) pain of appendicitis being referred to the umbilical region;
   (c) pain from the testis being referred to the infra-umbilical region;

4. Discuss the rationale of:
   (a) presacral neurectomy for intractable pain from the pelvic viscera;
   (b) lumbar sympathectomy for peripheral vascular disease.

Topic: Blood vessels and lymphatics

General objective

Comprehend the important clinical features of the blood supply and lymphatic drainage of the region.

Specific objectives

1. Enumerate the sites of arterial anastomoses in the gastrointestinal tract.
2. Enumerate the sites of portosystemic anastomoses.
3. Discuss the clinical significance of:
   (a) aberrant renal arteries;
   (b) renal artery stenosis;
   (c) relations of the uterine artery;
   (d) vascularity of the ureter.
4. Define the location of the primary lymph nodes draining:
   (a) the testis; (b) ovaries; (c) body of the uterus; (d) cervix of the uterus; (e) the rectum above the level of peritoneal reflection as well as below it; (f) the vagina; and (g) the anal canal.

Topic: Skeletal framework of abdomen

General objective

Comprehend the important features of the skeletal framework of the region.

Specific objectives

1. Identify the costal and transverse elements in a lumbar vertebra and in the sacrum.
2. Describe the important differences between the male and female pelves.
3. Discuss the functional importance of:
   (a) the large size of the lumbar vertebral bodies and intervertebral discs;

(b) lumbar lordosis;
(c) the basivertebral veins and the vertebral venous plexus;
(d) diameters of the pelvis;
(e) linea terminalis;
(f) iliolumbar, sacrotuberous, sacrospinous and sacroiliac ligaments.

4. Interpret the radiographs and ultrasounds of the lumbar vertebral column and pelvic girdle.

Section 5

HEAD AND NECK

Introduction

In most vertebrates, specialisations have occurred at the cranial end. As a result, the organs of special sense concerned with vision, hearing, balance, olfaction and taste are found in the head. The inflow of sensory input from these sense organs has caused an enormous development of the cranial end of the nervous system, resulting in the formation of the brain.

The brain and special sense organs are in close association with one another and have become enclosed in a common protective covering known as the skull. The part of the skull protecting the brain, internal ear, eye and nose is called the **neurocranium** while that part of the skeleton forming the face and lodging the organs of taste is known as the **viscerocranium**. These two components have fused to form the skull. However, the lower jaw or mandible, which is a part of the viscerocranium is still free to move at the temporomandibular joint. The two different parts of the skull have different developmental origins. Thus, the neurocranium is developed from paraxial mesoderm whereas the viscerocranium is derived from branchial mesoderm. The branchial mesoderm not only forms the facial skeleton but also gives rise to the branchial musculature which is concerned with mastication and facial expression. In addition, it gives rise to the pharyngeal and laryngeal musculature concerned with deglutition and phonation.

Owing to the dominance of vision in higher primates, including humans, the olfactory sense organs have undergone recession. Thus, the facial region has become more flattened and the eyes have shifted to the front so that there is a considerable increase in the range of binocular stereoscopic vision. Moreover, the erect posture of humans and their bipedal mode of progression have resulted in the shifting of the foramen magnum towards the centre of the base of the skull. This enables the skull to be balanced more easily without having recourse to the development of the large postvertebral neck muscles so characteristic of lower mammals.

Although the arrangement of structures in the neck appears complicated at first sight, it is built on the same general pattern as the trunk. However, the coelom represented by the pleural, pericardial and peritoneal cavities in the trunk is absent in the neck. In addition, both branchial and somatic musculature are found in the neck. The somatic muscles are concentrated in front of, and behind the vertebral column as the pre- and postvertebral muscle groups, as well as in the ventral midline as the superior continuation of the rectus abdominis mass. The branchial musculature is found around the pharynx and larynx. In the peripheral parts of the neck, it is represented by the trapezius, sternocleidomastoid and platysma.

Overview of Schedule 23

Before you begin dissection note:

POSTERIOR TRIANGLE OF THE NECK

Relevant skeletal features:

temporal bone — mastoid process;
mandible — angle; lower border; symphysis menti;
sternum — jugular notch;
clavicle — medial end; shaft; lateral end.

Subcutaneous structures:

platysma muscle; external jugular vein; lesser occipital nerve; great auricular nerve; transverse cutaneous nerve of neck; supraclavicular nerves.

Deep fascia:

superficial layer of deep cervical fascia (forming roof of posterior triangle); prevertebral fascia (covering floor of posterior triangle); axillary sheath.

Muscles:

platysma; sternocleidomastoid; trapezius; inferior belly of omohyoid; scalenus anterior; scalenus medius; levator scapulae; splenius capitis; semispinalis capitis.

Boundaries and floor of posterior triangle.

Nerves:

accessory nerve; brachial plexus; roots; trunks; suprascapular; long thoracic; cervical plexus; cutaneous branches; phrenic nerve.

Arteries:

occipital; suprascapular; subclavian.

Veins:

suprascapular; external jugular; anterior jugular; subclavian.

Lymph nodes:

superficial cervical nodes along external jugular vein.

Surface anatomy:

accessory nerve; external jugular vein.

Clinical anatomy:

injury to roots and trunks of brachial plexus.

Dissection Schedule 23

POSTERIOR TRIANGLE OF THE NECK

1. *With the body in the supine position make the following incisions*:
   (a) *from the* **jugular notch** *along the clavicle as far as the acromion process of the scapula* (*if not already made*);
   (b) *from the* **mastoid process** *of the temporal bone along the lateral side of the neck to the acromion process* (*if not already made*);
   (c) *from the mastoid process along the anterior margin of the* **sternocleidomastoid muscle** *to the jugular notch, taking care not to cut too deep.*

   Remove the skin flap.

2. *Try to identify* the fibres of the **platysma** muscle in the *superficial fascia*. This muscle passes from the skin and fascia below the clavicle towards the lower border of the **mandible**. *Divide the muscle about 2 cm above the clavicle and reflect the divided portions*. Avoid damaging the underlying **external jugular vein** and the **supraclavicular nerves**.

3. *Identify the external jugular vein* as it descends from behind the angle of the mandible towards the middle of the clavicle where it pierces the deep fascia to enter the **subclavian vein**. Note its formation by the union of the **posterior auricular vein** with the **posterior branch of the retromandibular vein** which emerges from the inferior margin of the **parotid gland**. The external jugular vein receives the **transverse cervical**, **suprascapular** and **anterior jugular veins** which will be seen later.

4. *Try to dissect the following cutaneous branches of the* **cervical plexus** radiating like the spokes of a wheel from *about the middle of the posterior border* of the sternocleidomastoid muscle:
   (a) **lesser occipital nerve** (C2) ascending along the posterior border of the sternocleidomastoid to reach the back of the scalp and the adjoining posterior surface of the auricle;
   (b) **great auricular nerve** (C2,3) passing superficial to the sternocleidomastoid towards the parotid gland and ear;
   (c) **transverse cutaneous nerve** of neck (C2,3) crossing the sternocleidomastoid superficially towards the midline of the neck;

(d) **medial, intermediate** and **lateral supraclavicular nerves** (C3,4) descending over the corresponding portions of the clavicle.

5. *Now turn your attention* to the *boundaries of the posterior triangle* formed in front by the sternocleidomastoid, behind by the **trapezius**, and below by the intermediate third of the clavicle. *Observe* that the lower boundary forms the base while the meeting point of the two muscles constitutes the apex of the triangle.

6. *Identify the* **superficial layer of deep cervical fascia** stretching between the sternocleidomastoid and trapezius and forming the *roof* of the triangle. *Secure the* **accessory nerve** (spinal part) lying in this deep fascia and issuing out from the posterior border of the sternocleidomastoid at the junction of the upper and middle third of the muscle. *Trace the nerve downwards* and note that it disappears under the anterior border of the trapezius . Note that the accessory nerve is the uppermost nerve running across the triangle. It supplies both the sternocleidomastoid and trapezius muscles on their deep surface.

7. *Cut the clavicular head of the sternocleidomastoid and displace the cut portion of the muscle medially to expose the underlying* **scalenus anterior muscle** *close to the root of the neck.* Note that this muscle and the muscles forming the floor of the posterior triangle are covered by the *prevertebral layer of deep cervical fascia. Identify the* **phrenic nerve** (C3,4,5) as it descends in front of the scalenus anterior deep to the prevertebral fascia. *Now clean the structures crossing in front of the muscle.* From above downwards these are:

   (a) **inferior belly of omohyoid**, a slender muscle running obliquely downwards and backwards across the posterior triangle about 1–2 cm above the middle third of the clavicle;

   (b) **suprascapular artery** running below the omohyoid and passing towards the middle of the clavicle to accompany the suprascapular nerve. The suprascapular artery is a branch of the **thyrocervical trunk** from the first part of the **subclavian artery**;

   (c) **anterior jugular vein** running deep to the sternocleidomastoid in the lower part of the neck and draining into the external jugular vein;

   (d) **subclavian vein** which receives the external jugular vein.

8. Behind the scalenus anterior, *identify* the **scalenus medius muscle**. Between these two muscles *look for the* **roots of the brachial plexus** formed by the *ventral rami* of C5-T1 and the subclavian artery.

   Secure the **upper trunk** formed by the union of C5,6 and the **middle trunk** formed by the ventral ramus of C7, both of which lie above the omohyoid muscle. *Clean the* **lower trunk** formed by C8,T1 below the muscle.

   Trace the following branches of the brachial plexus:

   (a) **suprascapular nerve** C5,6 arising from the *upper trunk* of the brachial plexus and running along the upper border of the omohyoid muscle;
   (b) **long thoracic nerve** from the back of C5,6,7 *roots* descending behind the brachial plexus. Note that roots C5,6 pierce the scalenus medius.

9. *Identify the muscles which form the floor of the posterior triangle*. From above downwards these are:

   (a) **semispinalis capitis** near the apex;
   (b) **splenius capitis**;
   (c) **levator scapulae**; and
   (d) **scalenus medius** and **posterior** lying behind the brachial plexus.

10. *Elevate the cut ends of the clavicle on the right side and clean the third part of the subclavian artery*. This part of the artery begins at the lateral border of the scalenus anterior and ends at the outer border of the first rib where it continues as the **axillary artery**. *Observe* the relationship of the lower trunk of the brachial plexus to the artery. *Clean the subclavian vein* which lies below and in front of the artery and is separated from it by the scalenus anterior. Note that the artery, vein and trunks of the brachial plexus are enclosed within a prolongation of the prevertebral fascia which is continued into the axilla as the **axillary sheath**. You will see that the subclavian artery arches above the clavicle while the vein is completely hidden by the bone.

Summary

It must be noted that the deep cervical fascia covers the neck like a collar. This superficial layer of deep cervical fascia splits to enclose the sternocleidomastoid and trapezius muscles. These muscles have possibly developed from the same premuscle mass. Consequently, it is not surprising that they are innervated by the same nerve, i.e. accessory nerve, which provides their *motor supply*. However, additional branches from the cervical plexus passing to these muscles are said to provide them with proprioceptive (sensory) fibres.

Other important structures in the posterior triangle are the brachial plexus and subclavian vessels. The plexus descends behind the lower fourth of the sternocleidomastoid muscle to enter the posterior triangle. Here the trunks of the brachial plexus course downwards and outwards behind the middle third of the clavicle. The lower trunk of the brachial plexus is closely related to the subclavian artery so that the groove behind the **scalene tubercle** of the first rib is produced not only by the subclavian artery but also by the lower trunk of the plexus. This close relationship of the vessel and the lower trunk (or more particularly the ventral ramus of the first thoracic nerve) implies that both of them can be affected when a **cervical rib** is present. Such a condition may lead to a compression of the subclavian artery which is the only vessel supplying the upper limb. It can also produce symptoms of compression of the ventral ramus of the first thoracic nerve.

Objectives for Dissection Schedule 23

Topic: Posterior triangle of the neck

General objective

Comprehend the arrangement of the structures in the region.

Specific objectives

1. Define the boundaries, roof and floor of the posterior triangle.
2. Describe the relationship of the superficial layer of deep cervical fascia to (a) the trapezius and sternocleidomastoid muscles; and (b) the accessory nerve.
3. Describe the relationship of the prevertebral fascia to the axillary sheath.
4. Test the integrity of the trapezius and sternocleidomastoid muscles.
5. Define the posterior border of the sternocleidomastoid muscle and use it to surface mark the accessory nerve and brachial plexus.
6. Identify the scalenus anterior muscle and the structures passing in front of and behind this muscle.
7. Illustrate: (a) the formation of the trunks of the brachial plexus from nerve roots C5–T1; and (b) the branches given off by the roots and trunks.
8. Trace the course of the neurovascular bundle of the upper limb from the posterior triangle into the axilla.
9. Enumerate the contents of the posterior triangle.
10. Identify, on a living subject, the surface landmarks of this region.
11. Discuss the anatomical basis of:
    (a) injuries to the subclavian artery and lower trunk of the brachial plexus;
    (b) damage to the accessory nerve during surgery in the posterior triangle; and
    (c) the cervical rib syndrome.

Questions for study:

1. What areas are drained by the superficial cervical lymph nodes?
2. The posterior triangle can be divided into a "carefree" portion above the accessory nerve and a "careful" portion below the accessory nerve. Why? What important structures may be damaged during surgery in the inferior portion of the posterior triangle?
3. What is torticollis?

Overview of Schedule 24

Before you begin dissection note:

ANTERIOR TRIANGLE OF THE NECK

Relevant skeletal features:

occipital bone — superior nuchal line;
temporal bone — mastoid process;
mandible — lower border; symphysis menti;
hyoid bone — body; lesser and greater horns;
thyroid cartilage — thyroid notch; oblique line;
cricoid cartilage — arch;
trachea — cartilaginous rings;
manubrium sterni — jugular notch.

Subcutaneous structures:

platysma; anterior jugular vein; cervical branch of facial nerve; transverse cutaneous nerve of neck; submental lymph nodes.

Deep fascia:

superficial layer of deep cervical; pretracheal; prevertebral; carotid sheath.

Ligaments:

median thyrohyoid; cricothyroid; cricotracheal.

Glands:

parotid; thyroid; parathyroid.

Trachea:

cervical part.

Oesophagus:

cervical part.

Muscles:

sternocleidomastoid; digastric; mylohyoid; sternohyoid; superior belly of omohyoid; sternothyroid; thyrohyoid; cricothyroid; inferior constrictor of pharynx.

Nerves:

external laryngeal; internal laryngeal; recurrent laryngeal; hypoglossal; ansa cervicalis; vagus; sympathetic trunk.

Arteries:

common carotid; internal carotid; external carotid; superior thyroid; lingual; facial; occipital; posterior auricular; inferior thyroid.

Veins:

internal jugular; superior thyroid; middle thyroid; inferior thyroid; brachiocephalic.

Lymph nodes:

anterior cervical; jugulodiagastric; juguloomohyoid.

Surface anatomy:

thyroid gland; common carotid artery.

Clinical anatomy:

tracheostomy; laryngostomy.

Dissection Schedule 24

ANTERIOR TRIANGLE OF THE NECK

1. *Make the following incisions*:
   (a) *from the* **symphysis menti** *along the midline to the* **jugular notch**;
   (b) *from the symphysis menti along the lower border of the mandible to the mastoid process.*

   Remove the skin flap.

2. Again note the fibres of the **platysma muscle** in the superficial fascia which pass obliquely upwards and medially from the skin and fascia below the clavicle to gain insertion into the lower border of the mandible. The **cervical branch of the facial nerve** passes from the lower end of the **parotid gland** to supply the platysma.

3. *Clean the* **anterior jugular vein** which arises from below the chin and descends close to the midline. *Observe* that this vein passes *deep* to the lower part of the sternocleidomastoid to drain into the external jugular vein.

4. *Clear away the remains of the superficial fascia of the anterior triangle* which is bounded by the sternocleidomastoid, the lower border of the mandible and the midline of the neck. *Trace the superficial layer of deep cervical fascia* passing forwards from the anterior border of the sternocleidomastoid to gain attachment to the lower border of the mandible, the **hyoid bone** and the upper border of the sternum.

5. *Clean the sternal head of the sternocleidomastoid arising from the sternum.* The clavicular origin of the muscle has already been seen. *Follow the muscle to its insertion into the* **mastoid process** *of the temporal bone and the* **superior nuchal line** *of the occipital bone. Preserve the parotid gland* which overlaps this muscle near its insertion. The muscle is supplied by the **accessory nerve** and C2(3) nerves.

6. *Remove the remnants of the deep fascia* and note the structures lying along or close to the midline of the neck. From above downwards these are:

(a) the symphysis menti;

(b) the anterior bellies of the **digastric muscles** arising from the lower border of the mandible close to the symphysis menti and passing posterolaterally;

(c) the **mylohyoid muscles** which are visible between the two diverging anterior bellies of the digastric;

(d) the **hyoid bone**;

(e) the **median thyrohyoid ligament** attached to the upper border of the **thyroid cartilage** and passing upwards *behind* the **body of the hyoid** to be attached to its upper border;

(f) the V-shaped **notch of the thyroid cartilage** below the hyoid bone;

(g) the **cricothyroid ligament** connecting the upper border of the **arch of the cricoid cartilage** to the lower border of the thyroid cartilage;

(h) the **isthmus of the thyroid gland** below the cricoid cartilage; *look for the* **pyramidal lobe** on the upper border of the isthmus. The pyramidal lobe may be continued upwards as a fibromuscular band known as the **levator glandulae thyroideae**. This is attached to the hyoid bone;

(i) **trachea**;

(j) jugular notch.

7. *Detach the sternocleidomastoid muscle from its sternal origin (if not already detatched) and turn it upwards. Clean the underlying* **infrahyoid muscles**:

(a) the **sternohyoid** which arises from the back of the **manubrium sterni** and medial end of the clavicle to be inserted into the lower border of the body of the hyoid bone;

(b) the **superior belly of the omohyoid** which is attached to the body of the hyoid bone lateral to the insertion of the sternohyoid. *Identify* the intermediate tendon connecting the superior and inferior bellies of the muscle;

(c) *cut the sternohyoid in the middle and reflect the two halves to study the attachments of the* **sternothyroid** *and* **thyrohyoid** which lie deep to the sternohyoid. The sternothyroid muscles arises from the back of the manubrium sterni and first costal cartilage and is inserted into the **oblique line** of the thyroid cartilage; the thyrohyoid muscle arises from the oblique line of the thyroid cartilage and is inserted into the lower border of the **greater cornu of the hyoid bone**.

8. *Trace the nerve supply of the infrahyoid muscles from a slender nerve loop called the* **ansa cervicalis** *which lies on the* **internal jugular vein** *at the level of the cricoid cartilage.* The thyrohyoid muscle is supplied by a twig from the **hypoglossal nerve** carrying C1 fibres.

9. *Detach the sternothyroid from its origin and turn it upwards to expose the thyroid gland.* Note that the thyroid gland is enveloped by a sheath of **pretracheal fascia** which is attached to the cricoid cartilage and the oblique line of the thyroid cartilage. *Remove this fascia* and study the gland which consists of *two* **lobes** connected by an **isthmus**. Note that each lobe extends from the oblique line of the thyroid cartilage above to the level of the fifth or sixth tracheal ring below. The isthmus lies on the second, third and fourth tracheal rings.

   Identify the **superior** *and* **middle thyroid veins** *draining into the internal jugular vein and the* **inferior thyroid veins** *of the two sides draining into the* **left brachiocephalic vein**. Near the upper end of the lateral lobe, *secure the* **superior thyroid artery**, a branch of the **external carotid artery**. Near the lower end of the lateral lobe, *identify the* **inferior thyroid artery**, a branch of the **thyrocervical trunk** of the subclavian artery. Occasionally, there is a **thyroidea ima artery**, a branch of the **brachiocephalic trunk** supplying the isthmus. *Above, identify the* **external laryngeal nerve** accompanying the superior thyroid artery. *Below, follow the* **recurrent laryngeal nerve** running upwards in the groove between the trachea and oesophagus and disappearing behind the lateral lobe of the thyroid gland. *Divide the isthmus and remove one lobe by cutting the blood vessels close to the gland taking care not to damage the nerves. Trace the external laryngeal nerve distally into the* **cricothyroid muscle**. *Follow it proximally* to its origin from the **superior laryngeal nerve**. *Trace the other branch of the superior laryngeal nerve*, the **internal laryngeal nerve**, which pierces the **thyrohyoid membrane** to enter the larynx. *Now trace the recurrent laryngeal nerve* passing beneath the lower border of the **inferior constrictor muscle of the pharynx** to enter the larynx. Both the superior laryngeal and the recurrent laryngeal nerves are branches of the **vagus nerve**.

10. *Next clean and examine the cervical portion of the trachea and oesophagus.* Note that the **trachea**, which commences at the lower border of the cricoid cartilage (at C6), lies in the midline. Anterior to the trachea are: (a) the infrahyoid muscles; (b) the isthmus of the thyroid gland; (c) the inferior thyroid veins; (d) the **thymus**; and (e) the **left brachiocephalic vein**.

    Note that the **oesophagus**, which lies behind the trachea, also commences at the level of the lower border of the cricoid cartilage.

11. *Detach the superior belly of the omohyoid from the hyoid bone. Next clean the* **common carotid artery** *and the* **internal jugular vein** which are enclosed in a fascial sheath known as the **carotid sheath**. *Look for the* **deep cervical lymph nodes** that are distributed along the length of the internal jugular vein. *Remove these lymph nodes and clean the contents of the carotid sheath.* As you do so *preserve the* **superior root of the ansa cervicalis** (from C1), a branch of the **hypoglossal nerve** which runs down on the common carotid artery to join the **inferior root** (C2,3) to form the **ansa cervicalis** which has already been dissected. *Separate the internal jugular vein from the common carotid artery and identify the vagus nerve which lies between the two vessels. Clean the common carotid artery up to its bifurcation into the* **external** *and* **internal carotid arteries**. *Note that the bifurcation occurs at the level of the upper border of the thyroid cartilage*, where the *external carotid artery* lies *anteromedial to the internal carotid artery*. *Observe* that the internal carotid artery, internal jugular vein and vagus nerve lie within the carotid sheath.

12. *Clean the lower branches of the external carotid artery.* From below upwards these are:
    (a) **superior thyroid artery** which descends beneath the superior belly of the omohyoid to supply the thyroid gland;
    (b) **ascending pharyngeal artery** which ascends medial to the internal carotid artery (this will be seen later);
    (c) **lingual artery** which arises near the tip of the greater cornu of the hyoid bone; observe that it describes an upward loop which is crossed by the hypoglossal nerve;
    (d) **facial artery** ascending deep to the posterior belly of the digastric;
    (e) **occipital artery** running backwards along the lower border of the posterior belly of the digastric;

(f) **posterior auricular artery** running along the upper border of the posterior belly of the digastric.

13. *Identify the* **sympathetic trunk** lying posterior to the common and internal carotid arteries.

Summary

The neck, like the trunk, is derived from the three primary germ layers — ectoderm, endoderm and mesoderm. The gut which is developed from the endoderm is the deepest structure and is surrounded by visceral or branchial mesoderm forming the musculature of the gut. Outside this is the somatic mesoderm giving rise to the various muscles. Thus, in the neck, the gut and its derivatives are represented by the pharynx and oesophagus running in the midline as well as by the larynx and trachea which arise as a ventral outgrowth from the foregut. The thyroid gland, which itself is formed from a median diverticulum arising from the ventral aspect of the primitive pharynx (foregut), lies ventral (anterior) to the lower part of the larynx and upper part of the trachea. Dorsolateral to the gut in the embryo are the neurovascular structures. Thus, the carotid sheath containing the common carotid artery, internal jugular vein and vagus nerve occupy a posterolateral position to the gut. These are overlapped by the lateral lobes of the thyroid gland. Lying ventral to the thyroid gland are the infrahyoid muscles which appear to be a cranial continuation of the same muscle mass as the rectus abdominis. The upward continuation of the infrahyoid muscles are the geniohyoids. All these muscles are supplied by segmental nerves just like the rectus abdominis. Superficial to the infrahyoid muscles are the sternocleidomastoid muscles which run obliquely upwards from the sternum and clavicle towards the lateral side of the neck to be inserted into the skull. The exact developmental status of the sternocleidomastoid is uncertain although on the basis of its innervation by the accessory nerve it may be of branchial origin. Lying superficial to the sternocleidomastoid and running in the opposite direction to it is the platysma which is also of branchial origin. It is supplied by the facial nerve which is the nerve of the second branchial arch.

The pretracheal fascia which envelopes the thyroid gland is attached to the cricoid cartilage and to the oblique line of the thyroid cartilage. Because of this attachment the gland moves up and down together with the larynx during deglutition. The close relationship of the external laryngeal and recurrent laryngeal nerves to the superior and inferior thyroid arteries must be borne in mind during thyroid surgery so as to avoid damage to the nerves.

Objectives for Dissection Schedule 24

Topic: Anterior triangle of the neck

General objective

Comprehend the arrangement of the structures in the region.

Specific objectives

1. Define the boundaries of the anterior triangle of the neck.
2. Describe the arrangement of the superficial layer of deep cervical fascia, the pretracheal fascia and the carotid sheath. Explain why a knowledge of this anatomy is of great importance.
3. Enumerate the midline structures of the neck from the mandible to the jugular notch.
4. Review the attachments and actions of the infrahyoid muscles and the formation and distribution of the ansa cervicalis.
5. Give an account of the topographical relationships of the thyroid gland.
6. Discuss the clinical importance of:
   (a) the blood supply and lymphatic drainage of the thyroid gland; and
   (b) the nerves in relation to this gland.
7. Outline the course, branches and area of distribution of the external carotid artery.
8. Outline the course of the vagus nerve and the sympathetic trunk in the anterior triangle.
9. Review the attachments and relations of the sternocleidomastoid muscle.
10. Demonstrate the pulsations of the common carotid artery and the internal jugular vein in the living and explain their clinical importance.
11. Identify the vertebral levels at which the following structures can be found: the thyroid cartilage, the cricoid cartilage, the beginning of the trachea, and the isthmus of the thyroid gland.

Questions for study:

1. What vascular structures in the lower neck are at risk during the performance of a tracheotomy?
2. What are the relationships of the external laryngeal nerve and the recurrent laryngeal nerve to the thyroid gland? What functional deficits would result from injury to these nerves during thyroid surgery?

Overview of Schedule 25

Before you begin dissection note:

FACE AND SCALP

FACE

Relevant skeletal features:

nasal bone — root of nose;
maxilla — body; processes; infraorbital foramen;
zygomatic bone — arch, zygomaticoorbital foramen;
mandible — ramus; angle; body; symphysis; mental foramen.

Subcutaneous structures:

palpebral branch of lacrimal, infratrochlear, external nasal, infraorbital, zygomaticofacial, buccal, mental and great auricular nerves.

Muscles:

orbicularis oculi; orbicularis oris; buccinator and other muscles of facial expression.

Nerves:

temporal; zygomatic; buccal; mandibular and cervical branches of facial nerve.

Arteries:

facial; transverse facial; buccal and infraorbital branches of maxillary artery.

Veins:

facial; deep facial.

Surface anatomy:

parotid duct; facial artery (pulse).

Clinical anatomy:

'dangerous area' of face; facial palsy.

SCALP

Relevant skeletal features:

skull	— vault; base;
individual bones	— frontal; parietal; temporal; occipital;
sutures	— sagittal; coronal; lambdoid;
meeting point of sutures	— bregma; lambda;
eminences	— frontal; parietal;
landmarks	— nasion; superior orbital margin; supraorbital notch; temporal lines; mastoid process; inion (external occipital protuberance); superior nuchal line;
emissary foramina	— parietal; mastoid; condylar.

Subcutaneous structures:

supratrochlear nerve and vessels; supraorbital nerve and vessels; zygomaticotemporal nerve; auriculotemporal nerve and superficial temporal vessels; great auricular nerve; lesser occipital nerve; greater occipital nerve and occipital vessels; third occipital nerve; posterior auricular vessels.

Deep fascia:

temporalis fascia.

Muscles:

occipitofrontalis muscle; epicranial aponeurosis.

Five layers of the scalp.

Nerves:

posterior auricular and temporal branches of facial.

Lymph nodes:

occipital; mastoid.

Clinical anatomy:

scalp wounds; 'dangerous area' of scalp.

Dissection Schedule 25

FACE AND SCALP

FACE

1. *Make the following incisions*:
   (a) *from the root of the nose* (**nasion**) *to the symphysis menti*;
   (b) *from the angle of the mouth towards the* **intertragic notch**;
   (c) *incisions encircling the orbital, nasal and oral apertures*;
   (d) *from* nasion *to* **inion (external occipital protuberance)** *along the midline*;
   (e) *coronal incision from ear to ear passing through the* **vertex**.
   Reflect all the skin flaps.

2. Note that the muscles of the face are attached to overlying skin and fascia and consequently function as muscles of *facial expression*. Moreover, the muscles surrounding the mouth and eyes have a sphincteric function.

3. *Try to identify the following sensory nerves* which are derived chiefly from the three divisions of the **trigeminal nerve**:
   (a) palpebral branch of the **lacrimal nerve**, supplying the lateral part of the upper eyelid;
   (b) **infratrochlear nerve**, a branch of the **nasociliary nerve** *emerging along the medial angle of the eye* to supply the upper half of the nose, lower eyelid, **lacrimal sac** and **lacrimal caruncle**;
   (c) **external nasal nerve**, the terminal part of the nasociliary nerve supplying the lower half of the nose;
   These three branches arise from the **ophthalmic division**.
   (d) **infraorbital nerve**, *emerging 1 cm below the lower margin of the orbit*, and supplying the lower eyelid, lower lateral part of the nose and upper lip;
   (e) **zygomaticofacial nerve**, *emerging from the zygomatic bone* to supply the skin over the upper part of the cheek;
   These two nerves are from the **maxillary division**.
   (f) **buccal nerve**, *emerging in front of the ramus of the mandible* to supply the skin over the cheek;

(g) **mental nerve**, a branch of the **inferior alveolar nerve** *emerging from the* **mental foramen** to supply the skin over the body of the mandible and lower lip;

These two nerves are from the **mandibular division**.

(h) **great auricular nerve** (C2,3) supplying branches to the skin over the angle of the mandible.

4. *Clean the* **orbital** *and the* **palpebral portions** *of the* **orbicularis oculi muscles** arising from the medial side of the orbit. Note that the fibres of the muscle encircle the orbit. A deep portion of the muscle, the **lacrimal part**, will be identified later.

5. *Clean the superficial facial muscles lying between the orbit and the mouth.* These are the **levator labii superioris alaeque nasi, levator labii superioris, zygomaticus minor** and **zygomaticus major**, which take origin in this order from the frontonasal region medially to the **zygoma** laterally. *Trace these muscles towards the upper lip*. An additional slip from the levator labii superioris alaeque nasi passes to the **ala of the nose**.

   Trace the **risorius muscle** *passing from the fascia over the* **parotid gland** *towards the angle of the mouth. Clean the* **depressor labii inferioris** *and the* **depressor anguli oris** taking origin from the mandible and passing upwards towards the lower lip and the angle of the mouth, respectively.

   Identify the superficial part of the **orbicularis oris** *surrounding the oral aperture*. This is formed by the fibres of the superficial muscles which pass into the lips.

6. *Clean the fascia over the parotid gland and look for the* **parotid duct** arising from the anterior border of the gland and passing forward 2 cm below the zygomatic arch.

7. *Try to secure the following branches of the* **facial nerve** *as they emerge from the anterior border of the parotid gland and radiate to supply the muscles of the face*:
   (a) **temporal** supplying the frontal belly of the **occipitofrontalis** (see later);
   (b) **zygomatic** supplying the orbicularis oculi;
   (c) **buccal** innervating the superficial group of muscles lying above the mouth as well as the **buccinator** and part of the orbicularis oris;

(d) **mandibular** supplying the lower part of the orbicularis oris, the depressor labii inferioris, depressor anguli oris and the risorius;
(e) **cervical** supplying the platysma;
(f) **posterior auricular** passing behind the ear and supplying the occipital belly of the occipitofrontalis.

Note that these nerves form plexuses with the sensory nerves supplying the face.

8. *Clean the following arteries which form a rich network in the face:*
   (a) **facial artery**, a branch of the **external carotid**, *curving round the lower border of the mandible in front of the* **masseter muscle** and giving off several branches to the face. It anastomes near the inner angle of the eye with the **dorsal nasal branch of the ophthalmic artery** which is given off by the **internal carotid artery** inside the cranial cavity;
   (b) **transverse facial artery**, a branch of the **superficial temporal artery**, *running above the parotid duct* to supply the face; the superficial temporal artery is one of the terminal branches of the external carotid artery;
   (c) **buccal** and **infraorbital branches of the maxillary artery**, accompanying the corresponding nerves; the maxillary artery is the other terminal branch of the external carotid artery.

9. *Identify the* **facial vein** *formed near the medial angle of the eye* by the union of the **supratrochlear** and **supraorbital veins**. It has communications with the **ophthalmic vein**.

   Observe that the branches of the facial nerve, artery and vein lie between the superficial and deep facial muscles (neurovascular plane).

10. *Identify the buccinator and the* **levator anguli oris muscles** which form the *deep facial muscles*. Note the origin of the buccinator muscles from the maxilla above and mandible below and from the **pterygomandibular raphe** posteriorly. The fascia covering the buccinator is known as the **buccopharyngeal fascia**. *Remove this fascia and trace the fibres of the buccinator towards the lips* where they form the *deep layer of the orbicularis oris muscle.*

    Identify the levator anguli oris lying deep to the zygomaticus minor and partly overlapped by the levator labii superioris.

SCALP

Now turn your attention to the scalp. The layers of the scalp are: (a) skin; (b) subcutaneous tissue which is tough and loculated; (c) **occipital** and **frontal bellies of the occipitofrontalis muscle** connected by the **epicranial aponeurosis**; (d) loose areolar tissue; and (e) **pericranium**.

1. *Try to identify the fibres of the frontal belly of the occipitofrontalis muscle in the frontal region.*
2. Note that the following structures lie in the anterior half of the scalp:
   (a) **supratrochlear nerve** from the **frontal branch** of the *ophthalmic division ascending close to the medial margin of the orbit* to supply the medial part of the upper eyelid and forehead. It is accompanied by the supratrochlear artery and vein;
   (b) **supraorbital nerve** also from the frontal branch of the *ophthalmic division emerging from the upper margin of the orbit* about 2–3 cm lateral to the supratrochlear nerve. It runs from the frontal region towards the **lambda**. It is accompanied by the **supraorbital artery** and **vein**.

   The supratrochlear and supraorbital arteries are branches of the **ophthalmic artery** which is given off by the internal carotid artery inside the cranium;
   (c) **auriculotemporal nerve** from the *mandibular division* ascending in front of the root of the ear. This nerve is accompanied by the **superficial temporal artery** and **vein**. Note that the superficial temporal artery divides into anterior and posterior branches. The superficial temporal vein disappears into the parotid gland where it joins the **maxillary vein** to form the **retromandibular vein**;
   (d) **temporal branches of the facial nerve** crossing the zygomatic arch to supply the frontal belly of the occipitofrontalis.
3. Note that the following structures lie in the posterior half of the scalp:
   (a) **great auricular nerve** (ventral rami of C2,3) behind the ear;
   (b) **lesser occipital nerve** (ventral ramus of C2) along the posterior border of the sternocleidomastoid muscle. This nerve supplies the cranial surface of the ear and the adjacent part of the scalp behind the ear;
   (c) **greater occipital nerve** (dorsal ramus of C2) ascending 2–3 cm lateral to the external occipital protuberance. Note that the nerve is

accompanied by the **occipital artery**, a branch of the external carotid artery;

(d) **third occipital nerve** (dorsal ramus of C3) medial to and below the greater occipital nerve;

(e) **posterior auricular branch of the facial nerve** behind the root of the ear where it supplies the occipital belly of the occipitofrontalis. This branch is accompanied by the **posterior auricular artery** and **vein.** The vein joins the **posterior branch of the retromandibular vein** to form the **external jugular vein**.

4. Note the lymph nodes in the region of the **external occipital protuberance** and mastoid process.

5. *Clean the* **frontal** *and* **occipital bellies of the occipitofrontalis** *and the* **epicranial aponeurosis** *connecting them.* The frontal belly originates from the skin over the region of the eyebrow and the occipital belly from the lateral part of the **highest nuchal line** of the occipital bone. Note that the epicranial aponeurosis is attached laterally to the **superior temporal line** and also sends an extension to the **zygomatic arch**.

6. *Incise the aponeurosis longitudinally and introduce the handle of the scalpel to explore the space deep to the aponeurosis containing loose areolar tissue.*

7. Note that the superficial layers of the scalp move as one unit over the underlying pericranium.

8. *Now examine the temporal region* and note that the **temporalis muscle** and the overlying **temporalis fascia** form additional layers of the scalp in this region. These are situated between the lateral extensions of the epicranial aponeurosis and the pericranium.

9. *Remove the temporalis fascia attached to the superior temporal line* and note the origin of the temporalis muscle from the **inferior temporal line** and **temporal fossa**. The insertion and other details regarding this muscle will be seen later.

Summary

The sensory innervation of the face is based on its development. The face is developed from three primordia — **frontonasal, maxillary** and **mandibular processes**. The frontonasal process gives rise approximately to the nasal and frontal regions. The maxillary and mandibular processes form the regions occupied by the maxilla and mandible, respectively. Each process has its own nerve supply. Thus, the frontonasal process is supplied by the ophthalmic division of the trigeminal nerve while the maxillary and mandibular divisions supply the areas developed from the corresponding processes. Consequently, branches from the *three divisions* of the *trigeminal nerve* provide the *sensory innervation* of the face. However, a small area over the angle of the mandible is supplied by C2 fibres of the great auricular nerve.

Although the facial muscles are known as the muscles of facial expression, they are generally **sphincters** and **dilators** of the oral, nasal and orbital cavities. Consequently, the facial muscles are developed in relation to these cavities. In humans, the sphincters and dilators are best developed around the oral cavity and least around the nares. Many of the muscles whose functions are alimentary and respiratory are used in speech, e.g. the muscles of the lips and cheeks.

All the facial muscles are developed from the second branchial arch and hence derive their motor supply from the facial nerve. During the course of evolution, the facial musculature has gradually differentiated into a number of components which are used for displaying different emotional states.

The sensory innervation of the scalp in front of the ear is by the three divisions of the trigeminal nerve. Both ventral and dorsal rami of cervical nerves supply the skin of the scalp behind the ear. These nerves run in the subcutaneous tissue which is dense and loculated. Hence, any infection of the subcutaneous tissue is localised and painful. Scalp infections are also dangerous since they could spread to the brain via emissary veins. The arteries of the scalp also run in the subcutaneous tissue and anastomose extensively. Injury to these vessels can cause profuse bleeding since their walls are prevented from collapsing by the adherent subcutaneous tissue.

Objectives for Dissection Schedule 25

Topic: Face and scalp

General objective 1

Comprehend the arrangement of the muscles and fasciae of the regions.

Specific objectives

1. Describe attachments of orbicularis oculi, orbicularis oris, buccinator and occipitofrontalis muscles and their actions.
2. Describe the layers of the scalp.
3. Discuss the clinical importance of:
   (a) the mobility of the superficial layers of the scalp on the pericranium;
   (b) the 'dangerous area' of the scalp.

General objective 2

Comprehend the principles of the arrangement of the nerves and blood vessels of the regions.

Specific objectives

1. Outline areas of the face and scalp supplied by the three divisions of the trigeminal nerve and the developmental basis for this arrangement.
2. Enumerate the nerves in each of the above areas.
3. Describe the relationship of the parotid gland to the motor branches of the facial nerve.
4. Discuss the anatomical basis for the clinical differentiation between upper and lower motor neuron types of facial nerve paralysis.
5. Describe the blood supply of the face and scalp emphasising the richness of their vascularity.
6. Discuss the anatomical basis for:
   (a) the spread of infection from the 'dangerous area' of the face into the cranial cavity;
   (b) profuse bleeding from scalp injuries; and
   (c) use of scalp flaps for tube grafts in plastic surgery.

Question for study:

1. At which points on the face can an arterial pulse be readily felt?
2. What is the arterial supply of the scalp? When the scalp is cut, between what layers would blood tend to accumulate? How could bleeding be stopped?
3. By what pathway could an infection of the scalp reach the brain?
4. What is Bell's palsy (facial paralysis)?

Overview of Schedule 26

Before you begin dissection note:

CRANIAL CAVITY

Relevant skeletal features:

skull — vault; inner and outer tables; diplöe.

Anterior cranial fossa:

ethmoid bone — cribriform plate; crista galli;
frontal bone — frontal crest; orbital plates;
sphenoid bone — lesser wing; anterior clinoid process;
foramina — olfactory; anterior and posterior ethmoidal; foramen caecum.

Middle cranial fossa:

sphenoid bone — body; hypophysial fossa; dorsum sellae; posterior clinoid process; basisphenoid; groove for cavernous sinus; greater wing;
temporal bone — anterior surface of petrous part; squamous part; groove for posterior branch of middle meningeal artery and vein;
parietal bone — anteroinferior angle; groove for anterior branch of middle meningeal artery and vein;
foramina — optic canal; superior orbital fissure; foramen rotundum; foramen lacerum; foramen ovale; foramen spinosum; hiatuses for greater and lesser petrosal nerves.

Posterior cranial fossa:

temporal bone — posterior surface of petrous part; squamous part; mastoid part; groove for sigmoid sinus;
occipital bone — groove for superior sagittal sinus; internal occipital protuberance; internal occipital crest; groove for transverse sinus;
parietal bone — posteroinferior angle; groove for sigmoid sinus;

foramina — internal acoustic meatus; jugular foramen; hypoglossal canal; foramen magnum.

Duramater:

outer (endocranial) and inner (meningeal) layers; falx cerebri; falx cerebelli; tentorium cerebelli; diaphragma sellae; cavum trigeminale.

Dural venous sinuses:

superior sagittal sinus; inferior sagittal sinus; straight sinus; occipital sinus sphenoparietal sinus; cavernous sinus (contents of its walls and its venous connections); superior petrosal sinus; inferior petrosal sinus; transverse sinus; sigmoid sinus.

Emissary foramina:

foramen caecum; parietal foramen; mastoid foramen; condylar canal.

Brain:

frontal, parietal, temporal and occipital lobes; diencephalon; three parts of brain stem; cerebellum.

Cranial nerves:

olfactory; optic; oculomotor; trochlear; trigeminal; abducent; facial; nervus intermedius; vestibulocochlear; glossopharyngeal; vagus; accessory; hypoglossal.

Arteries:

middle meningeal (extradural); internal carotid and branches; vertebral; basilar.

Surface anatomy:

middle meningeal artery.

Clinical anatomy:

subdural and extradural haemorrhage; fractures of base of skull.

Dissection Schedule 26

CRANIAL CAVITY

Before embarking on the dissection of the cranial cavity *it is useful to examine and familiarise yourself with the external and cranial cavity features of the skull.* Note the major bones that form the skull, the main sutures, and the fissures and foramina. Note also the main structures that pass through the latter two (see Appendix 1 and 2).

Removal of the brain

1. *Remove the remnants of the scalp. Mark a point 2 cm above the* **superior orbital margin** *in front and another point 2 cm above the* **external occipital protuberance** *behind. Connect these two points by a line passing round the skull. With care use a saw to cut the* **outer table** *of the bone along this line. Observe the* **diplöe** *and then with a chisel and a hammer gently break the* **inner table** *along the saw cut, taking care not to damage the underlying brain and its coverings.*

2. *Remove the vault of the skull and examine the outer layer of* **dura mater** *covering the brain.* This is the periosteum, the **endocranium**, covering the inside of the skull. Deep to this is the *inner layer of dura* which is adherent to the outer layer except where **dural venous sinuses** are situated.

3. *Observe the blood vessels seen on the surface of the dura.* These are the branches of the **middle meningeal artery** and accompanying veins. *Observe the grooves produced by these vessels on the inside of the* **vault**.

4. *Slit open the outer layer of dura in the midline longitudinally and observe the* **superior sagittal sinus** enclosed within the layers of the dura. This venous sinus extends from the **crista galli** in front to the **internal occipital protuberance** at the back. *Correlate the course of the sinus with the longitudinally-running groove in the middle of the inner aspect of the vault. Clean the sinus and note*: (a) the openings of the veins draining the cerebral hemispheres, and (b) projections of the **arachnoid** called **arachnoid granulations** (draining **cerebrospinal fluid**, CSF).

5. *Make an anteroposterior incision through the dura on either side of the superior sagittal sinus and observe the median fold extending between the two* **cerebral hemispheres**. This dural fold, called the **falx cerebri**, is formed by the inner layer of dura.

6. *Cut the anterior attachment of the falx cerebri close to the crista galli and pull it backwards. Observe* that the falx cerebri is sickle shaped and has a free inferior border enclosing the **inferior sagittal sinus** within its layers.

7. *Make a coronal incision in the dura on both sides starting from above the ear and passing towards the midpoint of the falx cerebri. Reflect the four triangular flaps downwards.* Note that the inner surface of the dura is smooth and that both outer and inner layers are fused.

8. *Allow the head to hang over the edge of the table to facilitate the removal of the brain. Pull the* **frontal lobes** *of the cerebral hemispheres gently backwards from the* **anterior cranial fossa**. *Identify and cut the following structures on either side close to the brain*:
   (a) **olfactory nerves** from beneath the **olfactory bulbs** which lie on the **cribriform plate** of the **ethmoid bone** on either side of the crista galli;
   (b) **optic nerves** close to the **optic canals**;
   (c) **internal carotid arteries** immediately behind the optic nerves;
   (d) **infundibulum of the pituitary gland** near the centre of the **hypophysial fossa**;
   (e) **oculomotor nerves** behind and lateral to the infundibulum;
   (f) the slender **trochlear nerves** behind the oculomotor nerves.

   Note that the **occipital lobes** of the brain rest on the **tentorium cerebelli**.

9. *Release the* **temporal lobes** *from the* **middle cranial fossa**. *Pass the knife along the upper surface of the tentorium cerebelli and cut across the* **midbrain** *up to the midline also severing the* **posterior cerebral artery**. *Repeat this procedure on the opposite side. Now the* **cerebrum** *and part of the midbrain can be removed together.* The rest of the **brain stem** and the **cerebellum** are retained in the **posterior cranial fossa**.

10. *Study the attachment of the tentorium cerebelli to the lips of the groove for the* **transverse sinus** *peripherally, the superior border of the* **petrous**

part of the temporal bone *and the* **posterior clinoid process** *medially.* This is the *attached border* of the tentorium. Now turn your attention to the *free border* of the tentorium and *trace its attachment to the* **anterior clinoid process**. *Examine the* **tentorial notch** *occupied by the midbrain.*

11. *Cut the tentorium along its attached margin. Next identify and cut the following structures close to the remaining part of the brain as they are encountered*:
    (a) **trigeminal nerves** near the apices of the petrous part of the temporal bones;
    (b) **abducent nerves** behind and medial to the trigeminal nerves;
    (c) **facial** and **vestibulocochlear nerves** near the **internal acoustic meati**;
    (d) **glossopharyngeal, vagus** and **accessory nerves** opposite the **jugular foramina**;
    (e) **hypoglossal nerves** close to the **hypoglossal canals**.

12. *Lift up the* **pons** *to bring into view* the **medulla oblongata** *and the two* **vertebral arteries** *related to it. Divide the arteries and the medulla oblongata at the level of the* **foramen magnum**. *Now remove the brainstem and cerebellum.*

Anterior Cranial Fossa

1. Note that the **anterior cranial fossa,** which contains the frontal lobe of the brain, is at a higher level than the **middle cranial fossa**. It is limited posteriorly by the sharp free border of the **lesser wings of the sphenoid** laterally and by the groove connecting the two optic canals in the middle.

2. In the midline of the fossa *observe the sharp keel of bone called the crista galli* as well as the raised ridge of bone running upwards on the frontal bone called the **frontal crest**. These give attachment to the falx cerebri.

3. At the junction of the frontal crest and the crista galli note the presence of the **foramen caecum** through which may pass an **emissary vein** connecting the superior sagittal sinus and the veins of the nasal cavity.

4. *Observe the numerous foramina in the cribriform plate on either side of the crista galli*. The olfactory nerves from the nose enter through these foramina to end in the olfactory bulbs which rest on the cribriform plate.

5. Note that the **anterior ethmoidal nerve**, a branch of the **nasociliary nerve**, and the **anterior ethmoidal artery**, a branch of the **ophthalmic artery**, come from the orbit and run along the lateral margin of the cribriform plate to enter the nasal cavity.
6. Note the sharp posterior border of the lesser wing of the sphenoid overhanging the middle cranial fossa. The dura along the free border contains a dural venous sinus called the **sphenoparietal sinus**.
7. *Trace the posterior border of the lesser wing of the sphenoid medially and identify the anterior clinoid process* to which the free border of the tentorium cerebelli is attached.

Middle Cranial Fossa

1. Note that the **middle cranial fossa**, which contains the temporal lobe of the brain, is at a higher level than the posterior cranial fossa. *Observe* that the posterior boundary of this fossa is formed by the sharp superior border of the **petrous temporal bone** posteriorly and the raised area of the **body of the sphenoid** with its **sella turcica** medially.
2. *Identify the optic canal* through which the **optic nerve** and **ophthalmic artery**, a branch of the internal carotid artery, pass into the orbit.
3. *Observe the concave depression in the body of the sphenoid called the sella turcica.* Note the fold of dura mater covering this depression is called the **diaphragma sellae** through which passes the stalk of the pituitary gland. This gland lies in the **pituitary fossa** within the sella turcica. *Dissect out the pituitary gland.* The posterior wall of the sella turcica is formed by the **dorsum sellae**.
4. *Examine the* **cavernous sinus** *situated on either side of the body of the sphenoid and dissect the following cranial nerves embedded in its lateral wall*:
   (a) **oculomotor nerve** which pierces the dura anterior to the crossing of the attached and free borders of the tentorium, slightly lateral to the posterior clinoid process;
   (b) **trochlear nerve** which pierces the dura at the crossing of the free and attached borders of the tentorium;

(c) **ophthalmic division** of the trigeminal nerve which lies below the trochlear nerve;

(d) **maxillary division** of the trigeminal nerve lying below the ophthalmic division.

Trace the latter two nerves backwards to the **trigeminal ganglion** situated in a depression near the apex of the petrous part of the temporal bone. *Cut the fold of dura called the* **cavum trigeminale** *to expose this ganglion.*

5. *Next expose the* **internal carotid artery** *and the* **abducent nerve** lying within the cavernous sinus.

6. *Identify the* **mandibular division** *of the trigeminal nerve arising from the lateral part of the ganglion and leaving the cranial cavity through the* **foramen ovale**.

7. *Peel off the dura over the anterior surface of the petrous part of the temporal bone and look for the* **greater petrosal nerve**, a branch of the **facial nerve** passing laterally beneath the trigeminal ganglion towards the **pterygoid canal**. It is joined by the **deep petrosal nerve** arising from the sympathetic plexus around the internal carotid artery.

8. *Look for the* **lesser petrosal nerve**, a branch of the **glossopharyngeal nerve** running anterolaterally to the greater petrosal nerve to leave the cranial cavity through the foramen ovale.

9. *Look for the* **middle meningeal artery**, a branch of the **maxillary artery**, which enters the middle cranial fossa through the **foramen spinosum** and divides into anterior and posterior branches. The anterior branch runs towards the **pterion** from where it ascends on to the vertex. This branch overlies the *motor area of the brain*. The posterior branch runs backwards and then upwards towards the **lambda**. This branch runs over the *auditory cortex*.

10. *Observe that the middle cranial fossa also lodges the ventral part of the* **diencephalon** *in the middle.*

Posterior Cranial Fossa

1. The **posterior cranial fossa** lodges the cerebellum, a part of the hindbrain. *Identify the following structures in this cranial fossa*:
   (a) **trigeminal nerve** which will be seen evaginating the dura below the tentorium near the apex of the petrous part of the temporal bone. *Look for the small motor root* on its under surface;
   (b) **abducent nerve** where it pierces the dura over the **clivus**;
   (c) **facial nerve** along with the **nervus intermedius**, the **vestibulocochlear nerve** and the **labyrinthine artery**, entering the **internal acoustic meatus**;
   (d) **glossopharyngeal**, **vagus** and **accessory nerves** passing through the middle compartment of the **jugular foramen**. Note that the anterior compartment transmits the **inferior petrosal sinus** while the **sigmoid sinus** passes through the posterior compartment to become the **internal jugular vein**;
   (e) **hypoglossal nerve** lying more medial to the preceding nerves and leaving the cranial fossa through the **hypoglossal canal**;
   (f) **medulla oblongata**, meninges, **vertebral arteries**, and **spinal roots of the accessory nerves** passing through the **foramen magnum**. Note that the vertebral arteries lie in front of the first pair of **ligamenta denticulata** while the spinal roots of the accessory nerves run behind them.

2. *Observe the following dural venous sinuses in the posterior cranial fossa*:
   (a) **superior petrosal sinus** along the superior border of the petrous temporal bone commencing from the posterior end of the cavernous sinus medially and draining into the junction of the transverse and sigmoid sinuses laterally;
   (b) **inferior petrosal sinus** in the groove between the **basiocciput** and the petrous temporal bone. This vein commences from the posterior end of the cavernous sinus and passes downwards through the anterior compartment of the jugular foramen to drain into the internal jugular vein;
   (c) **transverse sinus** lying in the attached margin of the tentorium and extending from the internal occipital protuberance to the base of the petrous temporal bone. Note that the right transverse sinus is a continuation of the superior sagittal sinus;

(d) **straight sinus** running in the junction of the falx cerebri and tentorium cerebelli. Note that it is formed by the union of the inferior sagittal sinus with the **great cerebral vein**. *Trace its continuity into the left transverse sinus*. At the internal occipital protuberance *verify* if there is a communication between the transverse sinuses of the two sides, i.e. **confluence of the sinuses**;

(e) **sigmoid sinus**, the continuation of the transverse sinus, entering the posterior compartment of the jugular foramen to become the internal jugular vein;

(f) **occipital sinus** within the **falx cerebelli**, a fold of dura separating the two cerebellar hemispheres and attached to the **internal occipital crest**. Note that it connects the transverse and sigmoid sinuses. This sinus also communicates with the vertebral venous plexus.

Slit open these sinuses and verify their communications.

Summary

The identification of the cranial nerves becomes easy if one remembers that the nerves arising from the forebrain (olfactory nerves) are found in the anterior cranial fossa, while the optic nerve (also from the forebrain) and the nerves arising from the midbrain (oculomotor and trochlear nerves) *pierce the dura* in the middle cranial fossa. The remaining cranial nerves arise from the pons and medulla of the hindbrain and pierce the dura in the posterior cranial fossa. However, the trigeminal and abducent nerves after piercing the dura in the posterior cranial fossa enter the middle cranial fossa where they are seen in relation to the cavernous sinus and internal carotid artery.

The functional components appear to determine the site at which a particular cranial nerve pierces the dura. Thus somatic efferent nerves, e.g. oculomotor, trochlear, abducent and hypoglossal nerves, pierce the dura close to the midline whereas those having entirely special somatic afferent components, e.g. the vestibulocochlear nerve, pierce the dura most laterally.

The internal carotid artery which supplies the cerebral hemispheres excepting the occipital lobe, has a sinuous course. It passes upwards and forwards through the carotid canal in the petrous part of the temporal bone to enter the middle cranial fossa where it pierces the dura mater and enters the cavernous sinus. It then passes forwards and gives off the important hypophyseal arteries. Thereafter, the internal carotid artery ascends medial to the anterior clinoid process and pierces the roof of the cavernous sinus. After giving off the ophthalmic artery it curves backwards. This tortuous course of the artery, and its passage through the bone and cavernous sinus are possible mechanisms which tend to reduce the pressure in the artery and its branches which supply the brain.

Objectives for Dissection Schedule 26

Topic: Cranial cavity

General objective

Comprehend the arrangement of the structures in the cranial cavity.

Specific objectives

1. Describe the reflections of the dura mater with special reference to the formation of the dural folds, viz. falx cerebri, falx cerebelli, tentorium cerebelli and diaphragma sellae.
2. Identify the major divisions of the forebrain, midbrain, and hindbrain.
3. Identify the twelve cranial nerves as they emerge from the brain and as they pass out of the skull.
4. Describe the formation and course of the dural venous sinuses.
5. Describe the walls and lining of a typical dural venous sinus.
6. Describe the contents of the cavernous sinus.
7. Name the vessels that drain into the cavernous sinus.
8. Describe the general arrangement of the three cranial fossae and enumerate the structures transmitted through the foramina in each fossa.
9. Discuss the anatomical basis of the signs and symptoms of fractures involving the anterior, middle or posterior cranial fossa.
10. What are the possible sequelae of a fracture of:
    (a) the cribriform plate of the ethmoid bone?
    (b) the squamous portion of the temporal bone?
11. Outline the nerve supply and blood supply of the dura mater.
12. Discuss the clinical importance of the middle meningeal artery and its branches.
13. Describe the course of the internal carotid artery from the carotid canal to the base of the brain.

Questions for study:

1. Into what major vein do the dural venous sinuses drain?
2. What is the difference between a diploic vein, an emissary vein and a dural venous sinus?
3. What arteries and nerves supply the meninges surrounding the brain?
4. What is the confluence of the sinuses?
5. By what pathway could (a) an infection on the skin of the cheek pass to the cavernous sinus; and (b) an infection travelling in the retromandibular vein pass to the cavernous sinus?
6. What might be one of the earliest symptoms of cavernous sinus thrombosis? Why?
7. How does cerebrospinal fluid drain into the venous system?

Overview of Schedule 27

Before you begin dissection note:

ORBIT AND LACRIMAL APPARATUS

Relevant skeletal features:

bony orbit — axis;
medial wall — frontal process of the maxilla; lacrimal; orbital plate of the ethmoid; body of the sphenoid;
floor — zygomatic; maxilla; orbital process of the palatine;
lateral wall — zygomatic; greater wing of the sphenoid;
roof — orbital plate of the frontal; lesser wing of the sphenoid;
openings — optic canal; superior orbital fissure; inferior orbital fissure; infraorbital foramen; supraorbital notch or foramen; nasolacrimal canal; anterior ethmoidal foramen; posterior ethmoidal foramen.

Fossa for lacrimal gland.

Fascial sheath of eyeball:

check ligaments; suspensory ligament.

Extraocular muscles:

levator palpebrae superioris; superior rectus; inferior rectus; medial rectus; lateral rectus; superior oblique; inferior oblique.

Nerves:

optic; ophthalmic division of trigeminal (lacrimal, frontal, nasociliary branches); oculomotor; trochlear; abducent; zygomatic; infraorbital; ciliary ganglion.

Arteries:

ophthalmic artery and its branches.

Veins:

superior and inferior ophthalmic.

Lacrimal apparatus:

lacrimal gland; lacrimal ducts; conjunctival sac; lacrimal papilla; lacrimal punctum; lacrimal canaliculus; lacrimal sac; nasolacrimal duct.

Surface anatomy:

supra- and infraorbital foramina.

Clinical anatomy:

spread of infection to cavernous sinus; occlusion of central artery of retina; lesions of ocular motor nerves.

Dissection Schedule 27

ORBIT AND LACRIMAL APPARATUS

1. *With a skull for reference* note that the orbit lies below the anterior cranial fossa and in front of the middle cranial fossa. *Now proceed as follows*:
   (a) *remove the superior wall of the orbit and the supraorbital margin by making two sagittal sawcuts through the frontal bone above the medial and lateral ends of the orbital margin*;
   (b) *carefully remove the supraorbital margin and the orbital plate of the frontal bone with bone forceps so as to expose the orbital periosteum. Take care not to damage the underlying nerves. Remove the bone back to and including the* **lesser wing of the sphenoid bone**. *In this way open the* **superior orbital fissure** *and* **optic canal**;
   (c) *with bone forceps remove the upper half of the lateral orbital margin.*

   See if there is an extension of the **frontal sinus** into the orbital plate.

2. *Remove the orbital periosteum taking care not to damage the nerves which lie immediately beneath it. Identify and clean*:
   (a) the **frontal nerve**, a branch of the ophthalmic division lying on the **levator palpebrae superioris muscle** in the middle of the orbit. *Trace this nerve forwards* where it divides into **supraorbital** and **supratrochlear branches** which have already been noted in the scalp;
   (b) the **trochlear nerve** running along the medial side of the orbit to supply the **superior oblique muscle** of the eyeball on its orbital surface;
   (c) the **lacrimal nerve**, a branch of the ophthalmic division running along the lateral aspect of the orbit.

3. *Clean the levator palpebrae superioris and* **superior rectus muscles**. The latter muscle lies deep to the levator. *Secure the upper division of the* **oculomotor nerve** supplying these muscles on their ocular surface.

4. *Clean the superior oblique muscle situated on the medial side of the orbit.* Note that its tendon passes through a pulley near the superomedial angle of the orbit where it turns backwards to pass deep to the levator palpebrae superioris and superior rectus to be inserted into the **sclera** of the eyeball.

5. *Divide the levator palpebrae superioris and the superior rectus about their middle sparing the overlying frontal nerve. Trace the* **optic nerve** *and the* **ophthalmic artery**. The artery crosses the optic nerve superiorly from the lateral to the medial side.

6. *Identify the* **nasociliary branch** of the ophthalmic division of the trigeminal nerve also crossing the optic nerve superficially from the lateral to the medial side after which it runs between the superior oblique and **medial rectus muscles**. *Clean this nerve and trace its branches*:
   (a) a slender twig to the **ciliary ganglion**. *Make use of this slender twig to try to identify* the ciliary ganglion which lies lateral to the optic nerve at the apex of the orbit. It is of the size of a pin head;
   (b) two **long ciliary nerves** which pass along with the optic nerve to pierce the sclera;
   (c) two **ethmoidal nerves** leaving the medial side of the orbit through the **posterior** and **anterior ethmoidal foramina**;
   (d) the **infratrochlear nerve** passing towards the medial angle of the eye where it supplies the root of the nose and the medial part of the upper eyelid.

7. *Trace the* **short ciliary nerves** *from the ciliary ganglion*. These run above and below the optic nerve towards the eyeball.

8. *Clean and trace the branches of the ophthalmic artery*, most of which are named according to the nerves which they accompany. *Secure the* **central artery of the retina**, the most important branch of the ophthalmic artery. It enters the optic nerve on its inferior surface. Note that it is an end artery.

9. *Secure the* **abducent nerve** running along the ocular surface of the **lateral rectus** to supply it.

10. *Identify the medial rectus muscle*, which lies below the superior oblique, and *trace its nerve supply* from the lower division of the oculomotor nerve.

11. *Cut the optic nerve and turn the eyeball forwards to see the* **inferior rectus muscle**. *Secure the nerve supply to this muscle from the lower division of the oculomotor nerve. Trace a twig from the branch to the inferior oblique towards the ciliary ganglion.*

12. *Observe the origin of the recti from the* **common tendinous ring** which extends between the medial side of the optic canal and the spicule of bone on the inferior margin of the superior orbital fissure. Note the oblique direction of the superior and inferior recti in relation to the axis of the eyeball. *Check the insertions of the recti* which are attached to the sclera *in front* of the **equator**. Note that the medial and lateral recti are anchored to their respective walls of the orbit by fascial thickenings called **check ligaments**.

13. *Observe the origins of the superior oblique and levator palpebrae superioris from the sphenoid medial to and above the optic canal respectively. Follow the tendon of the superior oblique to its insertion into the sclera* in the *upper lateral quadrant* of the eyeball *behind* the equator.

14. *Cut horizontally through the lower eyelid near its margin and lift the eyeball.* Note the origin of the **inferior oblique** from the floor of the orbit just lateral to the **nasolacrimal canal**. Note that the muscle passes below the inferior rectus to reach its insertion on to the sclera *behind* the equator in the *lower lateral quadrant* of the eyeball. *Trace the nerve supply to this muscle* from the inferior division of the oculomotor nerve, which enters it on its posterior border.

15. *Look for the* **lacrimal gland** *in the upper lateral part of the orbit where it causes a bulge in the* **conjunctiva**. *Carefully incise the upper eyelid along the superior orbital margin and divide the conjunctiva* at the **superior conjunctival fornix**. *With care remove the conjunctiva and examine the gland.* Note that some fibres of the levator palpebrae superioris are attached to the conjunctiva. *Trace the remaining part of the muscle into the* **tarsal plate**, the fascia and the skin of the upper eyelid.

16. *Examine the* **medial** *and* **lateral palpebral ligaments** which attach the medial and lateral extremities of the upper and lower tarsal plates to the respective orbital margins.

17. *Dissect carefully in the medial angle of the eye and identify the* **lacrimal sac** *lying in a depression called the* **lacrimal fossa** *on the medial wall of the orbit.*

18. *Define the attachment of the lacrimal part of the orbicularis oculi muscle to the posterior margin of the lacrimal fossa.*

19. *Remove the eyeball on one side and strip the periosteum off the floor of the orbit.* Note the **infraorbital nerve** and **artery** lying in the **infraorbital canal**.

Summary

The fascial sheath covering the eyeball, known as the **fascia bulbi**, extends up to the **sclerocorneal junction**. This fascial sheath is prolonged along the tendons to surround the muscle bellies of the recti.

From the lateral and medial recti, fascial extensions are attached to the adjacent parts of the orbit giving rise to the **check ligaments** which prevent undue backward displacement and compression of the eyeball. Between these check ligaments, the inferior part of the fascial covering of the eyeball is thickened so that it suspends the eyeball like a hammock. This is known as the **suspensory ligament**. Thus, the eyeball does not rest on the floor of the orbit.

All the extraocular muscles are supplied by the oculomotor nerve, except the superior oblique which is supplied by the trochlear nerve and the lateral rectus which is supplied by the abducens nerve — (LR6 SO4)3.

The action of the extraocular muscles are complicated. They provide the finer adjustments of the eyeball for visual activity whereas coarse adjustments are produced by reflex movements of the head and neck in the required direction.

In the neutral position with the visual axis directed forwards, the medial and lateral recti produce direct medial and lateral movements of the eyeball. The superior and inferior recti are, however, not simple elevators and depressors only. They cross the equator from the back to the front and their direction is oblique since they travel *forwards* and *laterally*. Hence, both superior and inferior recti also cause *medial deviation* of the globe. The superior and inferior oblique muscles cross the equator from the *front to the back* and their direction is also oblique since they travel *backwards* and *laterally*. Their oblique pull thus causes a *lateral deviation* in addition to their actions of depression and elevation respectively. Hence, in the normal movements it is said that the superior rectus acts in concert with the inferior oblique muscle of the same eye to produce the desired movement of pure elevation, while the inferior rectus in combination with superior oblique produces pure depression.

The structures passing through the superior orbital fissure deserve attention as this fissure is the passageway for a large number of structures entering or leaving the orbit. The fissure is divided by the common tendinous ring into three parts. The part above and lateral to the ring transmits the lacrimal, frontal and trochlear nerves and the superior ophthalmic vein. Within the ring and between the two heads of the lateral rectus pass the two divisions of the oculomotor nerve, and the nasociliary and abducent nerves. Below the ring lies the inferior ophthalmic vein.

The ciliary ganglion is a relay station for parasympathetic fibres reaching the ganglion via the oculomotor nerve. From the ganglion the short ciliary nerves run forward to supply the **ciliary muscle** concerned with accommodation and the **sphincter pupillae muscle** which constricts the pupil.

The lacrimal gland receives its secretomotor fibres from the **pterygopalatine ganglion** which receives *preganglionic fibres* via the greater petrosal branch of the facial nerve.

Objectives for Dissection Schedule 27

Topic: Orbit and lacrimal apparatus

General objective

Comprehend the arrangement of the structures in the orbit.

Specific objectives

1. Describe the constitution of the four walls of the bony orbit.
2. Describe the arrangement of orbital fat and orbital fascia.
3. Describe the origins and insertions of the extraocular muscles.
4. Define the visual axis and illustrate the actions of these muscles.
5. Summarise the sensory and motor nerves in the orbit and deduce the effects of lesions of the third, fourth and sixth cranial nerves both alone and in combination.
6. Discuss the clinical importance of:
   (a) the venous drainage of the orbit;
   (b) the central artery of the retina.
7. Identify, on a living subject, the surface anatomy features of the eye, eyelids, and lacrimal apparatus.
8. Describe the lacrimal apparatus, including the mechanisms by which tears are produced and drained via the puncta, lacrimal canaliculi, lacrimal sac and nasolacrimal duct.
9. Give an account of the distribution and function of each major branch of the ophthalmic division of the trigeminal nerve.

Questions for study:

1. Where would one find the superior tarsal muscle? What is its function? What is its innervation?

2. What structures pass through (a) the superior orbital fissure; (b) the optic foramen?

3. How would you test for the integrity of the trochlear nerve and the abducent nerve?

Overview of Schedule 28

Before you begin dissection note:

THE EYE

Relevant features:

outer coat — cornea, sclera;
middle coat — choroid, ciliary body; ciliary muscle and its nerve supply; iris, its muscles and their nerve supply;
inner coat — retina and its parts;
arterial supply — central artery of the retina;
anterior chamber;
posterior chamber;
lens;
aqueous humor;
vitreous body.

Dissection Schedule 28

THE EYEBALL

You will be unable to obtain a clear idea of the internal structure of the eyeball from the eyes of the cadaver you are dissecting. *You should therefore examine the fresh eyeball of an ox.*

Dissection of the eyeball of an ox

1. *Make also full use of demonstration material.*
2. *Students should work in pairs.* Each group should be provided with two ox eyes.
3. *Remove the muscles, fat, fascia, and* **conjunctiva** *from the ox's eyeball* with which you have been provided. *This is best done with a pair of scissors, starting behind where the* **optic nerve** *pierces the outer coat of the eyeball* (*the* **sclera**), *and working forward and round the globe.*
4. The centre of the cornea in front is called the **anterior pole** of the eyeball; the corresponding point at the back of the eyeball is the **posterior pole**; the line joining the poles coincides with the **optic axis** of the eyeball.
5. *One eye should be divided sagittally and the other equatorially* (*coronally*). *Examine the sections, and notice that there are three coats*:
   (a) an outer protective coat, formed by the **sclera** or "white" of the eye in the posterior five-sixths and the transparent **cornea** in the anterior sixth;
   (b) an intermediate vascular and pigmented coat, the **choroid**, which continues anteriorly into the **ciliary body** and **iris**;
   (c) a delicate nervous inner layer, the **retina**. This innermost coat is so thin that it tears with the slightest touch, and will be found to be opaque and wrinkled from the action of preservative agents.

   These three coats enclose three refractive media: the **aqueous humor**, the **crystalline lens** and **vitreous body** from before backwards.

Now examine these features more closely:

1. The **sclera** is reinforced posteriorly by the sheath of the optic nerve and anteriorly it joins with the cornea at the **sclerocorneal junction**.

2. The **cornea** is thicker near the sclerocorneal junction than at the **anterior pole** of the eye. Both parts of the outer coat are made of fibrous tissue, but in front all the component elements of this tissue have the same refractive index, and so the cornea is transparent. The cornea is covered in front with a layer of stratified epithelium directly continuous with the **conjunctiva**.

3. *If the sclerocorneal junction is examined carefully with a hand-lens, the small* **venous sinus of the sclera (canal of Schlemm)** *will be seen cut in section.* This venous sinus drains excess aqueous humor from the anterior chamber of the eye (see below).

4. The **choroid coat** is continued forwards into the iris and is pigmented. Posteriorly, it is perforated by the optic nerve, while anteriorly, it becomes folded to form the **ciliary body** (to be noted later) just before it joins the iris. It is essentially a vascular coat.

5. The **iris** is the diaphragm which — by varying the size of its opening, the **pupil** — can regulate the amount of light admitted to the eye. It lies very close to and just in front of the lens, although there is a small triangular space known as the **posterior chamber** of the eye between the two, which is bounded peripherally by the bases of the **ciliary processes**. *It is thus seen that only the pupillary margin of the iris is in contact with the lens capsule.* The **anterior chamber** of the eye lies between the cornea and the iris, and is about 3 mm from before backwards. These two chambers contain the **aqueous humor**.

6. *The* **retina** *is seen as a delicate, whitish membrane which easily separates from the choroid*, especially when the vitreous humour is removed. A similar "detachment of the retina" sometimes occurs in life as the result of a blow on the eye. Note that the whole of the retina is not present in the delicate white membrane, which is the true nervous layer, **pars optica retinae**, because there is a layer of cells containing a black pigment which developmentally belongs to the retina, but is left behind on the choroid when the retina separates from it. This pigmented layer, lined internally by columnar epithelium, is continued forwards over the inner surface of the ciliary processes. Here the epithelial cells play an important part in the secretion of the aqueous humor; this part of the retina is known as the

pars ciliaris retinae. On the back of the iris, the black pigment layer, together with the columnar cells, here also pigmented, is very marked and is called the **pars iridica retinae**. Where the inner nervous layer of the retina ends, i.e. at the junction of the pars optica and pars ciliaris retinae, it presents a scalloped edge, the **ora serrata**.

7. The **lens** in the dissecting laboratory is opaque, especially if it has been treated with spirit. It is enclosed in a structureless capsule, but this is not visible to the naked eye. In section it is biconvex, with the anterior surface a good deal flatter than the posterior. It is about 8 mm in diameter. The **vitreous body** fills the cavity of the eyeball behind the lens; it has the consistency of very thin jelly, and is enclosed by a delicate membrane called the **hyaloid membrane**. Extending from the back of the ciliary body to the margin of the lens all round its circumference is a membrane formed of fine radiating fibres which splits to enclose the lens. The anterior is the stronger of the two layers formed by the splitting and passes in front of the lens to blend with its capsule. It is known as the **suspensory ligament of the lens**, and, when the ciliary processes are drawn forward, it relaxes and allows the front of the lens to become more convex through its own elasticity. The posterior layer of the splitting continues to enclose the vitreous body, and lies in close contact with the back of the lens. Running right through the vitreous body from the entrance of the optic nerve to the middle of the back of the lens is the **hyaloid canal**. In the fetus this canal transmits a branch from the retinal artery to the back of the lens.

8. *Now take the posterior half of the eyeball which was divided transversely, and scoop out the* **vitreous body** *as gently and as carefully as possible. It will be seen to retain its shape if it is placed in a vessel of water due to the hyaloid membrane and to a minute and very delicate network in its interior. On examining the retina*, preferably with a magnifying lens, the **optic disc** will be seen opposite the point where the optic nerve enters (3 mm to the medial or nasal side of the **posterior pole of the eye**). It is a circular disc only 1.5 mm across, and in its centre the **retinal artery** breaks up into radiating branches supplying the retina. The variations in the appearance of the disc are of great clinical importance and may be examined with an ophthalmoscope in the living subject. The optic disc, which consists only of nerve fibres, corresponds to the "**blind spot**" of the eye.

9. Having removed the vitreous body from the eyeball note that there is no **macula lutea** (yellow spot) in the ox, since this only occurs in animals which use their eyes for binocular vision. On the other hand, an iridescent colouring, not found in humans, is present in the eye of the ox. This is caused by a layer of fine connective tissue fibres on the inner aspect of the choroid known as the **tapetum**. It is more particularly observed in nocturnal animals, especially in carnivores, and is the cause of the glare seen in the eye of a cat or dog, for example, in the dark.

10. *In the anterior half of the eye remove the vitreous humour and trace the retina forwards.* As already noted, a little behind the region of the ciliary body its nervous elements end in the scalloped edge called the ora serrata, though a pigmented and epithelial layer is continued forwards as the pars ciliaris and pars iridica retinae over the back of the ciliary processes and iris.

11. *Carefully remove the lens.* The ciliary body can now be seen from behind. The pigment of the retina which covers it makes it look black.

12. The ciliary processes form a delicate fringe of vascular glomeruli which is present on the convex surface of the ciliary body.

13. *Next cut through the cornea close to the sclerocorneal junction three-quarters of the way round and open it like a lid.* Lining the back of the cornea is the **posterior limiting membrane**, *which may be peeled away from the cut edge for a little*, and is continued on to the front of the iris as a series of delicate ridges with spaces in between. This is the **pectinate ligament**, and the spaces are the **spaces of the iridocorneal angle** (filtration angle). It is here that the aqueous humor, which is secreted at the surface of the ciliary body, percolates into the adjacent venous sinus of the sclera.

14. *The* **iris** *can now be seen from the front and back.* Behind, the iris has the black pigment of the pars iridica retinae, but seen from the front its colour may range from dark brown to light blue, according to the amount of interstitial pigment which is deposited in the stroma of the iris. The iris contains circular (**sphincter pupillae muscle**) and radiating (**dilator pupillae muscle**) muscular fibres, but they are impossible to demonstrate macroscopically.

15. *Lastly, in the ox eye, which was bisected sagitally, examine the cut surface carefully with a hand-lens to see the* **ciliary muscle** rising from the sclerocorneal junction, close to the venous sinus of the sclera, and running backwards into the ciliary body in a fan-like manner. Internal to these are some circular fibres, but it is very difficult to make them out without a microscope.

Summary

The eye is a highly specialised sense organ designed to transmit visual stimuli to the brain. An optical system of transparent refracting media brings images of external objects to focus on a complex light-sensitive membrane, the retina, at the back of the eyeball. From here nerve fibres pass to the brain through the optic nerve, conveying information about the images that have been received. Other parts of the eye are responsible for the focussing of the optical system, and for controlling the amount of light falling on the retina.

Note that:

(a) The **ciliary muscle** is supplied by preganglionic fibres from the oculomotor nerve which relay in the ciliary ganglion and continue as postganglionic **parasympathetic** fibres in the short ciliary nerves. The muscle draws the choroid forwards and slackens the suspensory ligament of the lens so that the lens can become more convex in accommodating for near vision.

(b) The **sphincter pupillae muscle** is supplied by preganglionic fibres from the oculomotor nerve which relay in the ciliary ganglion and continue as postganglionic **parasympathetic** fibres in the short ciliary nerves. The muscle contracts the pupil.

(c) The **dilator pupillae muscle** is supplied by preganglionic fibres from the first thoracic segment of the spinal cord which relay in the superior cervical ganglion and continue as postganglionic **sympathetic** fibres in the long ciliary nerves. The muscle enlarges the pupil.

Objectives for Dissection Schedule 28

Topic: The eye

General objective

Comprehend the arrangement of the layers and structures in the eye.

Specific objectives

1. Describe the layers of the eye.
2. Describe the smooth muscles in the eye and their innervation.
3. Describe the circulation of the aqueous humor.
4. What is the importance of the central artery of the retina?

Questions for study:

1. What is the difference between the orbital axis and the visual (optic) axis? How does this difference affect the way in which the individual extraocular muscles are tested?
2. What is diplopia?
3. What are the major features of the following reflexes:
   (a) the light reflex;
   (b) the accommodation reflex; and
   (c) the blink reflex?
4. What is glaucoma?
5. What is cataract?

Overview of Schedule 29

Before you begin dissection note:

PAROTID AND INFRATEMPORAL REGIONS AND TEMPOROMANDIBULAR JOINT

PAROTID AND INFRATEMPORAL REGIONS

Relevant skeletal features:

mandible — body; mylohyoid line and groove; mental foramen; angle; ramus; condylar process (head); neck; pterygoid fovea; coronoid process; mandibular notch; lingula; mandibular foramen;

temporal bone — squamous part; tympanic plate; styloid process; zygomatic process; external acoustic meatus; mastoid process; stylomastoid foramen; squamotympanic and petrotympanic fissures; mandibular fossa; articular tubercle;

sphenoid bone — greater wing; infratemporal crest; lateral and medial pterygoid plates; scaphoid fossa; spine; foramen ovale; foramen spinosum;

maxilla — tuberosity; posterior surface.

pterygomaxillary fissure; pterygopalatine fossa.

Deep fascia:

capsule of parotid gland.

Ligaments:

stylomandibular; sphenomandibular.

Parotid gland:

surfaces and relations; duct; facial nerve and branches; retromandibular vein; external carotid artery; lymph nodes; nerve supply of the gland.

Muscles:

masseter; temporalis; pterygoids.

Nerves:

mandibular and branches; chorda tympani; maxillary and branches; facial and branches.

Arteries:

external carotid; superficial temporal; maxillary and branches.

Veins:

retromandibular; pterygoid plexus.

Surface anatomy:

parotid duct.

Clinical anatomy:

facial palsy; parotid infections; parotid tumours.

TEMPOROMANDIBULAR JOINT

Muscles in relation to capsule:

lateral pterygoid.

Capsule:

attachments.

Ligaments:

lateral ligament.

Accessory ligaments:

sphenomandibular; stylomandibular.

Intraarticular structures:

articular disc.

Synovial membrane:

reflection.

Movements:

protraction; retraction; elevation; depression; side-to-side movements.

Nerve supply:

auriculotemporal; masseteric.

Blood supply:

superficial temporal artery.

Clinical anatomy:

dislocation; mandibular nerve palsy.

Dissection Schedule 29

PAROTID AND INFRATEMPORAL REGIONS AND TEMPOROMANDIBULAR JOINT

PAROTID AND INFRATEMPORAL REGIONS

1. *Remove the superficial layer of the deep cervical fascia covering the* **parotid gland**. Note that the gland lies below the **zygomatic arch**, in front of the **mastoid process** and **sternocleidomastoid muscle** and behind the **ramus of the mandible** which it overlaps. *Observe that a portion of the gland tissue lies above the* **parotid duct** over the surface of the masseter muscle. This is the **accessory parotid gland**. *Trace the duct forwards* and note that it pierces the **buccinator muscle** to open into the **vestibule of the mouth** opposite the **crown of the upper second molar tooth**.

2. *Try to look for lymph nodes* on the superficial surface of the gland.

3. *Remove the substance of the gland piecemeal and trace the following structures from superficial to deep*:
   (a) the branches of the **facial nerve** proximally to the parent trunk. Note that there are communications between the branches of the facial, **auriculotemporal** and **great auricular nerves**;
   (b) the **retromandibular vein** formed by the union of the **superficial temporal** and **maxillary veins**;
   (c) the **external carotid artery** which ends by dividing into the **superficial temporal** and **maxillary branches** at the level of the **neck of the mandible**.

4. *Remove the remains of the gland and study its deep relations formed by the* **styloid process, tympanic plate** *and* **posterior belly of the digastric muscle**. Note that the space occupied by the gland is wedge shaped and consequently the gland has lateral, anteromedial and posteromedial surfaces. It also has an upper and lower pole. *Observe the* **stylomandibular ligament** extending between the styloid process and the **angle of the mandible** and forming the lower limit of the gland.

5. *Clean the* **masseter muscle** arising from the zygomatic arch and gaining insertion into the outer surface of the ramus of the mandible. Note the

direction of the muscle fibres. *Cut the zygomatic arch at its root and anteriorly through the* **temporal process of the zygomatic bone** *using a saw and bone forceps. Reflect the cut arch and attached masseter muscle downwards.* Note the **mandibular notch.**

6. *Trace the insertion of the* **temporalis muscle** *into the* **coronoid process.**

7. *Cut the coronoid process along with the insertion of the temporalis and reflect the muscle upwards.* Note the deep temporal vessels and nerves running deep to the muscle. *Observe* that the anterior fibres of the muscle are vertical while the posterior fibres are almost horizontal.

8. *Remove the ramus of the mandible by two saw cuts, one through the* **neck of the mandible** *and the other, a shallow cut, obliquely across the body just anterior to the angle of the mandible. Carefully nibble away the bone between the two cuts with bone forceps so as to expose the contents of the* **mandibular canal.** *Remove the fragments of the ramus and thereby gain access to the* **infratemporal region.**

9. *Identify and carefully clean the following branches of the* **mandibular division of the trigeminal nerve:**
   (a) the **inferior alveolar nerve** entering the **mandibular foramen** together with the **inferior alveolar vessels.** Note that the nerve appears below the lower border of the **lateral pterygoid muscle** and gives off the **mylohyoid nerve** posteriorly, which pierces the **sphenomandibular ligament;**
   (b) the **lingual nerve** in front of the inferior alveolar nerve and running downwards and forwards on the **medial pterygoid muscle;**
   (c) the **buccal nerve** emerging between the two heads of the lateral pterygoid muscle and running forwards to pierce the **buccinator.** It supplies the mucous membrane of the cheek.

10. *Clean the pterygoid muscles and study their attachments. Observe* the origin of the *upper head* of the **lateral pterygoid muscle** from the roof of the infratemporal fossa and the *lower head* from the lateral surface of the **lateral pterygoid plate.** *Trace the fibres of the muscle backwards to their insertion* into the front of the neck of the mandible. The additional insertion of this muscle into the capsule and articular disc of the **temporomandibular joint** will be seen later.

11. *Now clean* the large *deep head* of the **medial pterygoid muscle** arising from the medial surface of the lateral pterygoid plate and the smaller *superficial head* from the **tuberosity of the maxilla**. *Follow the muscle downwards, backwards and laterally to its insertion* into the medial surface of the **angle of the mandible** and the adjoining area.

12. *Identify the* **maxillary artery** and note that its course is divided into three parts by the lateral pterygoid muscle. The second part of the artery may pass either deep or superficial to this muscle.

13. *On one side carefully remove the lateral pterygoid muscle leaving behind a small portion of the muscle close to its insertion into the neck of the mandible.*

14. *Clean the maxillary artery*. In its *first* part it gives off several branches of which the main ones are:
    (a) the **middle meningeal artery** entering the middle cranial fossa through the **foramen spinosum**. Note that the artery ascends between the two roots of the **auriculotemporal nerve**;
    (b) the **inferior alveolar artery** entering the mandibular foramen in company with the **inferior alveolar nerve** after giving off the **mylohyoid branch**. In the mandibular canal, the nerve supplies branches to the mandible and all the lower teeth. Its terminal part, the **mental nerve**, passes through the mental foramen and has already been seen;
    (c) other branches supply parts of the external ear, the middle ear and dura mater.

    The *first part* of the maxillary artery lies deep to the neck of the mandible, the *second part,* associated with the lateral pterygoid muscle, supplies the masseter, temporalis, pterygoid and buccinator muscles, and the *third part* of the artery enters the pterygopalatine fossa.

15. Note that the veins accompanying the branches of the maxillary artery form a plexus known as the **pterygoid plexus**. The plexus communicates with the **cavernous sinus** mainly through the **foramen ovale** and **foramen lacerum**. It also communicates with the **facial vein**.

TEMPOROMANDIBULAR JOINT

16. *Examine the* **temporomandibular joint** *on the same side where the lateral pterygoid has been removed. As you proceed with your dissection again verify the attachment of the tendon of the later pterygoid* to the neck of the mandible, the capsule and articular disc. *Clean the fibrous capsule* and note that it has a thickened **lateral ligament** which stretches downwards and backwards between the zygoma and the neck of the mandible.

17. *Open the joint cavity by cutting across the joint capsule and observe that it is subdivided into two parts by means of an* **articular disc** which is concavoconvex above to adapt to the **mandibular fossa** situated in the **squamous part of the temporal bone**. Note that the articular disc is attached anteriorly and posteriorly to the capsule and to the medial and lateral sides of the head of the mandible. *Now remove the head of the mandible.*

18. *Trace the auriculotemporal nerve from behind the joint to its origin from the mandibular nerve.* Note that it splits around the middle meningeal artery.

19. *Trace the* **chorda tympani nerve**, a branch of the facial nerve emerging from the **petrotympanic fissure** and joining the **lingual nerve** on its upper posterior aspect.

20. Note that the following additional branches are given off from the trunk of the mandibular division of the trigeminal nerve:
    (a) a **meningeal branch** which enters the cranial cavity through the foramen spinosum;
    (b) the **nerve to the medial pterygoid**.

Deep dissection of infratemporal fossa

21. *Clean the lateral surface of the lateral pterygoid plate on the same side where the lateral pterygoid muscle had previously been removed. Next remove the lateral plate and the medial pterygoid muscle with a bone foreceps. Cut the lingual and inferior alveolar nerves close to their origin and reflect the mandibular nerve trunk. Try to find the* **otic ganglion** which

lies on the medial side of the mandibular nerve trunk. *Carefully clean the exposed area.*

22. *Now identify the triangular* **tensor veli palatini muscle** which is attached to the base of the skull and lies on the side of the pharynx medial to the medial pterygoid muscle. The tensor veli palatini is supplied by the mandibular nerve.

23. *Follow the maxillary artery towards the* **pterygomaxillary fissure** *where it enters the pterygopalatine fossa* (the *third part* of the artery) to break up into the **infraorbital, posterior superior alveolar**, and branches supplying the pharynx, palate, nose, etc. Note that the infraorbital artery enters the orbit through the **inferior orbital fissure** together with the **infraorbital nerve**. The posterior superior alveolar branches enter the posterior surface of the maxilla along with the **posterior superior alveolar branches of the maxillary nerve**.

24. *Try to identify the* **maxillary nerve** *in the upper part of the pterygomaxillary fissure and trace its infraorbital and superior alveolar branches* which accompany the corresponding branches of the maxillary artery.

Summary

In the *parotid region*, the most important structure is the *facial nerve* which passes through the substance of the parotid gland. As the nerve lies superficial to the blood vessels, the nerve can be damaged before any serious bleeding is noticed during parotid surgery. Injury to the facial nerve produces a condition known as facial palsy which results in flaccid paralysis of the facial muscles. In this condition, the patient is unable to close the eyes and there is drooping of the angle of the mouth with dripping of saliva.

The *muscles of mastication* produce movements of the mandible and are consequently attached to this bone. Note that the pterygoids, temporalis and masseter — which are the muscles of mastication — are all attached to the ramus of the mandible. The medial and lateral pterygoid muscles which cause side-to-side movement of the lower jaw have a lateral inclination while passing from their origin to their insertion on to the mandible. Thus, the pterygoids of one side are able to protrude the lower jaw and rotate the chin to the opposite side. The attachment of the tendon of the lateral pterygoid to the articular disc and neck of the mandible ensures that the articular disc is also drawn forward, as the jaw is protracted by the contraction of this muscle so that the condyle can rest within the concavity of the disc. It must also be noted that both temporomandibular joints act in unison, i.e. they act as a single joint.

All muscles of mastication are developed from the *first branchial arch* and are therefore supplied by the *mandibular nerve* which is the nerve of the first arch. The mandibular nerve divides into anterior and posterior divisions after its exit through the foramen ovale. The branches of the anterior division are all motor except for the buccal branch, which is sensory, while the branches of the posterior division are all sensory except for the mylohyoid nerve, which supplies the mylohyoid and the anterior belly of the digastric muscle.

Objectives for Dissection Schedule 29

Topic: Parotid gland

General objective

Comprehend the clinical importance of a knowledge of the parotid gland.

Specific objectives

1. Define the surfaces of the gland and parotid 'bed'.
2. Describe the relations of the gland.
3. Describe the fascial relation of the gland.
4. Enumerate the structures inside the gland from superficial to deep stressing the importance of this arrangement in parotid surgery.

Topic: Infratemporal region and temporomandibular joint

General objective 1

Comprehend the arrangement of the nerves and blood vessels of the region.

Specific objectives

1. Compare the formation of the mandibular nerve trunk to that of a mixed spinal nerve.
2. Enumerate the branches from the trunk and divisions of the mandibular nerve.
3. Enumerate the main branches of the first two parts of the maxillary artery.
4. Analyse the role of the pterygoid venous plexus in the spread of sepsis into the cranial cavity.

General objective 2

Comprehend the functional anatomy of the temporomandibular joint.

Specific objectives

1. Define the articular surface of the condylar process of the mandible and the mandibular fossa.

2. Describe the capsule of the joint.
3. Ascribe the functional roles to:
   (a) the articular disc and the reciprocally concavoconvex nature of the articular surfaces;
   (b) the sphenomandibular and stylomandibular ligaments.
4. Deduce the line of pull of:
   (a) the vertical and horizontal fibres of the temporalis;
   (b) the medial pterygoid; lateral pterygoid and masseter.
5. Define the muscles taking part in protraction, retraction, elevation, depression and side-to-side movements of the mandible.
6. Discuss the functional significance of Hilton's law as applied to the joint with special reference to proprioception.
7. Describe the innervation of the teeth and gingivae.
8. Give an account of the chorda tympani.
9. Describe the innervation of the buccal mucosa and of the lower teeth.

Questions for study:

1. The parotid fascia is an upward continuation of which layer of deep fascia in the neck?
2. Why are infections of the parotid gland, such as mumps, so painful? What nerves are involved?
3. Why is the buccinator muscle referred to as an accessory muscle of mastication? To which other important muscle is it attached?
4. What structures must be avoided during surgical dissection of the parotid gland?
5. What is trismus?
6. During what movement is the mandible most easily dislocated?
7. Where would a dentist inject in order to anaesthetise the lower teeth?

8. Which branch of the trigeminal nerve receives cutaneous sensation from (a) the upper lip; (b) the dorsum of the nose; (c) the chin; and (d) the upper eyelid?
9. Which branch of the trigeminal nerve supplies general sensory innervation to: (a) the cornea; (b) the lower second molar tooth (c) the upper central incisor tooth; (d) the mucosa of the lateral wall of the nose; and (e) the mucosal lining of the cheek?
10. Which muscles are innervated by the motor root of the trigeminal nerve? How can this nerve be tested?
11. Which branch of the trigeminal nerve supplies the temporomandibular joint?
12. How could an infection involving the buccal pad of fat spread to the cavernous sinus?

Overview of Schedule 30

Before you begin dissection note:

SUBMANDIBULAR REGION AND DEEP DISSECTION OF THE NECK

SUBMANDIBULAR REGION

Relevant skeletal features:

mandible — lower border; digastric fossa; superior and inferior mental spines;
hyoid bone — body; lesser and greater horns;
temporal bone — mastoid and styloid processes.

Ligaments:

stylohyoid ligament.

Submandibular gland:

surfaces; relations; duct; nerve supply.

Muscles:

digastric; mylohyoid; hyoglossus; genioglossus; geniohyoid; styloglossus; middle and superior constrictors of pharynx.

Nerves:

lingual; inferior alveolar; facial; glossopharyngeal; hypoglossal; submandibular ganglion.

Arteries:

facial; lingual.

Veins:

facial; retromandibular.

Surface anatomy:

facial artery.

Clinical anatomy:

salivary calculi; veins and lymph nodes in relation to submandibular gland.

DEEP DISSECTION OF THE NECK

Relevant skeletal features:

cervical vertebrae — transverse processes; foramina transversaria;
first rib — head; neck; shaft; scalene tubercle.

Deep fascia:

prevertebral.

Muscles:

sternocleidomastoid; scalenus anterior; scalenus medius and scalenus posterior.

Nerves:

glossopharyngeal; vagus; accessory; hypoglossal; sympathetic trunk; cervical plexus; phrenic.

Arteries:

common carotid and level of bifurcation; internal carotid; external carotid; subclavian; vertebral; thyrocervical trunk.

Veins:

internal jugular; subclavian; brachiocephalic; vertebral.

Lymphatic ducts:

thoracic; right lymphatic.

Surface anatomy:

apex of lung and pleura; carotid arteries; subclavian artery; accessory nerve.

Clinical anatomy:

fascial spaces of neck; jugular venous pulse; vertebrobasilar insufficiency; thoracic duct at the root of the neck.

Dissection Schedule 30

SUBMANDIBULAR REGION AND DEEP DISSECTION OF THE NECK

SUBMANDIBULAR REGION

1. *Clean the two bellies of the* **digastric muscle** and note that the *posterior belly* arises from the **mastoid notch** of the temporal bone. The origin of the *anterior belly* from the **digastric fossa** of the mandible has already been noted. *Follow the two bellies to their intermediate tendon* which is attached to the hyoid bone by a loop of fibrous tissue. The nerve supply to the posterior belly comes from the facial nerve and to the anterior belly from the mylohyoid branch of the inferior alveolar nerve.

2. *Clean the* **stylohyoid muscle** which arises from the styloid process and runs along the upper border of the posterior belly of the digastric to be inserted into the hyoid bone. The nerve supply to this muscle comes from the facial nerve.

3. *Detach the anterior belly of the digastric from its origin and clean the* **mylohyoid muscle** *which arises from the* **mylohyoid line** *of the mandible* and is inserted into a median raphe and also into the hyoid bone. *Observe that the muscle has a free posterior border.* Its nerve supply comes from the mylohyoid nerve.

4. Note that the **facial vein** is joined by the anterior branch of the **retromandibular vein** and lies superficial to the **submandibular gland**. The facial vein drains into the **internal jugular vein**.

5. *Clean the submandibular gland and observe* that the major (superficial) part of the gland lies on the mylohyoid muscle while the deep portion passes deep to the muscle by curving round its posterior border. Note that the facial artery lies in a groove in the posterior part of the gland. *Trace the artery* as it descends between the gland and the mandible to appear at the anteroinferior angle of the masseter *where its pulsation can be felt in the living.*

6. *Now displace the gland laterally and carefully cut and reflect the thin mylohyoid muscle from the* **mandible** *to expose the* **hyoglossus** *and the* **genioglossus muscles**. *Define the origin of the hyoglossus* from the greater

horn as well as from the body of the hyoid bone and *its insertion* into the posterior part of the side of the tongue. *Observe that the* **genioglossus** *arises from the upper* **mental spine** from where it fans out to be inserted into the whole length of the tongue close to the midline. The most inferior fibres are inserted into the hyoid bone. Below the genioglossus, *identify the* **geniohyoid muscle** passing from the inferior mental spine to the hyoid bone.

7. *Clean the structures which lie on the hyoglossus muscle.* These are from above downwards:
   (a) the **lingual nerve**;
   (b) the **submandibular ganglion** suspended from the lingual nerve;
   (c) the **submandibular duct**;
   (d) the **hypoglossal nerve**.

   Note that the deep part of the submandibular gland also lies on the hyoglossus muscle. *Trace the lingual nerve* and note that it crosses the submandibular duct superficially and then recrosses the duct on its deep aspect further forwards.

8. *Identify and trace the* **styloglossus** muscle which takes origin from near the tip of the styloid process and the **stylohyoid ligament** and runs downwards and forwards to be inserted into the whole length of the side of the tongue. The nerve supply to the styloglossus, hyoglossus and genioglossus muscles comes from the **hypoglossal nerve**. *C1 fibres running along with the hypoglossal nerve supply the geniohyoid and thyrohyoid muscles.*

9. *Carefully cut the hyoglossus from the hyoid bone, raise the muscle upwards and trace the* **lingual artery**. Note that the course of the lingual artery is divided into three parts by the hyoglossus muscle. After giving off the **dorsal lingual branches** the artery continues as the **deep artery of the tongue**. *Identify the* **middle constrictor muscle of the pharynx** on which the proximal part of the lingual artery lies.

10. *Observe that the facial artery lies first on the middle constrictor and then on the* **superior constrictor muscle of the pharynx** where it gives off its **tonsillar branch** before reaching the posterior part of the submandibular gland.

DEEP DISSECTION OF THE NECK

11. *Trace the* **internal jugular vein** *downwards to the root of the neck* where it forms a dilatation known as the **inferior bulb**. *Observe* that this vein is joined by the **subclavian vein** to form the **brachiocephalic vein**. At the junction of the internal jugular and subclavian veins, *look for the entry of the* **thoracic duct** on the *left* side and the **right lymphatic duct** on the *right.*

12. *Cut the internal jugular vein near its termination and lift it upwards.* Note that the cervical part of the thoracic duct commences on the left side of the **oesophagus** and runs behind the **carotid sheath** to arch forwards in front of the subclavian artery, after which it descends to its termination.

13. *Divide the common carotid artery at the root of the neck and turn it upwards. Examine the subclavian artery* whose course is divided by the **scalenus anterior muscle** into three parts. Note that the *first part* which lies proximal to the muscle gives off:
    (a) the **vertebral artery**;
    (b) the **internal thoracic artery**;
    (c) the **thyrocervical trunk** which in turn gives off the **inferior thyroid**, **suprascapular** and **transverse cervical arteries**.

14. *Trace the* **right recurrent laryngeal nerve** which is given off by the right vagus as it descends in front of the subclavian artery. *Observe that this nerve curves under the subclavian artery* to ascend in the groove between the trachea and oesophagus where it has been dissected.

15. *Observe the* **costocervical trunk** arising from the *second part* of the subclavian artery which lies behind the scalenus anterior muscle. *Follow this trunk as it curves backwards over the apex of the lung* where it divides into the **superior intercostal** and **deep cervical branches** at the neck of the first rib. The superior intercostal artery enters the thorax across the neck of the first rib where it has been examined.

16. *Follow the third part of the subclavian artery from the lateral border of the scalenus anterior muscle to the outer border of the first rib where it continues as the* **axillary artery**.

17. *Now return to the upper part of the neck. Cut the sling which attaches the intermediate tendon of the digastric to the hyoid bone and reflect the muscle laterally. Carefully clean the* **stylopharyngeus muscle** which arises from the medial surface of the styloid process and *secure its nerve supply from the* **glossopharyngeal nerve** which winds round the posterior border of the muscle. Note that the muscle runs downwards and forwards *between* the **internal** and **external carotid arteries** to gain insertion into the inner aspect of the pharynx by passing through the interval between the superior and middle constrictors.

18. *Clean the glossopharyngeal nerve* and note that it emerges *between* the internal jugular vein and the internal carotid artery. It then follows the stylopharyngeus muscle *between* the internal and external carotid arteries to the side of the pharynx after which the nerve reaches the posterior part of the tongue where it breaks up into its terminal branches.

19. *Trace the stylohyoid ligament from the tip of the styloid process to the* **lesser horn of the hyoid bone**. Note its relationship to the glossopharyngeal nerve and lingual artery.

20. *Turn your attention to the* **vagus nerve** and note that it pursues a vertical course at first between the **internal jugular vein** and the **internal carotid artery** and then between the vein and the **common carotid artery**. *Identify the* **pharyngeal branch** passing *between* the internal and external carotid arteries and the **superior laryngeal nerve** passing *deep* to both the arteries. *Trace the vagus nerve upwards and look for the two ganglia* which contain the cell bodies of the sensory fibres of this nerve.

21. *Trace the* **accessory nerve** which descends *between* the internal jugular vein and internal carotid artery. *Observe* that the nerve inclines backwards superficial to the internal jugular vein before it enters the sternocleidomastoid. Its further course in the roof of the posterior triangle of the neck has already been seen.

22. *Now trace the* **hypoglossal nerve** which after emerging from the **hypoglossal canal** lies posteromedial to the internal carotid artery and internal jugular vein. *Observe* that it then winds round the vagus to emerge *between* the artery and the vein. Its further course has already been seen.

23. *Clean the internal carotid artery and trace it upwards* and note that it enters the cranial cavity through the **carotid canal**. *Observe that this artery does not give any branches in the neck.*

24. *Review the branches of the external carotid artery.* Note that the **ascending pharyngeal artery** runs upwards along the side of the pharynx. It supplies the pharynx and neighbouring structures near the base of the skull.

25. *Clean the internal jugular vein near the base of the skull* and note that it is a continuation of the **sigmoid sinus** and has a **superior bulb** in the jugular fossa. *Review its tributaries* which are the **inferior petrosal sinus, pharyngeal veins, facial vein, lingual veins** and **superior** and **middle thyroid veins.**

26. *Clean the* **sympathetic trunk** *which runs along the roots of the transverse processes of the cervical vertebrae. Identify the* **superior** *and* **middle cervical ganglia**. Note that the *superior ganglion* lies opposite the second and third cervical vertebrae and gives **grey rami communicantes** to the upper four cervical nerves. It continues superiorly as the **internal carotid nerve** which later gives rise to the **internal carotid plexus**. The superior ganglion also gives off **pharyngeal, external carotid** and **cardiac branches.**

27. *Identify the* **middle cervical ganglion** lying opposite the sixth cervical vertebra. Note that it gives off grey rami communicantes to the fifth and sixth cervical nerves, branches to the thyroid gland, a **cardiac branch** and the **ansa subclavia**. This ansa is a loop connecting the middle and **cervicothoracic ganglia** and passes round the subclavian artery.

28. *Replace the sternocleidomastoid in position and revise the deep relations of this muscle.*

29. *Divide the* **trachea** *and* **oesophagus** *near the root of the neck and separate them from the vertebral column. Clean the prevertebral fascia which covers the prevertebral muscles.* The fascial space between it and the pharynx is called the **retropharyngeal space**.

30. *Examine the* **cervical plexus** *which is in front of the* **scalenus medius muscle**. Note that this plexus is formed by the ventral rami of the upper four cervical nerves. Its branches are:

(a) a communicating branch from C1 to the hypoglossal nerve;
(b) the **lesser occipital**, **greater auricular**, **transverse cervical** and **supraclavicular nerves**;
(c) branches to the levator scapulae, sternocleidomastoid, trapezius and the prevertebral muscles;
(d) the **phrenic nerve** (C3, 4, 5) to the diaphragm;
(e) the **inferior root of the ansa cervicalis** (C2, 3) which joins the **superior root (C1)**, a branch of the hypoglossal nerve, to form the **ansa cervicalis**.

31. Quickly note the attachments of the prevertebral muscles on either side:
(a) **scalenus anterior** which arises from the transverse processes of the third, fourth, fifth and sixth cervical vertebrae and is inserted into the **scalene tubercle** of the first rib in front of the subclavian artery;
(b) **scalenus medius** which arises from the transverse processes of all the cervical vertebrae and is inserted into the upper surface of the first rib behind the **groove for the subclavian artery**;
(c) **scalenus posterior** which arises from the transverse processes of the lower cervical vertebrae and is inserted into the second rib;
(d) **rectus capitis anterior** and **lateralis** which are two small muscles extending between the atlas and occiput;
(e) **longus colli** muscle which is attached cranially to the anterior tubercle of the atlas and caudally to the bodies of the third, fourth, fifth and sixth cervical vertebrae and the bodies of the upper three thoracic vertebrae;
(f) **longus capitis** which arises from the transverse processes of the third, fourth, fifth and sixth cervical vertebrae and gains insertion into the basiocciput.

32. *Look at the following structures in relation to the* **cervical pleura** *at the root of the neck lying medial to the scalenus anterior muscles*:
(a) the **vertebral vein** which emerges from the **foramen transversarium** of the sixth cervical vertebra and passes in front of the subclavian artery to enter the **brachiocephalic vein**;
(b) the **vertebral artery** which arises from the subclavian artery and passes upwards behind the vertebral vein to enter the foramen transversarium of the sixth cervical vertebra. This is the *first part* of the artery;

(c) deep to the vertebral artery *look for the sympathetic* **cervicothoracic ganglion** which lies on the neck of the first rib. Note that it has a **cardiac branch** as well as branches to the **vertebral** and **subclavian plexuses**. The ganglion is a fusion of the inferior cervical and first thoracic ganglia;

(d) the **internal thoracic artery** which arises from the subclavian artery and passes downwards over the apex of the lung where it is crossed by the phrenic nerve.

33. Note that the *second part* of the vertebral artery passes through the foramina transversaria of the upper six cervical vertebrae. The further course of the vertebral artery will be seen in the **suboccipital triangle**.

Summary

In the submandibular region the mylohyoid muscles form the oral diaphragm separating the neck from the oral mucosa. Related to the muscle is the submandibular salivary gland. Its nerve supply is conveyed by the chorda tympani nerve from the facial nerve. The fibres of the chorda tympani contain *preganglionic* parasympathetic fibres which relay in the submandibular ganglion before supplying the gland with postganglionic secretomotor fibres. Note that salivary calculi are most common in the submandibular duct. The relationships of the facial artery and the adjacent veins must be borne in mind during surgical removal of the gland.

The *deep fascia* of the neck has important components, viz superficial, pretracheal and prevertebral layers. The superficial layer encloses both the trapezius and sternocleidomastoid muscles. The pretracheal fascia lies deep to the infrahyoid muscles and provides the fascial capsule for the thyroid gland. Between the superficial and pretracheal layers is a potential space of the neck which passes into the anterior mediastinum in front of the heart. The prevertebral fascia which is thick and well defined lies in front of the prevertebral muscles. Between the fascia and pharynx in front, is the retropharyngeal space which permits the movements of the pharynx during swallowing. Moreover, as the retropharyngeal space leads down into the thorax, retropharyngeal abscesses can track down from the neck into the mediastinum.

As in the rest of the body, the *lymphatics of the head and neck* can be conveniently divided into superficial and deep sets. The superficial lymphatics usually drain into the *superficial lymph nodes* which, in general, are distributed along the superficial veins. For example, the pericervical collar formed by the **occipital, posterior auricular, parotid, submandibular** and **submental lymph nodes** can all be regarded as being situated along the occipital, posterior auricular, superficial temporal, facial and anterior jugular veins. The superficial nodes distributed along the anterior jugular and external jugular veins are known as the **anterior** and **superficial cervical lymph nodes**, respectively. The lymphatics from the superficial regions of the head and neck, after reaching the superficial lymph nodes eventually pass to the *deep cervical nodes* distributed along the internal jugular vein. The *intermediate* set of lymph nodes draining various organs are found along the branches of arteries supplying these organs or the corresponding veins accompanying the arteries. For example, the **pre-** and **paratracheal nodes** draining the thyroid can be regarded as being situated along the tributaries of the superior and inferior thyroid veins. From these nodes they eventually pass along the superior and inferior thyroid veins into the **deep cervical** and **brachiocephalic nodes**. Thus, the deep lymphatics may be said to accompany the deep veins. However, there are exceptions to these generalisations, e.g. the tip of the tongue drains not only into the submental nodes but may also reach the **juguloomohyoid node** situated on the internal jugular vein where the vein is crossed by the omohyoid muscle. The remainder of the lymphatics of the tongue follow the veins of the tongue.

The lymphatics of the tongue, thyroid and larynx are important as these organs are common sites of cancer. Moreover, the cervical lymph nodes become enlarged in infections such as tuberculosis.

Objectives for Dissection Schedule 30

Topic: Submandibular region

General objective

Comprehend the basic anatomical features of the region.

Specific objectives

1. Define the extent and surfaces of the submandibular gland.
2. Demonstrate the relations of the gland surfaces.
3. Review the course of the facial artery.
4. Discuss the anatomical aspects of:
   (a) submandibular salivary calculi;
   (b) veins related to the submandibular gland.

Topic: Deep structures of the neck

General objective 1

Comprehend the arrangement of the large blood vessels in the neck.

Specific objectives

1. Surface mark the common and external carotid arteries.
2. Review the area of distribution of the branches of the external carotid artery.
3. Enumerate the branches of the subclavian artery.
4. Describe the course and relations of the internal jugular vein and enumerate its tributaries.

General objective 2

Comprehend the basic anatomy of the nervous structures in the region.

Specific objectives

1. Identify the carotid canal, jugular foramen and hypoglossal canal in the base of the skull.

2. Enumerate the structures traversing the above foramina and illustrate the relationships between the last four cranial nerves at the base of the skull.
3. Indicate the course of the last four cranial nerves enumerating their branches in sequence.
4. Deduce the effects of lesions of the last four cranial nerves both alone and in combination.
5. Identify the cervical sympathetic trunk and the superior, middle and cervicothoracic ganglia.
6. Illustrate the sympathetic innervation of the heart.
7. Illustrate the formation and branches of the cervical plexus.
8. Describe the relationships of the hypoglossal nerve, submandibular duct, lingual nerve, and lingual artery to the hyoglossus muscle.
9. Give an account of the main branches of the subclavian artery, including an account of the relationship of the artery to the scalene muscles.
10. Describe the course of the vertebral artery.
11. Give an account of the sympathetic innervation of the structures in the head and neck.
12. Describe the major fascial compartments of the neck, including the structures contained in each.
13. Describe the course of the thoracic duct from the cisterna chyli to its termination.

Questions for study:

1. Which muscle forms the floor of the mouth? What is the relationship of this muscle to the submandibular gland and its duct?
2. What functional components are found in the lingual nerve proximal to its union with the chorda tympani? Distal? What functional deficits would result from accidental sectioning of this nerve during surgery for removal of a lower third molar?

3. Extensive atherosclerosis of the internal carotid artery can be surgically treated by a procedure, termed a carotid endartectomy, during which the artery in the neck is opened and carefully cleaned. Which nerves in the neck may be at particular risk during such a procedure?
4. How do sympathetic nerve fibres reach their target organs in the head?
5. What is Horner's syndrome?
6. How might a chylothorax be produced in an attempted brachiocephalic venipuncture on the left side?
7. Where would one find the deep cervical lymph nodes? Where do efferent vessels from these nodes drain?

Overview of Schedule 31

Before you begin dissection note:

DEEP STRUCTURES OF THE BACK OF THE NECK AND THE TRUNK

DEEP DISSECTION OF THE BACK

Relevant skeletal features:

occipital bone — superior and inferior nuchal lines; foramen magnum;
temporal bone — mastoid process;
vertebral column — atlas; posterior tubercle; posterior arch; transverse processes; axis; dens of axis; spine; vertebral arch; typical vertebra; spinous process; laminae; pedicle; transverse processes; articular process; sacrum; sacral canal; coccyx.

Subcutaneous structures:

greater occipital nerve; occipital artery.

Deep fascia:

thoracolumbar.

Ligaments:

supraspinous; interspinous; ligamenta flava; anterior and posterior atlantooccipital membranes.

Muscles:

splenius capitis; semispinalis capitis; rectus capitis posterior major and minor; obliquus capitis superior and inferior;

erector spinae; transversospinalis.

Nerves:

suboccipital; dorsal rami of spinal nerves.

Arteries:

vertebral.

Veins:

suboccipital plexus.

Surface anatomy:

transverse process of atlas.

Clinical anatomy:

cisternal puncture.

SPINAL CORD AND MENINGES

Coverings:

spinal dura mater; spinal arachnoid; spinal pia mater and its processes.

Spaces:

epidural, containing vertebral venous plexus; subdural, containing lymph; subarachnoid, containing cerebrospinal fluid.

Spinal cord:

anteromedian sulcus; posteromedian fissure; antero- and posterolateral fissures; cervical and lumbar enlargements; conus medullaris.

Spinal nerves:

31 pairs; rootlets; roots; ganglia; trunk; cauda equina.

Arteries:

anterior and posterior spinal; spinal branches of intersegmental arteries.

Veins:

longitudinal venous channels.

Surface anatomy:

emergence of spinal nerves in relation to the vertebrae; conus medullaris.

Clinical anatomy:

lumbar puncture.

JOINTS OF THE SKULL, JOINTS OF THE VERTEBRAL COLUMN AND SACROILIAC JOINT

Joints of the skull:

sutural joints between skull bones; primary cartilaginous joint between basisphenoid and basiocciput; peg and socket joints between teeth and alveolus.

Joints of the vertebral column:

secondary cartilaginous joints between vertebral bodies;
synovial joints — between atlas and occiput; between dens of axis and atlas;
between articular processes of adjacent vertebrae.

Ligaments:

anterior and posterior atlantooccipital membranes; membrana tectoria; cruciate ligament; transverse ligament of atlas; apical; alar; anterior and posterior longitudinal ligaments.

Sacroiliac joint:

synovial type.

Ligaments:

ventral, dorsal and interosseous sacroiliac ligaments; iliolumbar;
sacrotuberous;
sacrospinous.

Clinical anatomy:

low back pain; whiplash injury.

Dissection Schedule 31

DEEP STRUCTURES OF THE BACK OF THE NECK AND TRUNK

DEEP DISSECTION OF THE BACK

1. *Place the body in the prone position. Remove the remains of the trapezius muscle.* Note that the **occipital artery** ascends across the superior nuchal line after emerging from under the cover of the **mastoid process** and the muscles attached to it. It supplies the back of the scalp.

2. *Next remove the latissimus dorsi and the rhomboid muscles. Identify the two thin sheets of muscles over the back of the trunk which belong to the second layer.* These are the **serratus posterior superior** deep to the rhomboids and the **serratus posterior inferior** under cover of the latissimus dorsi. *Remove these muscles and note the* **thoracolumbar fascia** *covering the third layer of muscles of the back.* The thoracolumbar fascia is thick in the lumbar region where it has **anterior, middle** and **posterior layers**. The anterior and middle layers enclose the **quadratus lumborum muscle**, while the middle and posterior layers enclose the **erector spinae muscle**. Lateral to these muscles, the thoracolumbar fascia gives partial origin to the muscles of the anterior abdominal wall. *Trace the posterior layer over the thoracic region* and note that it thins out and is replaced by the **splenius capitis muscle** over the back of the neck.

3. *Clean the splenius capitis muscle* taking origin from the upper six thoracic spines and the **ligamentum nuchae**. It gains insertion into the **transverse processes** of the upper two or three cervical vertebrae, the mastoid process and the adjoining **superior nuchal line**. *Detach this muscle from its origin and reflect it upwards.*

4. *Identify the massive* **semispinalis capitis muscle** which arises from the transverse processes of the upper cervical vertebrae to be inserted into the medial half of the area between the superior and **inferior nuchal lines**. *Observe the thick* **greater occipital nerve** which pierces this muscle. *Detach the semispinalis capitis from its insertion and carefully reflect the muscle downwards.* This exposes the **suboccipital triangle**.

5. *Examine the suboccipital triangle* bounded by the **rectus capitis posterior major** medially, the **obliquus capitis superior** above and laterally, and the **obliquus capitis inferior** below. The floor of the suboccipital triangle is made up of the **posterior atlantooccipital membrane** above and the **posterior arch of the atlas** below. Note that the greater occipital nerve (C2) winds round the lower border of the obliquus capitis inferior and that **rectus capitis posterior minor** lies medial to the rectus capitis posterior major.

6. *Study the attachments of the suboccipital muscles*:

   The *rectus capitis posterior major* arises from the **spine of the axis** while the *rectus capitis posterior minor* takes origin from the **posterior tubercle of the atlas**. Both these muscles are inserted into the area below the inferior nuchal line, the major being lateral to the minor.

   The *obliquus capitis inferior* arises from the spine of the axis and is inserted into the transverse process of the atlas.

   The *obliquus capitis superior* arises from the transverse process of the atlas and is inserted into the area between the nuchal lines lateral to the semispinalis capitis.

7. *Follow the third part of the* **vertebral artery** medially under the posterior atlantooccipital membrane. *Observe* the plexus of veins in the suboccipital region.

8. *Now turn your attention to the vertical muscle masses of the back, clean them and observe that*:
   (a) they form prominent vertical bulges on either side of the midline and are supplied segmentally by the **posterior primary rami of the spinal nerves**;
   (b) they are a discontinuous layer of muscles usually running in relays from below upwards;
   (c) they are arranged in *two* layers from superficial to deep;
   (d) the *superficial layer* is the **erector spinae** which is subdivided into medial, intermediate and lateral groups. These groups consist of a medial **spinalis** portion (composed of the spinalis thoracis, cervicis and capitis); an intermediate **longissimus** portion (composed of the

longissimus thoracis, cervicis and capitis); and a lateral **iliocostalis** portion (composed of the iliocostalis lumborum, thoracis and cervicis);

(e) the *deep layer*, the **transversopinalis**, consists of *three* layers, from superficial to deep they are the **semispinalis** group (composed of the semispinalis thoracis, cervicis and capitis); the **multifidus**; and the **rotatores** in the thoracic region. *Do not waste time on trying to identify this deep layer.*

9. *Remove all the muscles on the back of the vertebral column between the mid-thoracic and mid-lumbar region and identify*:
   (a) the **supraspinous** and **interspinous ligaments** in between the **spines**;
   (b) the **ligamenta flava** between the **laminae** of adjacent vertebrae.

10. *Next carefully remove the spines and laminae from the mid-thoracic to the mid-lumbar region of the vertebral column using a saw*. You are thus removing the posterior wall of the **vertebral canal**.

11. Note that the space now exposed is the interval between the vertebral canal and the **dura mater** of the **spinal cord** and is called the **epidural space**. *Observe* that this space contains fat and vertebral venous plexuses. These plexuses communicate with the suboccipital plexus of veins, venous sinuses inside the skull, posterior intercostal and lumbar veins.

12. *Examine the dura mater*. Note that it is a dense, tough, fibrous tube extending from the **foramen magnum** to the level of the second piece of the sacrum where it ends as a blind sac.

13. *Slit open the dural sheath in the midline avoiding damage to the underlying* **arachnoid**. The capillary interval between the dura and arachnoid is called the **subdural space** and contains lymph which facilitates movement between these layers.

14. *Examine the arachnoid* which forms a loose, delicate and transparent covering for the spinal cord and nerve roots. Superiorly it becomes continuous with the arachnoid of the brain through the foramen magnum; inferiorly it ends as a blind cul-de-sac at the level of the second piece of the sacrum and at the sides it is prolonged over the nerve roots. Note that the **subarachnoid space** is the wide interval between the arachnoid and **pia mater** (which covers the spinal cord) and becomes continuous with

the subarachnoid space of the cranial cavity. The space contains **cerebrospinal fluid** (C.S.F.) which in addition to its metabolic functions provides a fluid cushion for the brain and the spinal cord.

15. *Remove the arachnoid over a portion of the spinal cord to study the pia mater. Look at a complete specimen of a spinal cord* and note that the pia mater is a firm vascular membrane which adheres to the nervous tissue. The pia mater is continued beyond the lower end of the spinal cord as the **filum terminale** which anchors the spinal cord, the arachnoid and the dura mater to the back of the coccyx. *At the sides examine a few* of the 21 pairs of tooth-like projections of the pia mater known as the **ligamenta denticulata** separating the **dorsal** and **ventral spinal roots**.

16. *Examine the spinal cord of a complete specimen* and note that it tapers inferiorly to end as the **conus medullaris** around the lower border of the first lumbar vertebra. The spinal cord has two swellings called the **cervical** and **lumbar enlargements** in relation to the origins of the nerves supplying the upper and lower limbs.

17. Note that each of the 31 pairs of **spinal nerves** arises by dorsal and ventral roots. Each root is composed of a number of rootlets. *Observe the direction of the roots* and note that their obliquity increases from above downwards so that the lower roots are nearly vertical and form a bundle called the **cauda equina**.

18. *Follow a few of the spinal roots of your dissected specimen and study the position of the* **spinal ganglia**. The ganglia are on the dorsal roots and lie in the **intervertebral foramina** with the exception of the first two cervical, the sacral and coccygeal ganglia. The first and second cervical ganglia lie on the posterior arch of the atlas and vertebral arch of the axis respectively, while the ganglia of the sacral and coccygeal nerves are located in the **sacral canal**. All the ganglia except the sacral are within the dural sac.

Joints of the skull and vertebral column

Examine these joints on the relevant skeletal parts and on prosections.

1. *Observe* that the joints between the skull bones are mainly **sutures** (fibrous joints) where movements are extremely limited in adults. The joints between

the teeth and gums are of the peg and socket type of fibrous joint (**gomphosis**).

2. *Return to your cadaver:*
   (a) *Remove that part of the spinal cord which you have exposed. Examine the* **anterior** *and* **posterior longitudinal ligaments** running along the front and posterior surfaces of the vertebral bodies respectively. The ligamenta flava between the laminae of the adjacent vertebrae have already been examined.
   (b) *Remove the anterior and posterior longitudinal ligaments in relation to two adjacent vertebrae and observe* that the vertebral bodies are joined together by a fibrocartilaginous disc, the **intervertebral disc**, constituting a median **secondary cartilaginous joint**. The disc is composed of a peripheral **annulus fibrosus** and a central **nucleus pulposus**. Note that hyaline cartilage intervenes between the disc and the bony vertebral bodies.

3. *With the help of a skull and an articulated vertebral column:*
   (a) Note the presence of synovial joints between the **articular processes** of adjacent vertebrae. *Observe* the differences in the disposition of the opposing articular surfaces in the cervical, thoracic and lumbar regions. What are the functional implications?
   (b) Note that in the cervical region there are additional synovial joints at the sides of the vertebral bodies.
   (c) *Observe* that the synovial joints between the **atlas** and **occipital condyles (atlantooccipital joint)** permit anteroposterior flexion and extension as well as lateral flexion, while rotation of the head occurs at the joint between the **dens of the axis** and the atlas.
   (d) Note that the **anterior atlantooccipital membrane** passes between the anterior margin of the foramen magnum above and the **anterior arch of the atlas** below. This membrane is a continuation of the anterior longitudinal ligament.
   (e) The **posterior atlantooccipital membrane** passes between the posterior margin of the foramen magnum above and the posterior arch of the atlas below. Note that the membrane arches over the vertebral artery and the C1 nerve laterally. The membrane corresponds to the ligamenta flava.

(f) *Next examine the articulations between the atlas and axis*, the **atlantoaxial joint**. The joints between the **inferior facets of the atlas** and the **superior facets of the axis** are synovial joints.

(g) From each side of the **apex of the dens** an **alar ligament** passes upwards and laterally to the medial side of each occipital condyle. These two ligaments check excess rotation.

(h) The **apical ligament** ascends from the apex of the dens to the anterior edge of the foramen magnum. This ligament contains traces of the notochord.

(i) Posterior to the alar and apical ligaments is the **cruciform ligament**. This ligament consists of two parts: a **longitudinal band** which extends upwards from the posterior aspect of the dens to the anterior edge of the foramen magnum, and a **transverse ligament of the atlas** which passes behind the dens between the medial sides of the **lateral masses of the atlas**.

(j) Posterior to the cruciform ligament lies the upward continuation of the posterior longitudinal ligament, the **membrana tectoria**, which passes through the foramen magnum to be attached to the inner aspect of the occipital bone.

Sacroiliac joint

1. *Now turn your attention to the* **sacroiliac joints** which are of the synovial type. *Examine a hip bone and sacrum and study an articulated pelvis showing the various ligaments*. Note that the joints are formed by the union of the **auricular surfaces** of the sacrum and ilium on either side. These surfaces are reciprocally curved and have elevations and depressions that fit into corresponding irregularities of the opposed surface, thus providing greater stability.

2. An articular **capsule**, lined by synovial membrane, connects the sacrum with the ilium at the periphery of the auricular surfaces.

3. A strong **interosseous sacroiliac ligament** connects the posterolateral surface of the sacrum with the **tuberosity of the ilium** which lies above and posterior to the auricular articular surface of the ileum.

4. Anteriorly, a thin **ventral sacroiliac ligament** connects the **ala** and pelvic surface of the sacrum with the adjacent part of the ilium.

5. Posteriorly, the **dorsal sacroiliac ligament** is attached to the iliac tuberosity and the **posterior superior iliac spine** of the ilium. From here the fibres spread out to be attached to the posterolateral surface and lateral border of the sacrum.

6. *Next examine the two accessory ligaments, the* **sacrotuberous** *and* **sacrospinous ligaments**. These ligaments convert the **greater** and **lesser sciatic notches** into **greater** and **lesser sciatic foramina**, respectively.
   (a) The sacrotuberous ligament is attached to the posterior iliac spines, the posterolateral part of the sacrum and the lateral border of the upper part of the coccyx. From this broad attachment the fibres converge to be attached to the medial margin of the **ischial tuberosity**.
   (b) Note that the sacrospinous ligament is triangular in shape and lies in front of the sacrotuberous ligament. Its base is attached to the lateral margin of the lower part of the sacrum and the upper part of the coccyx. Its apex is attached to the **ischial spine**. The **coccygeus muscle** is coextensive with its pelvic aspect.
   (c) In addition, the **iliolumbar ligament** extends laterally from the fifth lumbar transverse process to the iliac crest.

Summary

The joints between the atlas and occiput and between the atlas and axis are specialised to meet the functional needs of nodding, lateral flexion and rotatory movements of the head. Flexion and extension or nodding movements occur between the atlas and occiput while rotatory movements take place between the dens of the axis and the anterior arch of the atlas. The dens is held in position by the transverse ligament of the atlas. This ligament is so strong that fracture of the dens is more liable to occur than a tear of the transverse ligament. During rotation, the alar ligaments become tight and thus their function is to limit excessive rotation of the head.

The superior and inferior articular processes of the atlas and the superior articular facets of the axis are developmentally different from the articular processes present in the other cervical vertebrae. Consequently, the ventral rami of C1 and C2 pass behind the articular processes whereas the ventral rami of the other cervical nerves pass in front of the corresponding articular processes. The homologues of the articular processes of the atlas and axis are to be found in the synovial joints occurring between the neurocentral lips of the cervical vertebrae 3–7 and the vertebral bodies overlying these neurocentral lips.

The spinal cord terminates at the level of L1 vertebra while the arachnoid is continued down to S2 vertebra, so that the subarachnoid space extends as far down as S2 vertebra. Therefore, a **lumbar puncture**, i.e. a procedure adopted to withdraw C.S.F. is usually performed by passing a lumbar puncture needle into the space between the L3 and L4 vertebrae. This space is chosen so as to avoid damage to the lower end of the spinal cord.

Sometimes a **cisternal puncture** is performed by passing a needle upwards and forwards in the interval between the atlas and the occiput. In this case the needle enters the **cerebellomedullary cistern**. This procedure entails a certain degree of risk as there is the danger of the needle causing damage to the part of the **medulla oblongata** which contains the vital centres such as the cardiac and respiratory centres.

The spinal cord receives its blood supply from a single **anterior spinal** and four **posterior spinal arteries**. However, the major part, i.e. about two-thirds of the substance of the spinal cord, is supplied by the anterior spinal artery while only the posterior part of the spinal cord and peripheral portions of the lateral and anterior white columns receive their blood supply via the posterior spinal arteries. The anterior and posterior spinal arteries are reinforced by branches from the vertebral, posterior intercostal, lumbar and lateral sacral arteries. These spinal branches pass through the intervertebral foramina and divide into anterior and posterior radicular arteries which accompany the corresponding nerve roots before joining the spinal arteries.

Having studied the sacroiliac joints, review the **mechanics of the pelvis**:

(a) the irregular elevations and depressions on the joint surfaces fit into one another and restrict movement and contribute to the strength of the joint;
(b) the two pubic bones and their connection in front act as a strut and prevent the sacroiliac joints from opening anteroinferiorly;
(c) resistance to downward pressure is due to the wedge-shaped sacrum between the two hip bones;

(d) resistance to inward pressure into the pelvis is due to the strong interosseous ligaments;

(e) and resistance to rotation pressure on the sacrum is due to the sacrotuberous and sacrospinous ligaments.

Objectives for Dissection Schedule 31

Topic: Deep structures of the back of the neck and trunk

General objective 1

Comprehend the arrangement of the muscles in the region.

Specific objectives

1. Enumerate the muscles of the medial, intermediate and lateral columns of the erector spinae from medial to lateral.
2. Trace the continuity of these muscles in relays and define the semispinalis capitis and longissimus capitis, which are the only muscles to reach the skull.
3. Explain the attachments and functions of the thoracolumbar fascia.
4. Define the muscular boundaries of the suboccipital triangle.
5. Discuss the more important actions of the erector spinae and suboccipital muscles.

General objective 2

Comprehend the arrangement of the nerves and blood vessels in the region.

Specific objectives

1. Explain the retention of the primitive segmental innervation of muscle by reference to the innervation of the erector spinae.
2. Describe the course of the second and third parts of the vertebral artery.
3. Explain the role of the vertebral venous plexus and its communications in the spread of cancerous secondary deposits to the skull.
4. Discuss the spread of infection into the cranial cavity from the suboccipital region.

Topic: Spinal cord and coverings

General objective

Appreciate the basic anatomical features of the spinal cord and meninges.

Specific objectives

1. Define the extent of the spinal cord.
2. Define the origin of the spinal nerves and the position of the dorsal root ganglia in the different regions.
3. Assign functional roles to:
   (a) the subdural space;
   (b) ligamenta denticulata;
   (c) filum terminale;
   (d) cerebrospinal fluid.
4. Indicate the anatomical basis of the sites chosen for aspiration of C.S.F.
5. Review the blood supply of the spinal cord.
6. Explain the anatomical basis of:
   (a) Queckenstedt's test;
   (b) myelography;
   (c) pneumoencephalography;
   (d) rhizotomy;
   (e) chordotomy.

Topic: Joints of the skull and vertebral column and the sacroiliac joint

General objective

Comprehend the functional anatomy of the various joints.

You should be able to:

1. Review the classification of joints with reference to examples chosen from the regions.
2. Explain the development and differentiation of the sclerotomes and notochord in terms of adult structures.

3. Define the parts of a typical vertebra.
4. Demonstrate the manner of articulation of the bodies and the articular processes of adjacent vertebrae.
5. Explain the formation of the primary and secondary curvatures of the vertebral column.
6. Define the attachments of the supraspinous, interspinous and intertransverse ligaments; the ligamenta flava; the anterior and posterior longitudinal ligaments; and the iliolumbar and sacroiliac ligaments.
7. Analyse the different types of movement exhibited in the different parts of the vertebral column with special reference to the role played by:
   (a) the intervertebral discs;
   (b) the plane of the joints between the articular processes;
   (c) the lumbosacral articulation;
   (d) the ribs.
8. Enumerate the muscles principally involved in flexion, extension and rotation of the vertebral column.
9. Explain the anatomical features of:
   (a) prolapsed intervertebral disc;
   (b) kyphosis, scoliosis and lordosis;
   (c) spondylolisthesis.
10. Interpret normal radiographs of the skull, vertebral column and pelvis.

Overview of Schedule 32

Before you begin dissection note:

NASAL CAVITY

Relevant features:

1. bony and cartilaginous parts of nasal septum;
2. superior, middle and inferior nasal conchae;
3. superior, middle and inferior nasal meatuses;
4. sphenoethmoidal recess and opening of sphenoidal sinus;
5. frontal sinus and frontonasal duct;
6. hiatus semilunaris of middle meatus and the opening of the maxillary sinus;
7. maxillary sinus and roots of upper molar teeth;
8. opening of nasolacrimal duct into the inferior meatus;
9. sphenopalatine foramen;
10. opening of auditory tube;
11. arterial supply of nasal cavity;
12. sensory nerve supply of nasal cavity.

Clinical anatomy:

epistaxis; sinusitis.

Dissection Schedule 32

NASAL CAVITY

1. *Examine sagittal and coronal sections of prosected specimens and models of the head and neck. Observe the* **external nose** *and the more deeply placed* **nasal cavity**. Note the air-containing extensions of the nasal cavity giving rise to the paired **paranasal sinuses**, namely, the **frontal, ethmoidal, sphenoidal** and **maxillary sinuses**.

2. *Examine the pyramid-shaped external nose in the cadaver* and note that it opens to the exterior by the **external nares** or nostrils. These are separated from each other by a **nasal septum**. This region is known as the **vestibule**. Note that the framework of the lower part of the external nose is cartilaginous.

3. *Identify the bony framework of the upper part of the bridge of the nose* formed by the two **nasal bones** articulating with each other. Lateral to these are the **frontal processes of the maxillae**, while above the nasal bones are the **nasal processes of the frontal bone**. *Verify this in the skull.*

4. *Next bisect the head and neck. For this the following instruments should be used*: a frame-saw, a small amputation-saw, bone-cutting forceps and a wooden block to support the head.
   (a) *Lay the body supine, with the neck on the block. In order to avoid debris falling on the floor make sure that the head does not overlap the edge of the table.*
   (b) *Stand at the head of the body.*
   (c) *The nose, which is often bent to one side, should be pushed back into the midline, and divided in the median plane with a scalpel as deeply as you can.*
   (d) *Insert the blade of the frame-saw into this incision and, keeping your saw slightly off the median sagittal plane, start sawing through the mandible and the bone of the forehead.*
   (e) *When you have divided the mandible, use a scalpel to continue the cut through the soft tissues of the floor of the mouth and upper part of the neck in the median plane. Divide the hyoid bone with bone-cutting forceps at its midpoint. Next divide the larynx and trachea and the*

pharynx and oesophagus in the neck in the median plane with a scalpel, the scalpel should reach the midline of the cervical part of the vertebral column. At this point start sawing again, with someone helping you by holding the head and neck and guarding the divided soft tissues from the saw.

(f) *Deepen the saw-cut as far as possible, until the handle of the saw meets the table on which the body is lying.*

(g) *Turn the body over, and incise the skin over the occiput with a scalpel, in line with the saw-cut. The soft tissues overlying the spinous processes should then be incised with a scalpel until you reach the bone. Having done so, insert the saw in the incision, and saw forward in the median plane as deeply as possible. The saw-cut should be extended into the spinous processes.*

(h) *Turn the body on its left side and transect all the soft tissues with a scalpel just above the line of the right first rib. The incision should pass between the subclavian vessels below and the lower end of the thyroid gland above. Use a saw to carry the section right through the vertebral column.*

(i) *Complete the median section of the bones of the skull and neck, where necessary, with a small amputation-saw, until you can separate the two halves.*

5. *In your half of the head and neck examine the nasal septum* and note that the upper part is lined by *olfactory mucosa*. In the lower part of the septum *identify the* **nasopalatine nerve** running along with the **sphenopalatine artery**.

6. *Remove the mucous membrane from the septum and examine its framework*, consisting of the **vomer** posteroinferiorly, the **perpendicular plate of the ethmoid** posterosuperiorly, and the **septal cartilage** which fits anteriorly into the angle between these two bones. *Carefully remove the skeletal framework of the septum leaving the mucous membrane of the opposite side intact* (submucous resection of the septum).

7. *Dissect the nasopalatine nerve in the intact mucosa of the septum. Follow the nerve backwards from the septum across the roof of the nasal cavity to the* **sphenopalatine foramen** *laterally and thence to the* **pterygopalatine**

ganglion *lying in the* **pterygopalatine fossa**. *Strip off the mucoperiosteum from the* **palatine bone** *with forceps, and carefully remove the bone with bone forceps. Follow the* **greater palatine nerve** *as it descends on the lateral side of the palatine bone to reach the* **palate** *at its posterolateral corner. Trace it upwards to the ganglion.*

8. *Remove the remains of the septum and examine the lateral wall of the nose. Identify the anteriorly situated vestibule* carrying stiff hairs or **vibrissae**. *Further posteriorly observe the three scroll-like* **conchae**. The **superior** and **middle nasal conchae** are parts of the ethmoid while the **inferior nasal concha** is a separate bony entity. Below each concha *identify* a **meatus** of the nose. Thus there are three meatuses, **superior, middle** and **inferior**. Above and behind the superior concha *identify the* **sphenoethmoidal recess** into which opens the **sphenoidal air sinus**. Note the *olfactory mucosa* in the upper third of the lateral wall.

9. *Identify the opening of the* **nasolacrimal duct** *into the inferior meatus.*

10. Note that the posterior ethmoidal sinus opens into the superior meatus and all other sinuses open into the middle meatus. The space leading into the middle meatus from the nasal vestibule is called the **atrium** of the middle meatus.

11. *Follow the middle concha backwards* and note that it leads to the sphenopalatine foramen. *Similarly follow the inferior concha posteriorly and observe that it leads to the opening of the* **auditory tube**.

12. *Remove the anterior half of the inferior nasal concha. Pass a probe through the* **nasolacrimal canal** *from the orbit above and locate its lower opening in the nasal cavity. Next remove the other conchae carefully with scissors and identify the prominent bulge towards the centre of the middle meatus caused by the underlying middle ethmoidal air cells.* This is the **bulla ethomoidalis**. Note the semicircular groove called the **hiatus semilunaris** lying below the bulla. *Identify the* **frontonasal duct** *at the anterior end of the hiatus.* Some of the anterior ethmoidal air cells and the frontal sinus drain by this common opening. The main opening of the anterior ethmoidal sinus is just behind this while the **maxillary sinus** opens further posteriorly in the middle of the hiatus.

13. *Make an attempt to trace the branches of the pterygopalatine ganglion and the branches of the* **maxillary** *and* **ethmoidal arteries** *supplying the lateral wall of the nose. Strip the mucoperiosteum off the lateral wall of the nose and study its skeletal framework. Observe* that the frontal process of the maxilla and the nasal bones are most anterior, the medial surface of the maxilla and perpendicular plate of the palatine bone lie behind and below. Note the bones covering the medial wall of the maxillary sinus. These are the lacrimal in front, ethmoid above, perpendicular plate of the palatine behind and inferior nasal concha below. *Finally, explore the maxillary sinus by breaking through the bones which constitute its medial wall. Try to see whether the tip of a root of a* **premolar** *or* **molar** *tooth projects into the sinus.*

Summary

The nose includes the external nose and the nasal cavity. The nasal cavity extends from the external nares in front to the **posterior nasal aperture**. Above, it is related to the anterior and middle cranial fossae. Below, it is separated from the oral cavity by the hard palate. Laterally, it is related to the exterior in front, and farther back to the orbit, the maxillary and ethmoidal sinuses, and the pterygoid processes. Posteriorly, the nasal cavity communicates with the nasopharynx. The nasal cavity is divided into right and left halves by the nasal septum.

The functions of the nose are: (a) to subserve the sense of smell, (b) to provide an airway for respiration, (c) to filter, warm and moisten the inspired air, and (d) to cleanse itself of foreign matter that is extracted from the air.

Objectives for Dissection Schedule 32

Topic: Nasal cavity

Specific objectives

1. Identify, on a living subject, the features of the surface anatomy of the nose.
2. Describe the bony skeletons of the nasal septum and nasal cavity.
3. Give an account of the paranasal air sinuses with particular reference to their purported functions and drainage.
4. Describe the general and special sensory innervation of the nasal mucosa.

Questions for study:

1. What is epistaxis? Which arteries are most commonly involved?
2. Why might a patient with maxillary sinusitis present with a toothache?
3. Why is the maxillary sinus particularly prone to infection?
4. What is an oro-antral fistula? Why might it result from an extraction of an upper premolar or molar tooth?
5. Why is the pterygopalatine ganglion known as the ganglion of hay fever?

Overview of Schedule 33

Before you begin dissection note:

ORAL CAVITY

Relevant features:

1. surface features of the dorsum of the tongue;
2. palatoglossal arch;
3. muscles of the tongue and their function;
4. motor and sensory nerve supply of the tongue;
5. submandibular ganglion;
6. sublingual gland;
7. deciduous and permanent teeth;
8. openings of parotid and submandibular ducts.

Dissection Schedule 33

ORAL CAVITY

1. *In the sagittal section of the head study the* **oral cavity** which is the most cranial part of the alimentary canal. *Also examine your own mouth. Observe that the teeth separate the oral cavity into two parts*. The larger part enclosed within the teeth is the **oral cavity proper**. The narrow space placed outside the teeth and limited externally by the lips and cheek is the **vestibule** into which the **parotid duct** opens *opposite the crown of the upper second molar tooth*.

2. *Observe that the oral cavity proper has a roof and a floor and that it continues posteriorly into the* **pharynx**. Note that the oral cavity proper is bounded *laterally and in front* by the **alveolar arches**, the teeth and gums. *Verify* that the *roof* is formed by the **hard palate** in front and the **soft palate** behind. In the middle of the soft palate identify the **uvula** hanging downwards from its posterior edge. *Posteriorly, observe* the anterior **palatoglossal** and the posterior **palatopharyngeal folds (arches)** passing down from the sides of the soft palate. The palatoglossal folds, which cover the **palatoglossus muscles**, pass to the sides of the tongue, and the palatopharyngeal folds, which cover the **palatopharyngeal muscles**, pass into the pharynx. The palatoglossal folds mark the posterior limit of the oral cavity, this is the **oropharyngeal isthmus**, the entrance to the pharynx. In between the palatoglossal and palatopharyngeal folds lies the **palatine tonsil**. The greater part of the *floor* of the mouth is formed by the anterior region of the tongue resting on the mylohyoid muscles.

3. *Examine the tongue*. Note that it has a **root**, the **pharyngeal part**, through which its extrinsic muscles gain entry into the tongue. That part of the tongue which projects into the oral cavity is called the **oral part**. The tongue has a tip, margins as well as dorsal and ventral surfaces. On the dorsum of the tongue note the inverted V-shaped sulcus called the **sulcus terminalis**. The oral part of the tongue lies in front of the sulcus while the pharyngeal part lies behind it. *Observe a midline fold*, the **median glossoepiglottic fold** as it runs from the dorsum of the tongue to the **epiglottis**, and a pair of **lateral glossoepiglottic folds** running from the lateral borders of the tongue to the sides of the epiglottis. Between the median and lateral folds *observe* the

shallow depression called the **vallecula**, one on each side. *Make a transverse section through the free part of the tongue and observe the closely packed,* **vertical, transverse** *and* **superior** *and* **inferior longitudinal muscles** *arranged on either side of a midline vertical septum*. These are the intrinsic muscles of the tongue.

4. In the median plane *observe a crescentic fold of mucous membrane*, the **frenulum linguae**, connecting the inferior surface of the anterior part of the tongue to the floor of the mouth. Note that the **submandibular duct** opens on either side of the lower part of the frenulum in the floor of the mouth. Lateral to the frenulum *observe the bulge in the mucous membrane caused by the* **sublingual gland**. The ducts of this gland open here by minute orifices.

5. *Remove the mucosa from the remainder of the tongue and follow the extrinsic muscles of the tongue into its substance*:
   (a) **genioglossus** originates from the **spine of the mandible** and radiates backwards and upwards into the whole tongue;
   (b) **hyoglossus** originates from the **greater horn** and adjacent part of the **body of the hyoid bone** and inserts into the posterior half of the side of the tongue;
   (c) **styloglossus** originates from the **styloid process** and passes downwards and forwards to insert into the side of the tongue; and
   (d) **palatoglossus** originates from the **palatine aponeurosis** and passes downwards to insert into the posterior part of the side of the tongue.

Summary

Note that all the intrinsic and extrinsic muscles of the tongue are supplied by the **hypoglossal nerve** except the palatoglossus which is supplied by the **cranial part of the accessory nerve** via the **vagus nerve** and **pharyngeal plexus**.

The *anterior two-thirds of the tongue* receives its sensory supply from the **lingual nerve** and taste from the **chorda tympani nerve**.

The *posterior one-third of the tongue* receives its sensory and taste supply from the **glossopharyngeal nerve**.

Note that the tongue is used in sucking, chewing and swallowing. It is important in speech and is also an organ of taste.

Objectives for Dissection Schedule 33

Topic: Oral cavity

Specific objectives

1. Identify the surface anatomical features of the lips, vestibule, oral cavity, palate, and tongue.
2. Give a complete account of the processes of chewing and swallowing.
3. Give a complete account of the innervation of the salivary glands.
4. Describe the muscles of the tongue and the movements they produce.
5. Describe the sensory, motor and taste innervation of the tongue.
6. Describe the lymphatic drainage of the tongue.
7. Identify the palatine and lingual tonsils on a living subject.

Questions for study:

1. Where would one look for the openings of the submandibular duct in the oral cavity?
2. What is a sialogram? What is a sialolith?
3. To which side would the tongue deviate if the right hypoglossal nerve was interrupted?
4. How does the lymphatic drainage of the anterior two-thirds of the tongue differ from that of the posterior one-third? Of what clinical significance is this difference?
5. In the case of infection of the palatine tonsils, which deep cervical lymph nodes are likely to be enlarged and tender?
6. Where would one find the valleculae?

Overview of Schedule 34

Before you begin dissection note:

SOFT PALATE AND PHARYNX

Relevant features:

1. three parts of the pharynx and their boundaries;
2. pharyngeal opening of the auditory tube and tubal elevation;
3. palatoglossal and palatopharyngeal arches, and palatine tonsil;
4. retropharyngeal space;
5. pharyngeal plexus on the surface of the buccopharyngeal fascia;
6. superior, middle and inferior constrictor muscles — their attachments and their innervation;
7. relationship of glossopharyngeal nerve to superior and middle constrictors;
8. levator veli palatini and tensor veli palatini muscles;
9. pterygoid hamulus and palatine aponeurosis;
10. greater palatine and nasopalatine nerves.

Dissection Schedule 34

SOFT PALATE AND PHARYNX

1. *In the sagittal section of the head and neck identify the* **pharynx**. *Verify* that the pharynx extends from the base of the skull to the level of the **cricoid cartilage** at C6.

   Identify the three subdivisions of the pharynx:

   (a) The **nasopharynx** is the part behind the nasal cavities and extends down to the level of the soft palate. Below this is the **oropharynx** lying behind the oral cavity. Most caudally is the **laryngopharynx** which lies behind the larynx.

   In the lateral wall of the **nasopharynx** *identify* the **opening of the auditory tube** once again. Note that the opening is bounded by an elevation — the **tubal elevation** — caused by the underlying cartilaginous part of the auditory tube. Behind the tube lies the **pharyngeal recess**. *Observe* that the fold of mucous membrane, the **salpingopharyngeal fold**, runs downwards from the tubal elevation. This fold contains the **salpingopharyngeus muscle**.

   (b) The **oropharynx** contains the **palatoglossal** and **palatopharyngeal arches** with the **palatine tonsil** in between them. Note that the medial surface of the tonsil is free while its lateral surface has a fibrous capsule separating it from the **superior constrictor muscle** which forms the lateral wall of the pharynx here. A **tonsillar branch** from the facial artery pierces the constrictor muscle to reach the tonsil. Between the tonsil and the muscle lie the large veins draining the tonsil.

   (c) *Now examine the* **laryngopharynx**. *Observe* that its anterior wall is composed of the **inlet of the larynx** with a depression on either side called the **piriform fossa** (deep to this fossa lies the **internal laryngeal nerve**); and the mucous membrane on the posterior surface of the **arytenoid** and **cricoid cartilages** below the level of the laryngeal inlet. Note that the boundaries of the laryngeal inlet are the **epiglottis** anterosuperiorly, the **interarytenoid fold** of mucosa posteroinferiorly and the **aryepiglottic folds** of mucosa on either side. Again note that on either side the piriform fossa lies between the aryepiglottic fold medially and the posterior part of the **lamina of the thyroid cartilage** laterally.

2. *Carefully strip off the mucosa from the superior and inferior aspects of the soft palate, as well as from the* salpingopharyngeal, **palatoglossal** and **palatopharyngeal folds** to expose the muscles (of the same name) contained within them. *Remove also the mucosa on the inner aspect of the pharynx and note the downward extension of the* **palatopharyngeus muscle**. Just below the opening of the auditory tube *identify the* **levator veli palatini muscle** *and trace it into the soft palate. Trace the* **tensor veli palatini muscle** *as it curves around the* **pterygoid hamulus** *and follow its tendon into the palate* where it forms the **palatine aponeurosis**, the framework of the soft palate.

3. *Remove the remains of the cervical part of the vertebral column. Examine the outer surface of the pharynx formed by the constrictor muscles of the pharynx.*

4. *Study the origin of the* **superior constrictor** from the pterygoid hamulus, **pterygomandibular raphe**, the side of the tongue and posterior end of the **mylohyoid line of the mandible**. *Verify the attachments of the pterygomandibular raphe.* Note that the anterior part of the raphe gives attachment to the **buccinator muscle**. *Clean the superior constrictor muscle and observe* how the **styloglossus muscle** enters the tongue by passing under the constrictor muscle near the mandible. Note the insertion of the superior constrictor muscle into a posterior **midline raphe** which extends to the **pharyngeal tubercle of the occipital bone** above. In the interval between the base of the skull and the superior constrictor, the auditory tube and levator veli palatini muscle enter the pharynx.

5. *Next observe the origin of the fan shaped* **middle constrictor** from the **stylohyoid ligament, lesser cornu of the hyoid**, and from the upper border of the **greater cornu**. Its fibres are inserted posteriorly into the median raphe. *Observe that the upper border of the middle constrictor overlaps the superior constrictor*, and that the **glossopharyngeal nerve** and the **stylopharyngeus muscle** enter the pharynx through this interval. On the outer surface of the middle constrictor note the **pharyngeal plexus** formed by branches of the glossopharyngeal, **vagus**, and **sympathetic nerves**.

6. *Examine the* **inferior constrictor** which arises from the cricoid cartilage and from the **oblique line of the thyroid cartilage**. *Follow its fibres*

backwards to its insertion into the midline raphe posteriorly. *Observe* how the upper border of the inferior constrictor overlaps the middle constrictor muscle, and in this interval identify the **internal laryngeal nerve** and the **superior laryngeal branch of the superior thyroid artery** as they enter the larynx. *Observe* how the lower fibres of the inferior constrictor (**cricopharyngeus**) become continuous with the inner circular muscle fibres of the **oesophagus**. Note that the **recurrent laryngeal nerve** and **inferior laryngeal branch of the inferior thyroid artery** ascend deep to its lower border before they enter the larynx while the **external laryngeal nerve** runs on its superficial surface.

Summary

The palate forms the roof of the mouth and the floor of the nasal cavity. It is divided into a larger anterior hard palate and a smaller posterior soft palate. The soft palate is elevated in swallowing, phonation (except nasal consonants) and in the act of blowing.

The pharynx represents the upper end of the digestive tube and is the common channel for deglution and respiration. It is a fibromuscular tube and from without inwards it is composed of **buccopharyngeal fascia**, muscles, a thin layer of fascia and a mucous membrane.

The pharynx lies behind the nasal cavity, the oral cavity and larynx and in front of the cervical part of the vertebral column. It extends from the base of the skull to the lower border of the cricoid cartilage at the level of the sixth cervical vertebra, where it is continuous with the oesophagus.

Note that:

(a) all the muscles of the *soft palate* are supplied by the cranial part of the accessory nerve via the vagus nerve and pharyngeal plexus except the tensor veli palatini which is supplied by the mandibular nerve;

(b) all the muscles of the *pharynx* are supplied by the cranial part of the accessory nerve via the vagus nerve and pharyngeal plexus except the stylopharyngeus which is supplied by the glossopharyngeal nerve.

Objectives for Dissection Schedule 34

Topic: Soft palate and pharynx

Specific objectives

1. Locate the retropharyngeal space.
2. Locate the three parts of the pharynx.
3. Identify the special characteristics of the nasopharynx, oropharynx and laryngopharynx.
4. Identify the arrangement of the muscles of the pharynx.
5. Discuss the significance of the motor and sensory innervation of the soft palate and pharynx.

Questions for study:

1. Which important nerve may be injured by a foreign body lodged in the piriform fossa? What danger would a patient face if this nerve were injured?
2. How can an enlargement of the pharyngeal tonsil (adenoid) be related to an infection of the middle ear?
3. What cranial nerves are involved in the pharyngeal (gag) reflex?

Overview of Schedule 35

Before you begin dissection note:

THE LARYNX

Relevant features:

1. skeleton of the larynx;
2. joints and ligaments of the larynx;
3. cricothyroid muscles and their function;
4. posterior cricoarytenoid muscles and their function;
5. vocalis muscles and their function;
6. inlet of the larynx formed by the epiglottis and aryepiglottic and interarytenoid folds;
7. vestibule of the larynx;
8. vestibular folds and rima vestibuli;
9. ventricle of the larynx;
10. vocal fold, vocal ligament, and the rima glottidis and vocalis muscle;
11. infraglottic part of the larynx;
12. submucous and mucous membrane layers;
13. internal and external branches of the superior laryngeal nerve;
14. recurrent laryngeal nerve.

Dissection Schedule 35

LARYNX

1. *Identify the* **larynx** *in the sagittal section of your head and neck specimen. For reference use also prepared specimens of the larynx. Verify* that the larynx extends from the **hyoid bone** and root of the tongue to the level of the **cricoid cartilage** (at C6) below which it continues as the **trachea**. It lies in front of the pharynx opposite the third, fourth, fifth and sixth cervical vertebrae. The larynx consists of a cartilaginous framework formed chiefly by the **thyroid**, **cricoid**, **artytenoid** and **epiglottic cartilages** which are covered with mucous membrane. *Look at models of the laryngeal cartilages and try to obtain a three-dimensional comprehension of the manner of articulation of these cartilages.* Note that the thyroid cartilage consists of the two quadrilateral **laminae** joined together in front by the **laryngeal prominence** and the **angle of the thyroid cartilage**. You saw that the laminae were covered by the thyroid gland and the infrahyoid muscles. The cricoid cartilage articulates with the **inferior cornua of the thyroid cartilage**. Posteriorly on the upper surface of the **lamina of the cricoid cartilage** are the two **arytenoid cartilages**. *Identify the* **apex** *and the* **vocal** *and* **muscular processes** *of each arytenoid cartilage.* The **vocal folds** pass from the vocal processes forwards to the inner aspect of the thyroid cartilage just on either side of the midline.

2. *Next look at the interior of the larynx. First examine the* **inlet of the larynx**. *Below the inlet identify the two horizontal folds on the lateral wall — the* **vestibular fold** *superiorly and the* **vocal fold** *inferiorly.* The space between the inlet of the larynx and the vestibular folds is the **vestibule**, and that between the vestibular folds and the vocal folds is known as the **ventricle**. The space below the vocal folds is the **infraglottic part of the larynx**. *Verify that the ventricle leads upwards into a recess lateral to the vestibular folds.* Note that the space between the right and left vestibular folds is the **rima vestibuli** and that between the two vocal folds is the **rima glottidis**. It is important to realise that the space between the two vocal folds is narrower than that between the vestibular folds.

3. *Now examine the posterior surface of the larynx. Dissect out the laryngeal muscles by removing the mucosa of the posterior wall. As you remove the mucosa try to identify the branches of the recurrent and internal laryngeal (sensory) nerves.* The muscles of the larynx are:
   (a) the **posterior cricoarytenoid muscle** arising from the posterior surface of the **lamina of the cricoid cartilage** and curving upwards and laterally to be inserted into the muscular process of the arytenoid of the same side;
   (b) the **lateral cricoarytenoid muscle** placed anteriorly and laterally in the interval between the cricoid and thyroid cartilages. It runs from the upper border of the **arch of the cricoid** and passes upwards and backwards to gain insertion into the muscular process of the arytenoid on the same side;
   (c) the **transverse arytenoid muscle** passing horizontally across from one arytenoid to the other;
   (d) the **oblique arytenoid muscle** forming an 'X' placed on the back of the arytenoids. *Some of these fibres can be traced into the* **aryepiglottic folds** *to become continuous with the* **aryepiglottic muscles** which are attached to the side of the epiglottis;
   (e) *re-identify the* **cricothyroid muscle** *on the external surface of the larynx and confirm its attachments to the arch of the cricoid and to the lower border of the thyroid cartilage*;
   (f) *carefully remove the lamina of the thyroid cartilage and identify the underlying* **thyroarytenoid muscle**. *Define its attachments to the arytenoid behind and to the inner aspect of the thyroid lamina in front.* Note that some fibres continue as the **thyroepiglottic muscle** superiorly; and
   (g) *medial to the thyroarytenoid muscle try to identify the fibres of the* **vocalis muscle** attached posteriorly to the **vocal process of the arytenoid** and anteriorly to the back of the thyroid cartilage near the midline. It lies along the lateral side of the **vocal ligament**.

4. *Remove the muscles to examine the ligaments connecting the laryngeal cartilages. Identify first the* **thyrohyoid membrane** passing from the upper border of the thyroid cartilage behind the hyoid bone to be attached to the superior border of the **body of the hyoid**. This part of the membrane is the

median thyrohyoid ligament. *Observe* the lateral thickening of the membrane which forms the **lateral thyrohyoid ligament**.

5. *Next identify the* **lateral cricothyroid ligament** which is attached to the upper border of the cricoid arch and sweeps upwards and medially to a free edge — the vocal ligament — which is attached anteriorly to the back of the thyroid cartilage near the median plane and posteriorly to the vocal process of the arytenoid cartilage. This ligament is the core of the vocal fold.
6. Note that the cricothyroid and cricoarytenoid joints are all synovial with loose capsules, thus permitting gliding and rotatory movements.
7. *Finally dissect the root of the epiglottis and define its attachment to the posterior surface of the thyroid cartilage below its notch.*
8. *Revise* the attachments and actions of the laryngeal muscles as sphincter, adductor and abductor groups.

Summary

The larynx connects the lower anterior part of the pharynx with the trachea. It is an air passage, an organ of phonation and has a sphincter mechanism.

The larynx has a skeleton consisting of supporting parts linked at joints and moved by muscles. Fascia, both well-defined and ill-defined, is present. And the larynx is covered by a mucous membrane on the inner aspect. The nerve supply and lymphatic vessels are of considerable clinical significance.

The muscles of the larynx consist of three functional groups: (a) those concerned with sphincteric action, (b) those that are adductors, and (c) the abductor group (this refers to the paired posterior cricoarytenoid muscles).

During quiet respiration the vocal folds are in mid-position between abduction and adduction, while in deep and forced respiration the vocal folds are widely abducted.

Voiced speech requires adduction of the vocal folds and sufficient forceful expiration. Adduction and abduction of the vocal folds in speech is due to expiratory air exerting sufficient pressure to separate the vocal folds.

Tension, length and thickness of the vocal folds affect the pitch of the voice and are varied by the laryngeal muscles.

Note the motor and sensory innervation of the larynx:

(a) All the muscles of the larynx are supplied by the **recurrent laryngeal nerve** with the exception of the cricothyroid muscle which is supplied by the **external laryngeal nerve**.

(b) The mucous membrane of the larynx is supplied by the **internal laryngeal nerve** down to the level of the vocal folds, below that level the supply comes from the **recurrent laryngeal nerve**.

Objectives for Dissection Schedule 35

Topic: The larynx

Specific objectives

1. Describe the skeleton and joints of the larynx.
2. Give an account of the major intrinsic muscles of the larynx that (a) act as sphincters to guard the entrance of the trachea and (b) change the position and length of the vocal folds.
3. Give an account of the motor supply of the muscles of the larynx.
4. Give an account of the sensory innervation of the mucosal lining of the larynx.
5. Describe the arrangement of the submucous layer in relation to oedema of the larynx.
6. Describe how the larynx moves during swallowing.

Questions for study:

1. In what position would you find the vocal folds during: (a) quiet respiration; (b) forced inspiration; and (c) production of a high note?
2. What are the differences between the vestibular and vocal folds?
3. What effects on breathing and speech would result from: (a) complete interruption of the external laryngeal nerve; (b) complete unilateral interruption of the recurrent laryngeal nerve; and (c) complete bilateral interruption of the recurrent laryngeal nerve?
4. A type of laryngotomy known as a cricothyroidectomy or coniotomy is an emergency procedure performed in order to relieve acute obstruction of the airway. How is it performed? What structures are at risk?
5. What is glottis (laryngeal) oedema?
6. What part of the thyroid gland may need to be moved or cut during a tracheotomy?

Overview of Schedule 36

Before you begin dissection note:

THE EAR

Relevant features:

1. external, middle and internal ear;
2. external acoustic meatus;
3. tympanic membrane;
4. walls, roof and floor of tympanic cavity;
5. mastoid cells and mastoid antrum;
6. auditory ossicles;
7. bony part of auditory tube, tensor tympani muscle and its canal;
8. fenestra vestibuli;
9. pyramidal eminence and stapedius muscle;
10. promontory and branches of tympanic plexus;
11. fenestra cochleae;
12. prominences of facial and semicircular canals;
13. chorda tympani nerve;
14. internal jugular vein and internal carotid artery related to floor of tympanic cavity;
15. internal acoustic meatus;
16. facial nerve in facial canal;
17. geniculate ganglion and origin of greater petrosal nerve;
18. orientation of the three semicircular canals;
19. cochlea;
20. greater and lesser petrosal nerves.

Dissection Schedule 36

THE EAR

Introduction

1. *In order to study the auditory and vestibular apparatus, the temporal bone and the adjacent parts of the sphenoid and occipital bones have to be removed and decalcified.*
2. *Remove the temporal bone from your specimen by making two saw-cuts:*
   (a) *make an anterior cut in the frontal plane through the articular tubercle of the temporal bone to the foramen spinosum and on to the median plane;*
   (b) *the posterior cut should pass from behind the mastoid process obliquely forwards to the anterolateral margin of the foramen magnum;*
   (c) *then break off the cut fragment.*
3. *Next decalcify the temporal fragment by immersing it in a 10 per cent solution of concentrated nitric acid for seven to 14 days, the solution should be changed twice weekly. To test for completion of decalcification, stick a needle into the bone. It should sink in when pressure is applied. When decalcification is complete, wash the specimen in running water for 24 hours and store it in a 50 per cent solution of alcohol in water.* This process makes dissection easier.

   Since decalcification takes about two weeks you may be supplied with a decalcified temporal bone taken from a cadaver dissected previously.

Dissection of the ear

1. The ear is divided into three parts: the **external ear**, which consists of the **auricle** and the **external acoustic meatus**; the **middle ear**, or **tympanic cavity**, which is a narrow air-filled chamber lying between the external and internal ear; and the **internal ear**, which comprises a complex system of canals in the **petrous part of the temporal bone** called the **bony labyrinth**. Within this labyrinth and surrounded by **perilymph** lie membranous tubes and sacs, the **membranous labyrinth**, which are filled with **endolymph**, and in which are located the receptors for the sensations of hearing and balance.

2. *Examine the skull and identify the following landmarks: the* **external acoustic meatus** *and* **suprameatal triangle** *externally; and the* **internal acoustic meatus** *and* **arcuate eminence** *on the temporal bone in the cranial cavity.*

3. *Examine a prosected specimen or a model of the ear and identify* the external, middle and inner ears. *Study the features of the external ear in the living.* Note that it consists of the auricle and the external acoustic meatus. *In the auricle identify the* **concha**, *the* **lobule, tragus, antitragus** *and the* **intertragic notch**. Note that the concha of the auricle leads into the external acoustic meatus. *Verify that the auricle has to be pulled upwards, backwards and laterally, to straighten the external acoustic meatus to enable one to look into the ear.*

4. *In your decalcified specimen remove the skin of the auricle and confirm that the auricle has a framework of elastic cartilage which makes it very pliable. Next try to identify the parts of the external acoustic meatus.* Note how tightly the skin is bound down to the wall of the meatus. The outer third of the meatus is cartilaginous while the rest is bony and the junction between the two is the narrowest part. *At the medial end of the external acoustic meatus identify the* **tympanic membrane**.

5. *Turn to the* **posterior cranial fossa** *aspect and identify the* **internal acoustic meatus**. *With a scalpel and a pair of forceps gently remove the roof of the internal acoustic meatus. Trace the* **facial** *and* **vestibulocochlear nerves** *laterally. The facial nerve is uppermost and can be traced towards the medial wall of the middle ear where it swells into the* **geniculate ganglion**. The ganglion contains the cell bodies of the sensory (taste) fibres that join the facial nerve in the **chorda tympani**. *Lever the facial nerve upwards and identify the divisions of the vestibulocochlear nerve*, and if possible the **labyrinthine artery**. *Very gently remove the bone between the* **hiatus for the greater petrosal nerve** *and the geniculate ganglion*; this will expose the course of the nerve and also the coils of the **cochlea**.

6. *Next with a pair of forceps carefully remove the* **tegmen tympani** which forms the *roof* of the middle ear. *As you do this the small* **auditory ossicles** *will come into view*. The most easily recognised ossicle is the **head of the malleus** which lies in the **epitympanic recess** (upper part) of the tympanic

cavity. Anteromedially, the tympanic cavity is continuous with the **bony part of the auditory tube**. *Try to pass a probe through the* **pharyngeal opening of the auditory tube** *into the tympanic cavity. Identify a small muscle, the* **tensor tympani**, which comes out of a canal just above the auditory tube and passes backwards to be attached to the **malleus** below its head.

Note that the malleus articulates with the **incus** and this in turn articulates with the **stapes**. The **base of the stapes** is applied to the medial wall of the tympanic cavity. The joints between the three ossicles are synovial joints.

7. *Now examine the lateral wall of the tympanic cavity*. Note the tympanic membrane to which the malleus is attached. *Above the insertion of the tensor tympani you should see a thread-like structure crossing the medial side of the malleus in an anteroposterior direction*. This is the **chorda tympani** which you saw joining the lingual nerve. The chorda tympani arises from the facial nerve.

8. *Next examine the medial wall of the tympanic cavity. Again identify the stapes in the medial wall*. Its base fits into a window, the **fenestra vestibuli**, which is covered by a membrane and lies above the **promontory** and below the **canal for the facial nerve**. The promontory forms a bulge of the medial wall due to the basal turn of the **cochlea**. *If you use a magnifying glass you may be able to see the thread-like tendon of the* **stapedius muscle**, which is attached to the stapes near its articulation with the incus. Posteriorly, the tendon emerges from the top of a very small projection of bone called the **pyramidal eminence**. In one of the depressions below and behind the promontory is another small window, the **fenestra cochleae**, which is closed by a membrane. *However, it is not easy to identify this window*.

9. The tympanic cavity opens *posteriorly* through the **aditus to the antrum** into the **mastoid antrum**.

10. *Now turn your attention to the bony labyrinth in the petrous part of the temporal bone. With the help of models and your atlas note the following*: the bony labyrinth consisting of the **vestibule**, the **cochlea** and the three **bony semicircular canals**. These form the internal ear.

The vestibule lies between the medial wall of the middle ear and the internal acoustic meatus. In its lateral wall is the fenestra vestibuli, which is closed by the periosteal lining and into which the base of the stapes fits. The vestibule communicates in front with the cochlea and behind with the semicircular canals.

The cochlea is a tapering spiral tube which makes about two and one-half turns around a central bony pillar, the **modiolus**. The first turn of the cochlea is responsible for the elevation on the medial wall of the tympanic cavity called the promontory.

Note the three semicircular canals. The **anterior semicircular canal** and the **posterior semicircular canal** are both vertical, the former at right-angles to, and the latter parallel with the long axis of the petrous part of the temporal bone. The anterior semicircular canal lies beneath an elevation, the **arcuate eminence**, on the upper surface of the petrous part of the temporal bone, about 1 cm behind the internal acoustic meatus. The **lateral semicircular canal** lies horizontal in the angle between the other two canals.

11. *Now return to the divisions of the vestibulocochlear nerve and attempt to trace the* **cochlear** *division into the modiolus and the* **vestibular** *division laterally into the vestibule.*

12. *You will not be able to study the more detailed anatomy of the membranous labyrinth on your specimen.* For this special preparations suitable for microscopic examination are required.

13. *Strip off all the muscles attached to the mastoid process and cut it open with a scalpel to expose the* **mastoid air cells** *contained within it. Remove the air cells and look for the mastoid antrum.* Again note that the antrum communicates with the tympanic cavity through the aditus to the antrum.

Summary

It is important to understand the functions of the auditory ossicles and their muscles. Sound waves pass from the external acoustic meatus and cause the tympanic membrane to vibrate. These vibrations are transmitted by the ossicles to the fenestra vestibuli and thence to the internal ear. Tensor tympani and stapedius muscles contract reflexly to dampen down excessive movements of the ossicles due to sounds of high intensity (sound mufflers) and allow soft sounds to be separated from irrelevant loud ones.

The main *sensory* and *motor* innervation of the external ear and middle ear is as follows:

(a) **Auricle**:

sensory — outer surface (lateral surface): mainly auriculotemporal nerve;
inner surface (cranial surface): mainly great auricular nerve;
concha: may be supplied by a sensory branch from the facial nerve and vagus nerve;

motor — facial nerve.

(b) **Tympanic membrane**:

sensory — outer surface: auriculotemporal and vagus nerves;
inner surface: glossopharyngeal nerve.

(c) **Tympanic cavity, mastoid antrum** and **auditory tube**:

sensory — glossopharyngeal nerve.

(d) **Tensor tympani muscle**: *motor fibres* from the mandibular nerve.

(e) **Stapedius muscle**: *motor fibres* from the facial nerve.

Objectives for Dissection Schedule 36

Topic: The ear

Specific objectives

1. Identify, on a living subject, the features of the surface anatomy of the external ear.
2. Describe the cutaneous sensory innervation of the external ear, tympanic membrane and tympanic cavity.
3. Give an account of the walls, roof and floor of the tympanic cavity.
4. Give a full account of the facial nerve.
5. Describe how sound is transmitted from the external ear to the fenestra vestibuli.

Questions for study:

1. Which nerve may be seen on the inner aspect of the tympanic membrane during an otoscopic examination?
2. What spaces communicate with the tympanic cavity? What is the clinical significance of these communications?
3. What is otitis media?
4. What functional components are represented in: (a) the greater petrosal nerve and (b) the chorda tympani?
5. What is the function of the tensor tympani and stapedius muscles? What is their innervation?
6. What kinds of cell bodies are found in the geniculate ganglion?

Additional Objectives for the Head and Neck

Topic: Muscles and fasciae of the head and neck

General objective 1

Comprehend the arrangement and actions of important muscles.

Specific objectives

1. Describe the relations of scalenus anterior, scalenus medius, posterior belly of digastric, sternocleidomastoid, hyoglossus, lateral pterygoid, obliquus capitis inferior and lateral rectus of the eyeball.
2. Analyse the movements and stability of the eyeball.

General objective 2

Comprehend the important features of the deep cervical fascia.

Specific objectives

1. Describe the attachments of the deep cervical fascia pointing out the continuity between the superficial layer, the carotid sheath and the pretracheal layers.
2. Explain why:
   (a) swellings of the thyroid gland move with swallowing;
   (b) swellings of the parotid gland are painful.
3. Review the attachments of the prevertebral fascia and explain:
   (a) the formation of the axillary sheath;
   (b) why it is an important landmark to the surgeon;
   (c) why an abscess from the cervical vertebrae points above the clavicle or tracks down into the posterior mediastinum.

Topic: Nerves of the head and neck

General objective

Comprehend the important principles in the nerves studied and their clinical applications.

Specific objectives

1. Describe the effects of lesions affecting the cranial nerves as well as the methods employed for testing their integrity.
2. Review the origin, course and distribution of the phrenic nerve.
3. Briefly describe the distribution of the branches of the superior, middle and cervicothoracic sympathetic ganglia.
4. Describe the location of the ciliary, pterygopalatine, submandibular and otic ganglia, and their connections.
5. Explain the anatomical basis of:
   (a) Horner's syndrome;
   (b) pain from teeth being referred to the ear and vice-versa;
   (c) bulbar palsy;
   (d) headache;
   (e) hiccup.

Topic: Blood vessels and lymphatics of the head and neck

General objective 1

Comprehend the general arrangement of the blood vessels of the head and neck.

Specific objectives

1. Review the areas of distribution of the branches of the external carotid artery.
2. Describe the structures supplied by the branches of the internal carotid artery.
3. Describe the sites of anastomoses between the external and internal carotid arteries.
4. Describe the area of distribution and course of the four parts of the vertebral artery giving the developmental reason for this arrangement.
5. Explain alternate routes of venous drainage when the internal jugular vein is ligated.

6. Explain: (a) the collateral circulation when the subclavian artery is ligated; (b) the importance of the tubercle on the transverse process of the sixth cervical vertebra (Chassaignac's tubercle); (c) the importance of the relationship of the subclavian artery to the first rib.

General objective 2

Comprehend the general arrangement of the lymphatics of the head and neck.

Specific objectives

1. Describe the location of: (a) the pericervical collar of lymph nodes; (b) the anterior cervical nodes; (c) the superficial and deep cervical nodes; (d) the retropharyngeal nodes. Indicate their territory of drainage.
2. Describe the formation and termination of the right lymphatic and thoracic ducts.

Topic: Viscera of the neck

General objective

Comprehend the important features of the viscera in the region.

Specific objectives

1. Describe the course and relations of the cervical part of the trachea.
2. Describe the course and relations of the cervical part of the oesophagus.
3. Enumerate the structures, from superficial to deep, encountered during a tracheostomy.
4. Indicate the clinical importance of the close relationship of:
   (a) the facial nerve and its branches to the parotid gland;
   (b) the inferior thyroid veins to the front of the trachea;
   (c) the lingual and facial veins to the submandibular gland;
   (d) the thoracic duct to the left internal jugular vein;
   (e) the cervical pleura to the structures in the root of the neck.
5. Describe the developmental basis for the occurrence of:
   (a) lingual and retrosternal thyroids;
   (b) branchial cysts and fistulae;

(c) thyroglossal fistulae;
(d) hare lip and cleft palate — unilateral and bilateral.

Topic: Skeleton of the head and neck

General objective

Comprehend the important anatomical principles seen in the skeletal framework of the region.

Specific objectives

1. Explain the development of the chondrocranium and viscerocranium paying attention to: (a) variation in their relative proportions; (b) the formation and closure of the fontanelles.
2. Explain the structure of: (a) a suture; (b) a flat bone of the skull.
3. Review the movements occurring between the occiput, atlas and axis and in the cervical vertebral column.
4. Indicate the muscles concerned in the above movements.
5. Discuss:
   (a) dangers of fracture of the dens;
   (b) dangers of fracture dislocations of the cervical vertebral column;
   (c) relationship between the neurocentral lip articulations and cervical spondylosis.

APPENDICES

Appendix 1

THE SKULL AND ITS SUBDIVISIONS

SKULL

The skull is the cranium plus the mandible. It is the total bony structure of the head including the mandible.

CRANIUM

The cranium is the skull minus the mandible, i.e. the bones of the head without the mandible.

CALVARIA

The calvaria is the cranium without the facial bones.

CALOTTE

The calotte is the skull cap.

MANDIBLE

The mandible is the lower jaw.

NEUROCRANIUM

The neurocranium is that part of the cranium that encloses the brain (the calvaria).

SPLANCHNOCRANIUM

The splanchnocranium consists of the orbits, facial bones and mandible.

CHONDROCRANIUM

The chondrocranium is that part of the skull that develops in cartilage.

Appendix 2

FORAMINA AND FISSURES OF THE SKULL AND THEIR PRINCIPAL CONTENTS

CRANIUM

A. View from above

Parietal foramen — emissary vein (from superior sagittal sinus to extracranial veins).

B. Front view

1. **Supraorbital foramen** (or **notch**) supraorbital vessels and nerve.
2. **Infraorbital foramen** — infraorbital vessels and nerve (continuation of maxillary vessels and nerve).

Orbit

1. **Optic canal** — optic nerve (with meningeal sheaths), ophthalmic artery.
2. **Nasolacrimal canal** — nasolacrimal duct.
3. **Inferior orbital fissure** — maxillary nerve, infraorbital vessels, zygomatic nerve.
4. **Superior orbital fissure** — *above the lateral rectus muscle*: trochlear, frontal and lacrimal nerves. *Between two heads of lateral rectus*: upper and lower divisions of the oculomotor nerve, nasociliary nerve, abducens nerve.
5. **Anterior** and **posterior ethmoidal foramina** — anterior and posterior ethmoidal nerves and vessels.

Nasal cavity

Openings into nasal cavity:

Sphenoethmoidal recess — sphenoidal sinuses.

Sphenopalatine foramen — posterior to superior nasal meatus, see C4.4.

Middle nasal meatus 1. Frontal sinus (upper part of hiatus semilunaris);
2. Maxillary sinus (lower part of hiatus semilunaris);

Inferior nasal meatus — nasolacrimal canal (nasolacrimal duct).

C. Lateral view

1. **Mastoid foramen** — emissary vein (from sigmoid sinus).
2. **External acoustic meatus.**
3. **Pterygomaxillary fissure** — maxillary artery and nerve.
4. **Pterygopalatine fossa** — maxillary nerve, pterygopalatine ganglion, terminal branches of maxillary artery and veins. Seven openings lead to, or from, the fossa:

Posterior wall: 4.1 **Foramen rotundum** — maxillary nerve.
4.2 **Pterygoid canal** — nerve of pterygoid canal (formed by deep petrosal and greater petrosal nerves).
4.3 **Palatovaginal canal** — pharyngeal branch of pterygopalatine ganglion.

Medial wall: 4.4 **Sphenopalatine foramen** — sphenopalatine artery and nasopalatine nerve (from pterygopalatine ganglion).

Anterior wall: 4.5 **Inferior orbital fissure** — see B: Orbit 3.

Lateral wall: 4.6 **Pterygomaxillary fissure** — see C3.

Inferior: 4.7 **Greater palatine canal** — greater and lesser palatine vessels and nerves.

5. **Posterior dental foramina** — posterior superior alveolar nerves and vessels.

D. Basal view

1. **Incisive fossa:** 1.1 *Anterior and posterior median incisive foramina* — nasopalatine nerves;
   1.2 *Right and left lateral incisive foramina* — greater palatine vessel and nerve.
2. **Greater palatine foramen** — greater palatine vessels and nerve.
3. **Lesser palatine foramina** (2) — lesser palatine vessels and nerve.
4. **Foramen ovale** — mandibular nerve and lesser petrosal nerve.
5. **Foramen spinosum** — middle meningeal vessels.
6. **Foramen lacerum** — small arteries and veins and lymph vessels.
7. **Carotid canal** — internal carotid artery, plexus of sympathetic nerves (from superior cervical ganglion).
8. **Jugular foramen** — (from before backwards) inferior petrosal sinus, glossopharyngeal nerve, vagus nerve, accessory nerve, sigmoid sinus (becoming internal jugular vein).
9. **Jugular fossa** — superior bulb of internal jugular vein.
10. **Petrotympanic fissure** — chorda tympani (coming from anterior canaliculus).
11. **Hypoglossal canal** — hypoglossal nerve.
12. **Stylomastoid foramen** — facial nerve.
13. **Foramen magnum** — lower end of medulla oblongata, dura mater, arachnoid, subarachnoid space, pia mater, spinal roots of accessory nerve, vertebral arteries and veins, membrana tectoria and apical ligament.

E. Interior cranium

Anterior cranial fossa

1. **Foramen caecum** — emissary vein (connects superior sagittal sinus with veins of frontal sinus and nose).
2. **Olfactory foramina** — olfactory nerves (with meningeal sheaths).

Middle cranial fossa

1. **Optic canal** — see B: Orbit 1.
2. **Superior orbital fissure** — see B: Orbit 4.
3. **Foramen rotundum** — maxillary nerve.
4. **Foramen ovale** — see D4.
5. **Foramen lacerum** — closed with cartilage. See D6.
6. **Foramen spinosum** — see D5.
7. **Hiatus for canal of greater petrosal nerve** — greater petrosal nerve.
8. **Hiatus for canal of lesser petrosal nerve** — lesser petrosal nerve.

Posterior cranial fossa

1. **Internal acoustic meatus** — facial nerve, vestibulocochlear nerve and labyrinthine artery (from basilar artery).
2. **Jugular foramen** — see D8.
3. **Hypoglossal canal** — see D11.
4. **Foramen magnum** — see D13.

MANDIBLE

1. **Mental foramen** — mental nerve.
2. **Mandibular foramen** — inferior alveolar vessels and nerve.

Appendix 3

PREFIXES COMMONLY USED IN ANATOMY
(G: Greek; L: Latin)

Prefix		Meaning	Example
a, an	G	lacking, without	asexual, anovulatory
ab	L	away from	abduction
ad	L	to, toward	adduction
af	L	to, toward	afferent
ana	G	up, back, again	anatomy
ante	L	forward, before	antebrachium
anti	G	against, opposed to	antitragus
bi	L	twice, double	bicipital
circum	L	around, about	circumduction
co, com, con	L	together, with	conjunctiva
de	L	away from, down	deglutition
di	G	double, twice	diaphysis
dis	L	apart, away	disarticulate
ecto	G	on outer side	ectoderm
endo	G	within	endocardium
epi	G	upon, over	epicardium
exo	G	outside	exoskeleton
extra	L	outside	extracellular
hyper	G	over, above, excessive	hypertrophy
hypo	G	under, deficient, below	hypothalamus
im, in	L	not	immature
infra	L	below	infraorbital
inter	L	between	intervertebral
intra	L	inside, within	intramuscular
intro	L	within, into	introspection
meta	G	change, after	metacarpal
para	G	by the side of	paravertebral

Prefix	Meaning	Example
peri	G around	peritoneum
post	L after, behind	postaxial
pre	L before	prenatal
pro	G before, for	pronation
re	L again, back	reflex
retro	L backward	retroperitoneal
semi	L half	semimembranosus
sub	L under	subclavius
supra	L above	supraspinatous
sym, syn	G together, with	symphysis, synostosis
trans	L across	transpyloric
ultra	L in excess, beyond	ultrasonic

www.ingramcontent.com/pod-product-compliance
Lightning Source LLC
Chambersburg PA
CBHW061614220326
41598CB00026BA/3758
* 9 7 8 9 8 1 0 2 3 5 6 9 7 *